Contents

Changes in this edition

The main changes in the 34th edition of Medicines, Ethics and Practice are as follows:

1.1 Introduction
Minor revisions to provide greater clarity. Additional definitions have been included for Contact lens specialist, Dental care professional register, Dental hygienist, Dental therapist and Registered dispensing optician.

1.2 Medicines for Human Use
1.2.2: Pharmacy medicines (P) The section on Personal control has been taken out and the section on The Responsible Pharmacist has had minor revisions to reflect the change in legislation.

1.2.3: Prescription-only medicines (POM) *Prescriptions for prescription-only medicines* has been updated to reflect the introduction of licensing for doctors.

To reflect changes in legislation paragraph (c) (iv) has been updated. From 26 July 2010 the legal requirement for a prescription issued by an EEA or Swiss doctor or dentist will change.

Additional information is provided on repeatable prescriptions for greater clarity.

Pharmacist Prescribers; Community practitioner nurse prescribers and nurse independent prescribers addition of information to reflect changes in legislation allowing pharmacist independent prescribers and nurse independent prescribers to prescribe any licensed or unlicensed medicine (with the exception of controlled drugs).

1.2.5: Sales of medicines to exempted organisations, healthcare professionals or other persons The section on *Midwives*, with regard to what they can sell, supply and administer, has been updated to reflect changes in legislation.

New sections on what a *Dispensing optician, Aircraft personnel* and *Her Majesty's armed forces* can sell, supply or administer, have been added to provide information on recent legislation changes.

1.2.13: Handling of waste medicines The section for *England and Wales* has been updated to reflect the Environment Agency's review of their waste exemptions.

1.2.14: Controlled Drugs Minor revisions have been made to the section on *Controlled Drugs in hospitals* and *Private controlled drug prescriptions* to provide greater clarity.

Instalment Prescriptions Additional Home Office approved wordings have been included.

Destruction of Controlled Drugs In England and Wales the Environment Agency is in the process of reviewing their waste exemptions. We are currently seeking clarification from the Environment Agency in relation to the destruction of returned controlled drugs which have been returned to a pharmacy in England or Wales as waste.

1.4: Non-medicinal poisons
Minor revision to update a reference.

1.6 Chemicals
Major changes to provide greater clarity on the new European Directives and legislation changes that come into force over an extended transition period.

1.7 Denatured alcohol
Minor revisions to reflect changes in legislation and to provide greater clarity.

1.7.3 Supply of denatured alcohol by authorised users Changes with respect to supply of CDA in Scotland.

1.8: Medicines for veterinary use Minor revisions to reflect changes in legislation and to provide greater clarity.

1.8.6 Sheep Dips Changes with respect to qualifications and certificates of persons authorised to use sheep dips.

2. Code of Ethics and Professional Standards and Guidance Documents
To avoid confusion during the impending transfer of the Society's regulatory function to the General Pharmaceutical Council, it has been decided not to publish any regulatory standards in this edition of *Medicines, Ethics and Practice*.

3. Professional Development and Training
This renamed section contains guidance on continuing professional development and pharmacy support staff training.

4. References
4.3 Headquarters telephone enquiries guide This has been amended to provide contact details for the current Society's main functions both before and after the transfer of the regulatory function to the General Pharmaceutical Council.

Published by the Royal Pharmaceutical Society of Great Britain, 1 Lambeth High Street, London SE1 7JN

New editions of *Medicines, Ethics and Practice: A Guide for Pharmacists and Pharmacy Technicians* are distributed free of charge to all practising and non-practising pharmacists and registered pharmacy technicians, to all preregistration trainees and in bulk to UK schools of pharmacy. Copies are not distributed to pharmacy premises. Additional copies are available at a cost of £34.99 each from Pharmaceutical Press, c/o MPS, The Macmillan Building, 4 Crinan Street, London N1 9XW, UK (Tel: +44 (0) 203 318 3141; Fax: +44 (0) 203 318 3139; e-mail: pharmpress@macmillansolutions.com), or you can order online at www.pharmpress.com

The Royal Pharmaceutical Society's Legal and Ethical Advisory Service is responsible for producing Part 1 of *Medicines, Ethics and Practice*. The content of *Medicines, Ethics and Practice* is collated and edited by Mary Snell
© Royal Pharmaceutical Society of Great Britain, 2010
All reproduction, including photocopying, rights reserved
ISBN: 978 0 85369 863 0
ISSN: 0955-4254
A catalogue record for this publication is available from the British Library
Printed in the UK by Precision Colour Printing, Haldane, Halesfield 1, Telford, Shropshire TF7 4QQ

1: General Legal Requirements

1.1 Introduction

Part 1 of *Medicines, Ethics and Practice* is intended primarily as a practical guide to the legal restrictions on the sale or supply of medicinal products and poisons.

While every possible care has been taken in the compilation of this guide, no responsibility can be accepted for any errors or for any consequences of such errors. The aim has been to present as clear and concise a summary of the law as possible, and to interpret the various orders and regulations so as to decide the categories into which individual products should be classified. On any question of interpretation, however, it should be borne in mind that only the courts can give a legally binding decision.

Part 1 is primarily intended for the guidance of hospital and community pharmacists who are concerned with the retail sale or supply of medicines and poisons.

The Medicines Act 1968, the Poisons Act 1972 and the Veterinary Medicines Regulations 2009, together with the Misuse of Drugs Act 1971, regulate all retail and wholesale dealings in medicines and poisons. Certain non-medicinal poisons and chemicals are also subject to the labelling requirements of chemicals legislation including the Chemicals (Hazard Information and Packaging for Supply) Regulations 2009; *see* Section 1.6. It is important to appreciate at the outset that the Medicines Act 1968 applies only to substances when they are used as medicinal products or as ingredients in medicinal products. Carbon tetrachloride, for example, when administered for a medicinal purpose is a prescription-only medicine under the Medicines Act 1968, but when it is not used as a medicine it is not subject to the Medicines Act 1968. It is also important to grasp that there is no statutory list of pharmacy medicines, that is, medicines which may be sold over the counter only in registered pharmacies.

The basic principle of the Medicines Act 1968 is that all medicines may be sold or supplied by retail from registered pharmacies. Another principal statutory list is the list of prescription-only medicines which can be supplied from pharmacies, only in accordance with an appropriate practitioner's prescription.

Medicines which are not prescription-only medicines and which are not included in the general sale list are pharmacy medicines, that is, medicines which may only be sold from a registered pharmacy under the supervision of a pharmacist.

The Medicines Act 1968 applies to all medicines for human use. The Veterinary Medicines Regulations 2009 replaced the Medicines Act 1968 as far as veterinary legislation is concerned. Veterinary medicines are dealt with in Sections 1.8 and 1.9.

Similarly, there are substances used in medicines which also have non-medicinal uses. Several of these substances are included (together with other non-medicinal poisons) in the poisons list made under the Poisons Act 1972. Non-medicinal poisons are dealt with in Sections 1.4 and 1.5.

Keys to the annotations used in the list of medicines for human use (Section 1.3) and the list of medicines for veterinary use (Section 1.9) appear on the first page of each list.

1.1.1 Definitions

The following are definitions of terms used in the Medicines Act 1968 and the Misuse of Drugs Regulations 2001, as amended, or are interpretations of terms used in these sets of legislation, that are not explained in the main text of this guide:

Accountable officer is a fit, proper and suitably experienced person appointed or nominated by a designated body to ensure the safe, appropriate and effective management and use of Controlled Drugs within organisations subject to their oversight. The role and responsibilities of an accountable officer are defined under the Health Act 2006 and under the Controlled Drugs (Supervision of Management and Use) Regulations 2006 and the Controlled Drugs (Supervision of Management and Use) (Wales) Regulations 2008.

Additional supply optometrist means a person who is registered as an optometrist, and against whose name particulars of the additional supply speciality have been entered in the relevant register (*See* p22).

Appropriate date means:
(a) in the case of a health prescription, the date on which it was signed by the appropriate practitioner giving it or a date indicated by him as being the date before which it shall not be dispensed, and
(b) in every other case, the date on which the prescription was signed by the appropriate practitioner giving it; and, where a health prescription bears both the date on which it was signed and a date indicated as being that before which it shall not be dispensed, the appropriate date is the later of those dates.

Appropriate non-proprietary name means, briefly:
(a) any name, or abbreviation, or suitable inversion of such name, at the head of a monograph in a "specified publication" (*see* below); or
(b) where the product is not described in a monograph, the British approved name; or
(c) where there is no monograph name or British approved name, the international non-proprietary name (INN); or
(d) where there is no monograph name, British approved name or INN, the accepted scientific name or any other name descriptive of the true nature of the product.

Appropriate practitioner *See* p13, under "Prescriptions for prescription-only medicines".

Appropriate quantitative particulars means, briefly, the quantity of each active ingredient (or that part of the active molecule responsible for the therapeutic or pharmacological activity) identified by its appropriate non-proprietary name and expressed in terms of weight, volume, capacity or, for certain products, in units of activity or as a percentage.
   The quantity to be shown is:
(a) the quantity in each dosage unit (for pastille and lozenges only it can be shown as a percentage), or
(b) if there is no dosage unit, the quantity of each active ingredient in the container, or
(c) if the product contains any active ingredient which cannot be definitively characterised, the quantity of the ingredient present in the highest proportion (diluents, excipient, etc, need not be stated).

   The quantity of antimicrobial preservative added to a biological medicinal product must be stated. This applies to antigens, toxins, antitoxins, sera, antisera and vaccines.
   The quantity can be expressed in terms of the dilution of the unit preparation for a homoeopathic product (ie, a product prepared in accordance with the methods of homoeopathic medicine or similar system which is sold or supplied as a homoeopathic product and is so described by the person who sells or supplies it).

Care home in relation to:
(a) England and Wales has the same meaning as in the Care Standards Act 2000; and
(b) Scotland means the accommodation provided by a care home service.
   Care home service has the same meaning as in the Regulation of Care (Scotland) Act 2001.

Clinical management plan means a written plan (which may be amended from time to time) relating to the treatment of an individual patient agreed by:
(a) the patient to whom the plan relates,
(b) the doctor or dentist who is a party to the plan, and
(c) any supplementary prescriber who is to prescribe, give directions for administration or administer under the plan.

Common name in relation to a relevant medicinal product means the international non-proprietary name, or, if one does not exist, the usual common name.

Community practitioner nurse prescriber means a person:
(a) who is a registered nurse or a registered midwife, and
(b) against whose name is recorded in the professional register an annotation signifying that he is qualified to order drugs, medicines and appliances from the Nurse Prescribers' Formulary for Community Practitioners in the current edition of the *British National Formulary*.

Contact lens specialist means a person who is a registered dispensing optician and against whose name particulars of the contact lens speciality have been entered in the register of dispensing opticians maintained under section 7(b) of the Opticians Act 1989.

Container means, briefly, the inner receptacle which holds the medicinal product. A package is every other outer receptacle.

Cosmetic means any substance or preparation intended to be applied to the various surfaces of the human body including epidermis, pilary system and hair, nails, lips and external genital organs, or the teeth and buccal mucosa wholly or mainly for the purpose of perfuming them, cleansing them, protecting them, caring for them or keeping them in condition, modifying their appearance (whether for aesthetic purposes or otherwise) or combating body odours or normal body perspiration.

Dental care professionals register means the dental care professionals register established under section 36B of the Dentists Act 1994.

Dental hygienist means a person whose name is registered under the title of dental hygienist in the dental care professionals register.

Dental therapist means a person whose name is registered under the title of dental therapist in the dental care professionals register.

Dispensed medicinal product includes a medicinal product prepared or dispensed by a practitioner (doctor, dentist or veterinarian) or prepared or dispensed in accordance with a prescription given by a practitioner and a medicinal product prepared or dispensed in a registered pharmacy by or under the supervision of a pharmacist, either in accordance with a specification furnished by the purchaser (for example, a customer's recipe) or in accordance with the pharmacist's own judgement as to the treatment required for a person present in the pharmacy (ie, counter-prescribing).

Dosage unit means:
(a) where a medicinal product is in the form of a tablet or capsule or is an article in some other similar pharmaceutical form, that tablet, capsule or other article, or
(b) where a medicinal product is not in any such form as aforesaid, the unit of measurement which is used as the unit by reference to which the dose of the medicinal product is measured.

EEA healthcare professional means:
(a) a doctor who is lawfully engaged in medical practice in a relevant European state, or
(b) a dentist who is lawfully engaged in dental practice in a relevant European state (including a person whose formal qualifications as a doctor are recognised for the purposes of the pursuit of the professional activities of a dental practitioner under Article 37 of the European Directive 2005/36/EC)

where "relevant European state" means an EEA state, other than the United Kingdom, or Switzerland.

Effervescent in relation to a tablet, means containing not less than 75 per cent, by weight of the tablet, of ingredients included wholly or mainly for the purpose of releasing carbon dioxide when the tablet is dissolved or dispersed in water.

Expiry date means the date after which, or the month and year after the end of which, the medicinal product should not be used, or the date before which or the month and year before the beginning of which, the medicinal product should be used.

External use means application to the skin, hair, teeth, mucosa of the mouth, throat, nose, ear, eye, vagina or anal canal when a local action only is intended and extensive systemic absorption is unlikely to occur; and references to medicinal products for external use shall be read accordingly except that such references shall not include throat sprays, throat pastille, throat lozenges, throat tablets, nasal drops, nasal sprays, nasal inhalations or teething preparations.

Food includes beverages, confectionery, articles and substances used as ingredients in the preparation of food, and includes any manufactured substance to which there has been added any vitamin and which is advertised as available and for sale to the general public as a dietary supplement.

General Sale List medicine means a medicine for which all active ingredients are listed in the Medicines (Products Other Than Veterinary Drugs) (General Sale List) Order 1984 or are so classified in their marketing authorisation.

Health prescription means a prescription issued by a doctor, a dentist, a supplementary prescriber, a community practitioner nurse prescriber, a nurse independent prescriber, an optometrist independent prescriber or a pharmacist independent prescriber under or by virtue of:
(a) in England and Wales, the National Health Service Act 1977,
(b) in Scotland, the National Health Service (Scotland) Act 1978, and
(c) in Northern Ireland, the Health and Personal Social Services (Northern Ireland) Order 1972.

IRME practitioner means, in relation to a medical exposure, a practitioner for the purposes of the Ionising Radiation (Medical Exposure) Regulations 2000.

Maximum daily dose (mdd) means the maximum quantity of a substance contained in the amount of a medicinal product which it is recommended should be taken or administered in any period of 24 hours.

Maximum dose (md) means the maximum quantity of a substance contained in the amount of a medicinal product which it is recommended should be taken or administered at any one time.

Maximum strength (ms) means either:
(i) the maximum quantity of a substance by weight or volume contained in a dosage unit of a medicinal product; or
(ii) the maximum percentage of a substance contained in a medicinal product calculated in terms of weight in weight (w/w), weight in volume (w/v), volume in weight (v/w) or volume in volume (v/v) as appropriate; and if the maximum percentage calculated in those ways differs, the higher or highest such percentage.

Medicinal product means any substance or article (not being an instrument, apparatus or appliance) which is manufactured, sold, supplied, imported or exported for use wholly or mainly in either or both of the following ways, that is to say:
(a) use by being administered to one or more human beings for a medicinal purpose;
(b) use as an ingredient in the preparation of a substance or article which is to be administered to one or more human beings for a medicinal purpose.

Medicinal purpose means any one or more of the following purposes, that is to say:
(a) treating or preventing disease;
(b) diagnosing disease or ascertaining the existence, degree or extent of a physiological condition;
(c) contraception;
(d) inducing anaesthesia;
(e) otherwise preventing or interfering with the normal operation of a physiological function, whether permanently or temporarily, and whether by way of terminating, reducing or postponing, or increasing or accelerating, the operation of that function or in any other way.

Nurse independent prescriber means a person:
(a) who is a registered nurse or a registered midwife, and
(b) against whose name is recorded in the professional register an annotation signifying that he is qualified to order drugs, medicines and appliances as a nurse independent prescriber or a nurse independent/supplementary prescriber.

Operating department practitioner means a person who is registered under the Health Professions Order 2001 as an operating department practitioner.

Optometrist independent prescriber means a person:
(a) who is a registered optometrist, and
(b) against whose name is recorded in the relevant register an annotation signifying that he is qualified to order

drugs, medicines and appliances as an optometrist independent prescriber.

Parenteral administration means administration by breach of the skin or mucous membrane.

Pharmacist independent prescriber means a person:
(a) who is a pharmacist, and
(b) against whose name is recorded in the relevant register an annotation signifying that he is qualified to order drugs, medicines and appliances as a pharmacist independent prescriber.

Prescriber identification number means the number recorded against a person's name by the relevant National Health Service agency for the purposes of that person's private prescribing.

Prescription-only medicine means a medicinal product of a description or falling within a class specified in Article 3 of the Prescription Only Medicines (Human Use) Order 1997.

Private prescribing means issuing prescriptions other than health prescriptions.

Professional register means the register maintained by the Nursing and Midwifery Council under Article 5 of the Nursing and Midwifery Order 2001.

Professional registration number means the number recorded against a person's name in the register of any body that licenses or regulates any profession of which that person is a member.

Radioactive medicinal product means a medicinal product which is, which contains or which generates a radioactive substance and which is, contains or generates that substance in order, when administered, to utilise the radiation emitted therefrom.

Radiopharmaceutical means a medicinal product which, when ready for use, contains one or more radionuclides included for a medicinal purpose.

Registered chiropodist means a person who is registered in Part 2 of the register maintained by the Health Professions Council under Article 5 of the Health Professions Order 2001.

Registered dietitian means a person who is registered in Part 4 of the register maintained by the Health Professions Council under Article 5 of the Health Professions Order 2001.

Registered dispensing optician means a person registered in the register of dispensing opticians maintained under section 7(b) of the Opticians Act 1989.

Registered midwife means a person registered in the Midwives' Part of the professional register.

Registered nurse means a person registered in the Nurses' Part or Specialist Community Public Health Nurses' Part of the professional register.

Registered occupational therapist means a person who is registered in Part 6 of the register maintained by the Health Professions Council under Article 5 of the Health Professions Order 2001.

Registered optometrist means a person whose name is registered in the register of optometrists maintained under Section 7(a) of the Opticians Act 1989, or in the register of visiting optometrists from relevant European States maintained under Section 8B(1)(a) of the Act.

Registered orthoptist means a person who is registered in Part 7 of the register maintained by the Health Professions Council under Article 5 of the Health Professions Order 2001.

Registered orthotist and prosthetist means a person who is registered in Part 10 of the register maintained by the Health Professions Council under Article 5 of the Health Professions Order 2001.

Registered paramedic means a person who is registered in Part 8 of the register maintained by the Health Professions Council under Article 5 of the Health Professions Order 2001.

Registered pharmacy means premises for the time being entered in the register required to be kept under the Medicines Act 1968 by the Registrar of the Royal Pharmaceutical Society of Great Britain (or of Northern Ireland, as appropriate).

Registered physiotherapist means a person who is registered in Part 9 of the register maintained by the Health Professions Council under Article 5 of the Health Professions Order 2001.

Registered radiographer means a person who is registered in Part 11 of the register maintained by the Health Professions Council under Article 5 of the Health Professions Order 2001.

Registered speech and language therapist means a person who is registered in Part 12 of the register maintained by the Health Professions Council under Article 5 of the Health Professions Order 2001.

Relevant medicinal product means, except in Regulation 3A and paragraph 1A of Schedule 3 (of the Medicines for Human Use [Marketing Authorisations Etc.] Regulations 1994, as amended) a medicinal product for human use to which the provisions of the 2001/83/EC Directive apply other than:
(a) a traditional herbal medicinal product, or (b) a homoeopathic medicinal product that fulfils the conditions laid down in Article 14(1) of the 2001 Directive.
(This definition is taken from the Medicines for Human Use (Marketing Authorisations Etc.) Regulations 1994, as amended.)

Repeatable prescription means a prescription which contains a direction that it may be dispensed more than once.

Retail pharmacy business means a business (not being a professional practice carried on by a practitioner) which consists of or includes the retail sale of medicinal products other than medicinal products on a general sale list (whether medicinal products on such a list are sold in the course of that business or not).

Specified publication means the European Pharmacopoeia, the British Pharmacopoeia, the British Pharmaceutical Codex, the International Pharmacopoeia, the Cumulative List of Recommended International Nonproprietary Names, the British National Formulary, the Dental Practitioners' Formulary (or other official compendia which may in the future be produced under the Medicines Act 1968, Section 99) and the list of names prepared and published under Section 100 of the Medicines Act 1968.

Strength in relation to a relevant medicinal product means the content of active ingredient in that product expressed quantitatively per dosage unit, per unit volume or by weight, according to the dosage form.

Supplementary prescriber means:
(a) a registered nurse,
(b) a pharmacist,
(c) a registered midwife, or
(d) a person whose name is registered in the part of the register maintained by the Health Professions Council in pursuance of Article 5 of the Health Professions Order 2001 relating to:
  (i) chiropodists and podiatrists;
  (ii) physiotherapists;
  (iii) radiographers: diagnostic or therapeutic; or (e) a registered optometrist
against whose name is recorded in the relevant register an annotation or entry signifying that he is qualified to order drugs, medicines and appliances as a supplementary prescriber or, in the case of a nurse or midwife, as a nurse independent/supplementary prescriber.

Unit preparation means a preparation, including a mother tincture, prepared by a process of solution, extraction or trituration with a view to being diluted tenfold or one hundredfold, either once or repeatedly, in an inert diluent and then used either in this diluted form or, where applicable, by impregnating tablets, granules, powders or other inert substances.

Veterinary medicinal product means:
(a) any substance or combination of substances presented as having properties for treating or preventing disease in animals; or
(b) any substance or combination of substances that may be used in, or administered to, animals with a view either to restoring, correcting or modifying physiological functions by exerting a pharmacological, immunological or metabolic action, or to making a medical diagnosis.

Veterinary requisition means a requisition which states, in accordance with Article 14 paragraph (2)(ii) of the Misuse of Drugs Regulations 2001, as amended, that the recipient is a veterinary surgeon or veterinary practitioner.

1.2 Medicines for human use

Section 1.2 covers the following:

Classes of medicinal products

There are three classes of products under the Medicines Act 1968, namely:
(1) General sale list medicines (GSL)
(2) Pharmacy medicines (P)
(3) Prescription-only medicines (POM).

The legal requirements which apply to the sale, supply, dispensing and labelling of each class are dealt with separately below.

Meaning of "retail sale" and "wholesale dealing"

The selling of a medicinal product constitutes "wholesale dealing" if it is sold to a person for the purpose of:

(a) selling or supplying it, or
(b) administering it, or causing it to be administered to one or more human beings;
the sale, supply or administration being in the course of a business carried on by the purchaser.

Any sale which does not fall within this definition of "wholesale dealing" is a retail sale. The restrictions on the retail sale of medicinal products also apply to supply and to supplying "in circumstances corresponding to retail sale," which includes the dispensing of prescriptions under the National Health Service.

1.2.1 General sale list medicines (GSL)

GSL medicines are those medicinal products which in the opinion of the appropriate Ministers can, with reasonable safety, be sold or supplied otherwise than by or under the supervision of a pharmacist. These are listed in the Medicines (Products Other than Veterinary Drugs) (General Sale List) Order 1984 (GSL Order). GSL medicines can also be classified as such as a result of their marketing authorisation.

All GSL medicines, except those that have been designated as foods or cosmetics, must be licensed products (it should be noted that a medicinal product made up in a pharmacy for sale from that pharmacy without a marketing authorisation, is classified as a pharmacy medicine even though all its ingredients are in the GSL Order).

Products not on general sale

Part of the GSL Order specifies certain classes of medicinal products for human use which shall not be available on general sale. They are medicinal products promoted, recommended or marketed:

(a) for use as anthelmintics,
(b) for parenteral administration,
(c) for use as eye drops,
(d) for use as eye ointments,
(e) for use as enemas,
(f) for use wholly or mainly for irrigation of wounds or of the bladder, vagina or rectum, or,
(g) for administration wholly or mainly to children being a preparation of aloxiprin or aspirin.

Foods and cosmetics

Medicinal products which are for sale or supply either for oral administration as a food or for external use as a cosmetic are general sale list medicines. This does not include products which are prescription-only medicines, eye drops or eye ointments, or any product that contains either:

(a) vitamin A, vitamin A acetate or vitamin A palmitate with a maximum daily dose equivalent to more than 7,500 international units of vitamin A or 2,250 micrograms of retinol; or
(b) vitamin D with a maximum daily dose of more than 400 units of antirachitic activity.

Retail sale of GSL medicines

Medicinal products on a general sale list may only be sold by retail, offered or exposed for sale by retail, or supplied in circumstances corresponding to retail sale either at registered pharmacies, or in circumstances where the following conditions are fulfilled:

(a) The place at which the medicinal product is sold, offered, exposed for sale or supplied, must be premises at which the person carrying on the business is the occupier and which he is able to close so as to exclude the public. Sales from automatic machines should only be made from machines located in premises which the occupier is able to close so as to exclude the public.
(b) The medicinal product must have been made up for sale in a container elsewhere and not have been opened since the product was made up for sale in it.

Pharmacy Only (PO)

A PO medicine is a product that is licensed as a GSL medicine, but is restricted to sale through pharmacies only. PO medicines do not need to be sold under the supervision of a phar-

but when in the form of a licensed product, for which the indications fall within the terms specified for an exemption, the product is licensed as a pharmacy medicine. No other hydrocortisone products can be sold without prescription, and the licensed products must only be sold within the terms of their licence (they cannot, for example, be mixed with other medicinal products, even where they are pharmacy only or even general sale list medicines). For examples, refer to the alphabetical list of medicines for human use (Section 1.3).

Some medicinal products are exempted from prescription-only status when sold or supplied for the treatment of specified conditions, and at dosages not exceeding stated maxima. However, the labelling of such products is complex, and pharmacists are advised to sell or supply only licensed products specially packed for over the counter sale.

Exemption for products consisting of or containing pseudoephedrine salts or ephedrine base or salts

It is unlawful to sell or supply a product or products containing more than 720mg of pseudoephedrine salts or more than 180mg ephedrine base (or salts) to a person at any one time (ie, in one transaction) except in accordance with a prescription.

A sale or supply without a prescription may be made of more than one product containing only one of these substances, provided that the total amount sold does not exceed the above limit. However, it is unlawful to sell or supply a pseudoephedrine-containing product at the same time as an ephedrine-containing product in one transaction.

Administration of prescription-only medicines

The legislation provides that no one may administer a parenteral prescription-only medicine otherwise than to himself, unless he is an appropriate practitioner or is acting in accordance with the directions of an appropriate practitioner.

Administration of parenteral medicines for the purpose of saving a life in an emergency

The legislation provides that no-one may administer a parenteral prescription-only medicine otherwise than to himself, unless he is an appropriate practitioner or is acting in accordance with the directions of an appropriate practitioner.

The following list of medicines for use by parenteral administration, are exempt from this restriction when administered for the purpose of saving life in an emergency.

Adrenaline injection 1 in 1000 (1mg in 1ml)
Atropine sulphate injection
Atropine sulphate and obidoxime chloride injection
Atropine sulphate and pralidoxime chloride injection
Atropine sulphate, pralidoxime mesilate and avizafone injection
Chlorphenamine injection
Dicobalt edetate injection
Glucagon injection
Glucose injection 50%
Hydrocortisone injection
Naloxone hydrochloride
Pralidoxime chloride injection
Pralidoxime mesilate injection
Promethazine hydrochloride injection
Snake venom antiserum

Sodium nitrite injection
Sodium thiosulphate injection
Sterile pralidoxime

Administration of smallpox vaccine

The legislation provides that no one may administer a parenteral prescription-only medicine otherwise than to himself, unless he is an appropriate practitioner or is acting in accordance with the directions of an appropriate practitioner. Smallpox vaccine for parenteral administration to human beings is exempt from this restriction where either:

1. (a) the vaccine has been supplied by, or on behalf of, or under arrangements made by:
(i) the Secretary of State,
(ii) the Scottish Ministers,
(iii) the National Assembly for Wales,
(iv) the Department of Health, Social Services and Public Safety,
(v) an NHS body; and
(b) the vaccine is administered for the purpose of providing protection against smallpox virus in the event of a suspected or confirmed case of smallpox in the United Kingdom, OR:
2. (a) the vaccine has been supplied by, or on behalf of, or under arrangements made by Her Majesty's Forces;
(b) the vaccine is administered for the purpose of providing protection against smallpox virus to:
(i) members of Her Majesty's Forces; or
(ii) other persons employed or engaged by those Forces.

For the purposes of this section, "NHS body" means:
(a) the Common Services Agency,
(b) a Strategic Health Authority, Health Authority or Special Health Authority,
(c) a Primary Care Trust,
(d) a Local Health Board, or
(e) an NHS Trust or NHS foundation trust.

Administration by operators

The legislation provides that no-one may administer a parenteral prescription-only medicine otherwise than to himself, unless he is an appropriate practitioner or is acting in accordance with the directions of an appropriate practitioner. This restriction does not apply to:

1. a radioactive medicinal product, administration of which results in a medical exposure; or,
2. any other prescription only medicine if it is being administered in connection with a medical exposure.
The following conditions must be satisfied:
(a) The radioactive medicinal product or other prescription only medicine is administered by an operator acting in accordance with the procedures and protocols referred to in regulation 4(1) and 4(2) of the Ionising Radiation (Medical Exposure) Regulations 2000;
(b) The medical exposure has been authorised by an IRME practitioner or, where this is not practicable, by an operator acting in accordance with written guidelines issued by an IRME practitioner;
(c) The IRME practitioner is the holder of a certificate granted under the Medicines (Administration of Radioactive Substances) Regulations 1978;
(d) The radioactive medicinal product or other prescription only medicine is not a Controlled Drug; and

(e) In the case of a prescription only medicine which is not a radioactive medicinal product, it is specified in the protocols (as referred to in subsection [a]) in connection with a medical exposure.

Administration of prescription-only medicines in hospital

The Medicines Act 1968 does not specify that the directions of an appropriate practitioner need be in writing, in order to authorise administration. Nevertheless, it is good practice to ensure that whenever a prescription-only medicine is administered it has been authorised in writing by an appropriate practitioner before administration takes place.

Some hospitals have formulated policies to permit administration in an emergency on the telephoned or verbal request of an appropriate practitioner, usually involving two nurses checking one another. Some hospitals have also formulated policies for the routine administration of prescription-only (and pharmacy and general sale list) medicines. Such a policy should be carefully considered and agreed by medical, nursing and pharmaceutical staff, to ensure that patients are not put at risk. If in doubt, the Department of Health should be consulted, where the hospital is in England, along with the legal advisors of the hospital. Hospitals in Scotland should contact the Scottish Executive and hospitals in Wales should contact the Department of Health and Social Services.

Prescriptions for prescription-only medicines

A prescription-only medicine may be sold or supplied by retail only in accordance with a prescription given by an appropriate practitioner (see pp14-15 for changes to this legislation in the event of a pandemic).

Appropriate practitioners include United Kingdom registered doctors, dentists, nurse independent prescribers, pharmacist independent prescribers, optometrist independent prescribers, veterinary surgeons and veterinary practitioners, supplementary prescribers, EEA or Swiss doctors and EEA or Swiss dentists (see below).

The General Medical Council (GMC) has introduced a licence to practise for doctors, in addition to the requirement for them to be registered with the GMC. In order to practise medicine in the UK and have the legal authority to carry out professional activities (e.g. issuing prescriptions), doctors will be required by law both to be registered with the GMC and to hold a licence to practise. Supplementary prescribers can issue prescriptions for any prescription-only medicine when acting in accordance with a clinical management plan (see p16).

Until additional changes to the Misuse of Drugs Regulations 2001 take place, pharmacist independent prescribers will not be able to prescribe Controlled Drugs, and nurse independent prescribers will continue to be limited to the range of Controlled Drugs they can currently prescribe for particular indications.

A prescription issued by an EEA or Swiss healthcare professional is legally valid in the UK. EEA healthcare professional refers only to doctors or dentists who are registered to practise in an EEA country or in Switzerland. UK registered doctors and dentists are excluded as they are already covered by current medicines legislation. EEA or Swiss healthcare professionals are not permitted to issue prescriptions for Schedule 1-5 Controlled Drugs and medicines that do not have a UK marketing authorisation.

Further information on dispensing prescriptions issued by EEA or Swiss healthcare professionals can be found on the Society website, *www.rpsgb.org*.

Pharmacists can telephone the General Medical Council (0845 357 3456 or 0161 923 6602) to confirm the registration and licensing status of a doctor.

Pharmacists can telephone the General Dental Council (020 7887 3800) to confirm that a dentist is registered.

Pharmacists can telephone the Nursing and Midwifery Council (020 7333 9333) to confirm a nurse's registration status.

Pharmacists can telephone the Society's Registration Department (020 7572 2532) to confirm a pharmacist's registration status.

Supplementary prescriber or independent prescriber status can be checked against the relevant register held by the appropriate professional or regulatory body. Contact details for medical and dental regulatory authorities in EEA states and Switzerland can be found on the Society's website (*www.rpsgb.org*).

To be valid, a prescription issued by an appropriate practitioner:

(a) shall be signed in ink with his own name by the appropriate practitioner giving it;

(b) shall be written in indelible ink (this includes typewriting and computer generated prescriptions). A health prescription, which is not for a Controlled Drug specified in Schedule 1, 2 or 3 to the Misuse of Drugs Regulations, can be written by means of carbon paper or similar material but must be signed in indelible ink by the practitioner giving it;

(c) shall contain the following particulars:

(i) the address of the appropriate practitioner giving it,

(ii) the appropriate date,

(iii) such particulars as indicate whether the appropriate practitioner giving it is a doctor, dentist, supplementary prescriber, community practitioner nurse prescriber, nurse independent prescriber, optometrist independent prescriber, pharmacist independent prescriber, EEA or Swiss doctor or an EEA or Swiss dentist,

(iv) where the appropriate practitioner giving it is a doctor, dentist, supplementary prescriber, community practitioner nurse prescriber, nurse independent prescriber, optometrist independent prescriber, pharmacist independent prescriber, EEA or Swiss doctor or an EEA or Swiss dentist, the name, address and the age, if under 12, of the person for whose treatment it is given; (From 26 July 2010, where the appropriate practitioner giving it is an EEA or Swiss doctor or an EEA or Swiss dentist the address and the age, if under 12, of the person for whose treatment the prescription is given is no longer legally required.)

(d) shall not be dispensed after the end of the period of six months from the appropriate date, unless it is a repeatable prescription in which case it shall not be dispensed for the first time after the end of that period nor otherwise than in accordance with the direction contained in the repeatable prescription;

(e) in the case of a repeatable prescription that does not specify the number of times it may be dispensed, shall not be repeated on more than one occasion unless it is a prescription for oral contraceptives in which case it may be dispensed a total of six times (ie five repeats) before the end of the period of six months from the appropriate date. Once a repeatable prescription has been dispensed for the first time within the six month period, there is no time period in which the prescription must be repeated. The exception to this is where the prescription falls under the NHS repeat dispensing scheme or the prescriber has specified otherwise. NB. Where the prescription is for a Schedule 4 Controlled Drug, the validity period for the purposes of (d) and (e) above will be 28 days not six months. For information on Controlled Drugs see p38.

A private prescription must be retained for two years from the date on which the prescription only medicine was sold or supplied, or, for a repeat prescription, the date on which the medicine was supplied for the last time.

A prescription, other than a prescription for a Controlled Drug listed in Schedule 1, 2 or 3 of the Misuse of Drugs Regulations 2001, may still be valid where it is created in an electronic form, is signed with an advanced electronic signature of the person prescribing it, and is sent to the person who is dispensing it as an electronic communication.

Advanced electronic signature means an electronic signature which is uniquely linked to the signatory, capable of identifying the signatory, created using means that the signatory can maintain under their sole control and which is linked to the data to which it relates in such a manner that any subsequent change of data is detectable. Signatory means the appropriate practitioner issuing the prescription.

When a prescription-only medicine is also a Controlled Drug listed in Schedule 2 or 3 of the Misuse of Drugs Regulations 2001, a prescription must also be written in accordance with the requirements of those Regulations. Note: repeat prescriptions are not permitted for Schedule 2 and 3 Controlled Drug prescriptions (see Section 1.2.14).

Validity of dental prescriptions

A dentist is an appropriate practitioner for the purpose of prescribing prescription-only medicines. A prescription written by a dentist is valid under the Medicines Act 1968 even where the item prescribed is not in the Dental Practitioners' Formulary. Under the terms of service, an FP10(D) prescription written by a dentist is valid only if the medicinal products ordered are in the Dental Practitioners' Formulary, but a private prescription can order any prescription-only (or pharmacy or general sale list) medicine. A pharmacy will be reimbursed for any drug that is on an FP10(SS) prescription form unless that drug is not prescribable on the NHS. This is regardless of who has written it, eg, hospital doctor or hospital dentist. Dentists are required by their registration body to restrict their prescribing to areas in which they are competent, and this would therefore mean that a dentist should generally prescribe only medicines which have uses in dentistry.

Facsimile transmission of prescriptions

A "fax" of a prescription does not fall within the definition of a legally valid prescription (see above), because it is not written in indelible ink, and has not been signed by an appropriate practitioner. A fax can, however, confirm that at the time of receipt, a valid prescription is in existence.

Any pharmacist who decides to dispense a prescription-only medicine against a fax, without sight of the original prescription, must ensure that adequate safeguards exist to ensure that the integrity of the original prescription is maintained, and that the prescription will be in his possession within a short time. Any doubt as to the content of the original prescription, caused by poor reproduction, must be overcome before the medicine is supplied. As it is possible to fax a prescription many times, the pharmacist is advised to ensure that no dispensing against a fax takes place unless the system used for the sending or receipt of faxes is secure. Under no circumstances can medicines listed in Schedules 2 or 3 of the Misuse of Drugs Regulations 2001 be dispensed against a fax.

Forged prescriptions

It can be extremely difficult to detect a forged prescription, but every pharmacist should be alert to the possibility that any prescription calling for a product liable to misuse could be a forgery. In many instances, the forger may make a fundamental error in writing the prescription or the pharmacist may get an instinctive feeling that the prescription is not genuine because of the way the patient behaves.

If the prescriber's signature is known, but the patient has not previously visited the pharmacy, or is not known to be suffering from a condition which requires the medicinal product prescribed, the signature should be scrutinised and, if possible, checked against an example on another prescription known to be genuine. Large doses or quantities should be checked with the prescriber in order to detect alterations to previously valid prescriptions.

If the prescriber's signature is not known, the prescriber must be contacted and asked to confirm that the prescription is genuine. The prescriber's telephone number must be obtained from the telephone directory, or from directory enquiries, not from the headed notepaper, as forgers may use false letter headings.

A list of matters that should alert a pharmacist to making further checks is given below. This list is not exhaustive.
(1) Unknown prescriber.
(2) New patient.
(3) Excessive quantities.
(4) Uncharacteristic prescribing or method of writing prescription by a known doctor.
(5) Dr before or after prescriber's signature.

These precautions should be applied to all prescriptions for drugs liable to misuse and not only for Controlled Drugs. The dispensing of a forged prescription for a Controlled Drug or prescription-only medicine can constitute a criminal offence.

Exemptions to medicines legislation in the event of a pandemic

The Department of Health will announce when a pandemic situation is imminent or has arisen, at which time the following provisions will apply.

Emergency supply

In the event of a pandemic, or in anticipation of a disease being imminently pandemic which poses a serious or potentially serious risk to human health, the conditions for making an emergency supply at the request of a patient are relaxed in that the pharmacist will not need to interview the person who requests the medicine.

The pharmacist will still be required to satisfy himself/herself that the treatment had been prescribed on a previous occasion by an appropriate practitioner and that the dose is appropriate for the person to be treated to take.

Currently, a dentist is not included as being an appropriate practitioner for this particular change to emergency supply legislation. In the event of a pandemic, or a disease being imminently pandemic, the legislation does not remove the requirement to interview the person requesting the medicine, if the patient was originally prescribed the medicine by a dentist. However, it is important to remember that in normal circumstances an emergency supply can be made at the request of a patient if the medicine was originally prescribed by a dentist. This is an anomaly in the legislation and the Medicines and Healthcare products Regulatory Agency (MHRA) does intend to amend the legislation so that this relaxation will also apply at the request of a patient previously prescribed a medicine by a dentist in the future. The MHRA and the Home Office are also considering whether an expanded range of Controlled Drugs should be available via the emergency supply provisions during a pandemic. Further guidance will be issued in the pharmaceutical press to inform pharmacists of any changes. Also *see* Emergency supplies of prescription-only medicines (pp17-18).

Supply of prescription-only medicines against a prescription

In the event, or in anticipation, of pandemic disease, the requirement whereby prescription-only medicines are only sold or supplied (in circumstances corresponding to retail sale) in accordance with a prescription given by an appropriate practitioner, will not apply.

This change will only apply when a disease is pandemic, or in anticipation of a disease being imminently pandemic, and a serious or potentially serious risk to human health. In such an event, supplies will be made from designated collection points in accordance with a specific protocol. In England, the Department of Health will announce when supplies under such a protocol can be made. In Scotland and Wales the relevant government departments will make the announcements.

The protocol must be approved by Ministers, an NHS body or the Health Protection Agency.

The protocol must contain criteria as to:
(i) symptoms of, and treatment for, that disease;
(ii) the recording of the name of the person who supplies the prescription only medicine to the person to be treated (or to a person acting on that person's behalf) and of the evidence that the medicine was supplied to the person to be treated (or to a person acting on that person's behalf).

Further guidance will be issued on protocols when more information is available.

Conditions under which the retail sale or supply of medicines can occur

In the event, or in anticipation, of a pandemic disease, the requirement for prescription-only medicines and pharmacy medicines to be sold or supplied from registered pharmacy premises, and the requirement that such transactions are made by or under the supervision of pharmacist, will not apply. This change will only apply while a disease is, or in anticipation of, a disease being imminently pandemic and a serious risk, or potentially serious risk, to human health and is in accordance with a specific protocol. The requirements for the protocol are the same as described above.

Labelling of certain children's medicines

The MHRA has temporarily authorised the distribution of unlicensed oseltamivir powder and an unlicensed oral liquid formulation of oseltamivir for administration to infants under one year of age in the prevention or treatment of influenza. The oral solution will be prepared in designated licensed NHS manufacturing units.

Linked to this authorisation, in the event of a disease being imminently pandemic or pandemic and a serious or potentially serious risk to human health, the labelling requirements for antiviral medicines in the form of a solution intended for the treatment of a child under the age of one year, will be simplified. Under such circumstances the container of the product only needs to be labelled with the following:
(i) the name of the person to whom the medicine is to be administered;
(ii) the date on which the medicine is dispensed; and
(iii) the necessary and usual instructions for proper use.

Written directions to supply (in hospitals)

The legislation allows a hospital to sell or supply a prescription-only medicine in the course of its business, against a patient specific "written direction" of a person (other than a veterinary surgeon or veterinary practitioner) who is an appropriate practitioner in relation to that medicine, instead of a prescription. The written direction does not need to comply with the requirements specified for prescriptions, but does need to relate to a specific patient. The intention is to permit the sale or supply of medicines against the patient's bed card or patient notes.

Most entries on a patient's bed card are directions to administer. However, providing the wording is clear, the entry can be taken as authority to make a supply, for example as take home medication. Providing the entry fulfils the requirements the details can be transposed onto an order form, to be used in pharmacy to prepare the take home medication. It is good practice for the transposition to be carried out by a pharmacist. By carrying out this transcription the pharmacist is not prescribing, as the original written direction to supply was made by a practitioner.

Patient group directions

The legislation also permits the supply of prescription-only medicines under a patient group direction (PGD).

A PGD is a written direction relating to supply and/or administration of a prescription-only medicine to persons generally (subject to specified exclusions), and is signed by a doctor or a dentist, and by a pharmacist.

The following is a list of the persons who are permitted under the Regulations to supply or administer under a PGD:
Dental hygienists;
Dental therapists;
Registered paramedics or individuals who hold a certificate of proficiency in ambulance paramedic skills issued by, or with the approval of, the Secretary of State;
Pharmacists;
Registered dietitians;
Registered midwives;
Registered nurses;
Registered occupational therapists;
Registered optometrists;

not apply to the sale, offer for sale or supply of any such medicinal product by a doctor or dentist to a patient of his, or to a person under whose care such a patient is.

Midwives

The wholesale of medicines to a midwife from a registered pharmacy for the midwife to SELL OR SUPPLY to their patients

Registered midwives can sell or supply the following medicines. Therefore, they can obtain these medicines by wholesale from a registered pharmacy:

(a) all general sale list medicines;

(b) all pharmacy medicines;

(c) prescription-only medicines containing any of the following substances:

Diclofenac

Ergometrine maleate (only when contained in a medicinal product which is not for parenteral administration)

Hydrocortizone Acetate

Lignocaine (Lidocaine)

Lignocaine (Lidocaine) hydrochloride

Miconazole

Nystatin

Phytomenadione

A midwife can only sell or supply these medicinal products, under certain conditions. These conditions are:

(i) the sale or supply shall be only in the course of their professional practice;

(ii) in the case of ergometrine maleate they can only sell or supply a medicinal product that is not for parenteral administration.

A supply made by a registered pharmacy to a midwife under this exemption is a wholesale transaction. For the requirements concerned with wholesale transactions *see* Section 1.2.4.

The wholesale of medicines to a midwife from a registered pharmacy for the midwife to ADMINISTER to their patients

Registered midwives can administer prescription only medicines for parenteral administration containing any of the following substances but no other substance. Therefore, they can obtain these medicines by wholesale from a registered pharmacy:

Adrenaline

Anti-D Immunoglobulin

Carboprost

Cyclizine hydrochloride

Diamorphine

Ergometrine maleate

Gelofusine

Haemaccel

Hartmann's solution

Hepatitis B vaccine

Hepatitis immunoglobulin

Lignocaine (Lidocaine)

Lignocaine hydrochloride (Lidocaine hydrochloride)

Morphine

Naloxone hydrochloride

Oxytocins, natural and synthetic

Pethidine hydrochloride

Phytomenadione

Prochloperazine

Sodium chloride 0.9%

A midwife can only administer the above parenteral medicines under certain conditions. These conditions are:

(i) the administration is in the course of their professional practice.

(ii) in the case of lignocaine and lignocaine hydrochloride it shall only be administered while attending on a woman in childbirth.

A supply made by a registered pharmacy to a midwife under this exemption is a wholesale transaction. For the requirements concerned with wholesale transactions *see* Section 1.2.4. Any pharmacist who is asked for advice or wishes to check on the legality of supplying any of the Controlled Drugs listed above, ie, diamorphine, morphine or pethidine to a midwife should contact the Society's Legal and Ethical Advisory Service for advice.

Chiropodists

The wholesale of medicines to a chiropodist from a registered pharmacy for the chiropodist to SELL OR SUPPLY to their patients

Registered chiropodists can obtain these medicines by wholesale from a registered pharmacy:

(a) General sale list medicines which are for external use;

(b) Any of the following pharmacy medicines for external use:

(i) potassium permanganate crystals or solution;

(ii) ointment of heparinoid and hyaluronidase; and

(iii) products containing as their only active ingredients, any of the following substances, not exceeding the strength specified in each case:

Borotannic complex 9.0%

Buclosamide 10.0%

Chlorquinaldol 3.0%

Clotrimazole 1.0%

Crotamiton 10.0%

Diamthazole hydrochloride 5.0%

Econazole nitrate 1.0%

Fenticlor 1.0%

Glutaraldehyde 10.0%

Griseofulvin 1.0%

Hydrargaphen 0.4%

Mepyramine maleate 2.0%

Miconazole nitrate 2.0%

Phenoxypropan-2-ol 2.0%

Podophyllum resin 20.0%

Polynoxylin 10.0%

Pyrogallol 70.0%

Salicylic acid 70.0%

Terbinafine 1.0%

Thiomersal 0.1%

The registered chiropodist can only sell or supply these medicinal products, under certain conditions. These conditions are:

(i) the sale or supply shall be only in the course of their professional practice;

(ii) the medicinal product has been made up for sale and supply in a container elsewhere than at the place at which it is sold or supplied.

Registered chiropodists who have the relevant annotation in the Health Professions Council register signifying that they are qualified to use the medicines specified below, can obtain these medicines by wholesale from a registered pharmacy:

(a) Any of the following prescription-only medicines:

(i) Co-dydramol 10/500 tablets;

(ii) Amorolfine hydrochloride cream where the maximum strength of the amorolfine in the cream does not exceed 0.25 per cent by weight in weight;

(iii) Amorolfine hydrochloride lacquer where the maximum strength of the amorolfine in the lacquer does not exceed 5 per cent by weight in volume;

(iv) Topical hydrocortisone where the maximum strength of the hydrocortisone in the medicinal product does not exceed 1 per cent by weight in weight;

(v) Amoxicillin;

(vi) Erythromycin;

(vii) Flucoxacillin;

(viii) Tioconazole 28%;

(ix) Silver sulfadiazine;

(b) Preparations which are not prescription-only medicines:

(i) Ibuprofen.

The chiropodist can only sell or supply these medicinal products under certain conditions. These conditions are:

(i)   the sale or supply shall be only in the course of their professional practice;

(ii) the medicinal product has been made up for sale and supply in a container elsewhere than at the place at which it is sold or supplied;

(iii) in the case of co-dydramol 10/500 tablets the quantity sold or supplied to a person at any one time shall not exceed the amount sufficient for 3 days' treatment to a maximum of 24 tablets; and

(iv) in the case of ibuprofen the maximum dose is 400mg, the maximum daily dose is 1,200mg and the maximum pack size is 3,600mg for 3 days treatment.

A supply made by a registered pharmacy to a registered chiropodist under this exemption is a wholesale transaction. For the requirements concerned with wholesale transactions *see* Section 1.2.4.

Pharmacists can only supply original and complete packs to chiropodists as this is a wholesale transaction. Pharmacists should therefore consider which pack size they wholesale to chiropodists especially in the case of co-dydramol and ibuprofen as chiropodists are limited to the quantity they can supply to their patients and are unable to alter the pack size once it has been supplied to them from the pharmacy.

The wholesale of medicines to a chiropodist from a registered pharmacy for the chiropodist to ADMINISTER to their patients

Registered chiropodists, who have the relevant annotation in the Health Professions Council register signifying that they are qualified to use the medicines specified below, can obtain these medicines by wholesale from a registered pharmacy:

Adrenaline

Bupivacaine hydrochloride

Bupivacaine hydrochloride with adrenaline where the maximum strength of the adrenaline does not exceed 1mg in 200ml of bupivacaine hydrochloride

Levobupivacaine hydrochloride

Lignocaine (Lidocaine) hydrochloride

Lignocaine (Lidocaine) hydrochloride with adrenaline where the maximum strength of the adrenaline does not exceed 1mg in 200ml of lignocaine (lidocaine) hydrochloride

Mepivacaine hydrochloride

Methylprednisolone

Prilocaine hydrochloride

Ropivacaine hydrochloride

A chiropodist can only administer the above parenteral prescription only medicines if the administration is in the course of their professional practice.

A supply made by a registered pharmacy to a registered chiropodist under this exemption is a wholesale transaction. For the requirements concerned with wholesale transactions *see* Section 1.2.4.

Optometrists

The wholesale of medicines to a registered optometrist from a registered pharmacy for the optometrist to SELL OR SUPPLY to their patients

Registered optometrists can sell or supply the following medicines. Therefore, they can obtain these medicines by wholesale from a registered pharmacy:

(a) all general sale list medicines;

(b) all pharmacy medicines.

(c) Certain prescription-only medicines which are not for parenteral administration. These medicines include:

Eye drops or eye ointments that are prescription-only medicines by reason only that they contain:

(i) mafenide propionate, or

(ii) not more that 30% sulphacetamide sodium, or

(iii) sulphafurazole diethanolamine equivalent to not more than 4% sulphafurazole, or

Eye drops that are prescription-only medicines by reason only that they contain no more than 0.5% chloramphenicol, or

Eye ointments that are prescription-only medicines by reason only that they contain no more than 1% chloramphenicol, or

Prescription-only medicines because they contain any of the following substances:

Cyclopentolate hydrochloride

Fusidic acid

Tropicamide

A registered optometrist can only sell or supply these medicinal products, under certain conditions. These conditions are:

(i)   In the case of general sale list medicines and pharmacy medicines the sale or supply must be in the course of their professional practice.

(ii) In the case of prescription-only medicines the sale or supply must be in the course of their professional practice and in an emergency.

A supply made by a registered pharmacy to a registered optometrist under this exemption is a wholesale transaction. For the requirements concerned with wholesale transactions *see* Section 1.2.4.

A pharmacist may supply the prescription only medicines (listed above) directly to a patient under the care of a registered optometrist on presentation of a signed order issued by the registered optometrist. It is not, however, a prescription, as a prescription is an authority to supply prescription-only medicines issued by an appropriate practitioner, and an optometrist does not come under this definition.

In making such a supply, pharmacists must ensure that they comply with the professional requirements of the Code of Ethics, in that the product supplied must be labelled accordingly, a patient information leaflet must be provided and the sale or supply must be recorded in the prescription-only register. The pharmacist must also be satisfied that the optometrist has provided sufficient information and advice to enable safe and effective use of the medicine and has made a follow-up appointment where necessary.

Registered optometrists can also obtain the following medicines by wholesale from a registered pharmacy:

Amethocaine hydrochloride
Lignocaine (Lidocaine) hydrochloride
Oxybuprocaine hydrochloride
Proxymetacaine hydrochloride

A supply made by a registered pharmacy to a registered optometrist under this exemption is a wholesale transaction. For the requirements concerned with wholesale transactions *see* Section 1.2.4.

Additional supply optometrists

The wholesale of medicines to a registered additional supply optometrist from a registered pharmacy for the additional supply optometrist to SELL OR SUPPLY to their patients

Registered additional supply optometrists can sell or supply the following medicines so long as they are not for parenteral administration. Therefore, they can obtain these medicines by wholesale from a registered pharmacy:

Acetylcysteine
Atropine sulphate
Azelastine hydrochloride
Diclofenac sodium
Emedastine
Homotropine hydrobromide
Ketotifen
Levocabastine
Lodoxamide
Nedocromil sodium
Olopatadine
Pilocarpine hydrochloride
Pilocarpine nitrate
Polymyxin B/ bacitracin
Polymixin B/ trimethoprim
Sodium cromoglycate

A registered additional supply optometrist can only sell or supply these medicinal products, under certain conditions. The condition is that:

(i) In the case of prescription only medicines the sale or supply must be in the course of their professional practice and in an emergency.

A pharmacist may supply the prescription only medicines listed above directly to a patient under the care of a registered additional supply optometrist on presentation of a signed order issued by the additional supply optometrist. The signed order is not, however, a prescription, as a prescription is an authority to supply prescription-only medicines issued by an appropriate practitioner, and an additional supply optometrist does not come under this definition.

In making such a supply, pharmacists must ensure that they comply with the professional requirements of the Code of Ethics, in that the product supplied must be labelled accordingly, a patient information leaflet must be provided and the sale or supply must be recorded in the prescription-only register. The pharmacist must also be satisfied that the additional supply optometrist has provided sufficient information and advice to enable safe and effective use of the medicine and has made a follow-up appointment where necessary.

Registered additional supply optometrists can also obtain the following medicines by wholesale from a registered pharmacy:

Thymoxamine hydrochloride

A supply made by a registered pharmacy to a registered additional supply optometrist under this exemption is a wholesale transaction. For the requirements concerned with wholesale transactions *see* Section 1.2.4.

Dispensing optician

The wholesale of medicines to a registered dispensing optician from a registered pharmacy for the registered dispensing optician to SELL OR SUPPY to their patients

Registered dispensing opticians can sell or supply the following medicines. Therefore, they can obtain these medicines by wholesale from a registered pharmacy:

(a) pharmacy medicines for external use containing chloramphenicol at a strength not exceeding:
0.5% in eye drops or 1% in ointment

A registered dispensing optician can only sell or supply these medicinal products, under certain conditions. These conditions are:

(i) the sale or supply shall be only in the course of their professional practice.

A supply made by a registered pharmacy to a registered dispensing optician under this exemption is a wholesale transaction. For the requirements concerned with wholesale transactions *see* Section 1.2.4.

Registered dispensing opticians can also obtain medicines which contain any one or more of the following substances by wholesale from a registered pharmacy, for use by registered optometrists and doctors attending the registered dispensing optician's practice:

Amethocaine hydrochloride
Chloramphenicol
Cyclopentolate hydrochloride
Fusidic acid
Lignocaine (Lidocaine) hydrochloride
Oxybuprocaine hydrochloride
Proxymetacaine hydrochloride
Tropicamide

A supply made by a registered pharmacy to a registered dispensing optician under this exemption is a wholesale transaction. For the requirements concerned with wholesale transactions *see* Section 1.2.4.

Registered dispensing opticians can also obtain medicines which contain any one or more of the following substances by wholesale from a registered pharmacy, for use by the registered dispensing optician in the course of their professional practice as a contact lens specialist:

Lignocaine (Lidocaine) hydrochloride
Oxybuprocaine hydrochloride
Proxymetacaine hydrochloride

A supply made by a registered pharmacy to a registered dispensing optician under this exemption is a wholesale transaction. For the requirements concerned with wholesale transactions *see* Section 1.2.4.

Drug treatment services

The wholesale of medicines to persons employed or engaged in the provision of lawful drug treatment services from a registered pharmacy for the drug treatment service to SUPPLY (BUT NOT SELL) to their patients

A person employed or engaged in the provision of lawful drug treatment service may supply the following medicinal product. Therefore, they can obtain this medicinal product by wholesale from a registered pharmacy:

> Ampoules of sterile water for injection containing not more than 2 ml of sterile water.

A person employed or engaged in the provision of lawful drug treatment service can only supply these medicinal products, under certain conditions. The condition is that:

(i) The supply shall be only in the course of provision of lawful drug treatment services.

A supply made by a registered pharmacy to a person employed or engaged in the provision of a lawful drug treatment service under this exemption is a wholesale transaction. For the requirements concerned with wholesale transactions *see* Section 1.2.4.

Shipping personnel

The wholesale of medicines to the owner or the master of a ship (including masters of foreign ships) which does not carry a doctor on board from a registered pharmacy for the SUPPLY (BUT NOT SALE) to persons on the ship

The owner or master of a ship (which does not carry a doctor on board) may supply the following medicines. Therefore, they can obtain these medicines by wholesale from a registered pharmacy:

(a) all general sale list medicines;

(b) all pharmacy medicines;

(c) all prescription-only medicines (including Controlled Drugs (*see* p34).

The owner or master of a ship (which does not carry a doctor on board) can only supply these medicinal products, under certain conditions. The condition is that:

(i) The supply is necessary for the treatment of persons on the ship.

A supply made by a registered pharmacy to a owner or master of a ship under this exemption is a wholesale transaction. For the requirements concerned with wholesale transactions *see* Section 1.2.4.

The wholesale of medicines to the owner or the master of a ship which does not carry a doctor on board from a registered pharmacy for the ADMINISTRATION to persons on the ship

The owner or master of a ship (which does not carry a doctor on board) may administer the following medicines. Therefore, they can obtain these medicines by wholesale from a registered pharmacy:

(a) All prescription only medicines that are for parenteral administration.

The owner or master of a ship (which does not carry a doctor on board) can only administer these medicinal products, under certain conditions. The condition is that:

(i) That the supply is necessary for the treatment of persons on the ship.

A supply made by a registered pharmacy to an owner or master of a ship under this exemption is a wholesale transaction. For the requirements concerned with wholesale transactions *see* Section 1.2.4. Pharmacists who receive a request for a supply of medicines from the owner or master of a ship would then need to establish the identity of the owner or master of the ship and ensure that the request is genuine. The company owning the ship could be contacted for confirmation or the Lloyds Register of Shipping could be checked. The pharmacist should also check that the prescription only medicines which have been requested are appropriate for the category of ship by contacting the Maritime and Coastguard Agency (MCA) on 0870 600 6505.

Royal National Lifeboat Institution

The wholesale of medicines to the Royal National Lifeboat Institution and certified first aiders of the Institution from a registered pharmacy for the SUPPLY (BUT NOT SALE) to sick and injured persons

The Royal National Lifeboat Institution and certified first aiders of the Institution may supply the following medicines. Therefore, they can obtain these medicines by wholesale from a registered pharmacy:

(a) all general sale list medicines;

(b) all pharmacy medicines;

(c) all prescription-only medicines.

The Royal National Lifeboat Institution and certified first aiders of the Institution can only supply these medicinal products, under certain conditions. These conditions are:

(i) In the case of general sale list medicines and pharmacy medicines the supply is necessary for the treatment of sick and injured persons.

(ii) In the case of prescription-only medicines the supply is necessary for the treatment of sick or injured persons in the exercise of the functions of the Institution.

A supply made by a registered pharmacy to Royal National Lifeboat Institution and certified first aiders of the Institution under this exemption is a wholesale transaction. For the requirements concerned with wholesale transactions *see* Section 1.2.4.

Aircraft personnel

The wholesale of medicines to the operator or commander of an aircraft from a registered pharmacy for the SUPPLY (BUT NOT SALE) to persons on the aircraft

The operator or commander of an aircraft may supply the following medicines. Therefore, they can obtain these medicines by wholesale from a registered pharmacy:

(a) all general sale list medicines;

(b) all pharmacy medicines;

(c) all prescription-only-medicines which are not for parenteral administration.

The operator or commander of an aircraft can only supply these medicinal products, under certain conditions. These conditions are:

(i) That the supply is necessary for the immediate treatment of sick or injured persons on the aircraft
(ii) That the supply shall be in accordance with the written instructions of a doctor as to the circumstances in which prescription-only medicines of the description in question are to be used on the aircraft.

The supply of prescription only medicines requires the pharmacist to be presented with an order in writing signed by a doctor. A supply made by a registered pharmacy to the operator or commander of an aircraft under this exemption is a wholesale transaction. For the requirements concerned with wholesale transactions *see* Section 1.2.4.

The wholesale of medicine to the operator or commander of an aircraft from a registered pharmacy for the ADMINISTRATION to persons on the aircraft

The operator or commander of an aircraft may administer the following medicines. Therefore, they can obtain these medicines by wholesale from a registered pharmacy:

(a) All prescription only medicines that are for parenteral administration,

The operator or commander of an aircraft can only administer these medicinal products, under certain conditions. These conditions are:

(i) That the administration is necessary for the immediate treatment of sick or injured persons on the aircraft and
(ii) That the administration shall be in accordance with the written instructions of a doctor as to the circumstances in which prescription-only medicines of the description in question are to be used on the aircraft.

The supply of prescription only medicines for parenteral administration requires the pharmacist to be presented with an order in writing signed by a doctor. A supply made by a registered pharmacy to the operator or commander of an aircraft under this exemption is a wholesale transaction. For the requirements concerned with wholesale transactions *see* Section 1.2.4.

First aid organisations

The wholesale of medicines to the British Red Cross Society, St John Ambulance Association and Brigade, St Andrew's Ambulance Association and the Order of Malta Ambulance Corps from a registered pharmacy for the SUPPLY (BUT NOT SALE) to sick and injured persons

The British Red Cross Society, St John Ambulance Association and Brigade, St Andrew's Ambulance Association and the Order of Malta Ambulance Corps may supply the following medicines. Therefore, they can obtain these medicines by wholesale from a registered pharmacy:

(a) all general sale list medicines;
(b) all pharmacy medicines.

The British Red Cross Society, St John Ambulance Association and Brigade, St Andrew's Ambulance Association and the Order of Malta Ambulance Corps can only supply these medicinal products, under a certain condition. This condition is that:

(i) The supply is necessary for the treatment of sick and injured persons.

A supply made by a registered pharmacy to these first aid organisations under this exemption is a wholesale transaction. For the requirements concerned with wholesale transactions *see* Section 1.2.4.

Occupational health schemes (OHSs)

The wholesale of medicines from a registered pharmacy to a person operating an OHS for the SUPPLY (BUT NOT SALE) in the course of the OHS

The person operating an OHS may supply the following medicines. Therefore, they can obtain these medicines by wholesale from a registered pharmacy:

(a) all general sale list medicines;
(b) all pharmacy medicines;
(c) all prescription-only medicines.

The person operating an OHS can only supply these medicinal products, under certain conditions. These conditions are:

(i) That the supply shall be in the course of the OHS;
(ii) That the individual supplying the prescription-only medicine, if not a doctor, shall be a registered nurse acting in accordance with the written instructions of a doctor as to the circumstances in which prescription-only medicines of the description in question are to be used in the course of the OHS.

In the case of prescription-only medicines the pharmacist must have an order in writing signed by a registered doctor or a registered nurse.

A supply made by a registered pharmacy to an OHS under this exemption is a wholesale transaction. For the requirements concerned with wholesale transactions *see* Section 1.2.4.

The wholesale of medicines from a registered pharmacy to a person operating an OHS for the ADMINISTRATION in the course of the OHS

The person operating an OHS may administer the following medicines. Therefore, they can obtain these medicines by wholesale from a registered pharmacy:

(a) All prescription-only medicines that are for parenteral administration.

The person operating an OHS can only administer these parenteral medicinal products, under certain conditions. These conditions are:

(i) That the administration is in the course of the occupational health scheme;
(ii) That the individual administering the prescription-only medicine, if neither a doctor nor acting in accordance with the directions of a doctor, is a registered nurse acting in accordance with the written instructions of a doctor as to the circumstances in which prescription-only medicines of the description in question are to be used in the course of the OHS.

The pharmacist must have an order in writing signed by a registered doctor or a registered nurse, to supply parenteral prescription-only medicines to a person operating an OHS.

A supply made by a registered pharmacy to an OHS under this exemption is a wholesale transaction. For the requirements concerned with wholesale transactions *see* Section 1.2.4.

Offshore installations - First aid personnel

The wholesale of medicines to the person employed as the qualified first-aider on offshore installations for the SUPPLY (BUT NOT SALE) to persons on the installation

The person employed as the qualified first-aider on offshore installations may supply the following medicines. Therefore, they can obtain these medicines by wholesale from a registered pharmacy:
(a) all general sale list medicines;
(b) all pharmacy medicines;
(c) all prescription-only medicines.

The person employed as the qualified first-aider on offshore installations can only supply these medicinal products, under certain conditions. The condition is that:
(i) The supply shall be only so far as is necessary for the treatment of persons on the installation.

A supply made by a registered pharmacy to a person employed as the qualified first-aider on offshore installations under this exemption is a wholesale transaction. For the requirements concerned with wholesale transactions *see* Section 1.2.4.

The wholesale of medicines to the person employed as the qualified first-aider on offshore installations for the ADMINISTRATION to persons on the installation

The person employed as the qualified first-aider on offshore installations may administer the following medicines. Therefore, they can obtain these medicines by wholesale from a registered pharmacy:
(a) all prescription-only medicines that are for parenteral administration.

The person employed as the qualified first-aider on offshore installations can only administer these medicinal products, under certain conditions. The condition is that:
(i) The administration shall be only so far as is necessary for the treatment of persons on the installation.

A supply made by a registered pharmacy to a person employed as the qualified first-aider on offshore installations under this exemption is a wholesale transaction. For the requirements concerned with wholesale transactions *see* Section 1.2.4.

Paramedics

The wholesale of medicines to persons who hold a certificate of proficiency in ambulance paramedic skills issued by, or with the approval of, the Secretary of State or persons who are registered paramedics to be ADMINISTERED to sick or injured persons

A registered paramedic may administer the following parenteral medicines. Therefore, they can obtain these parenteral medicines by wholesale from a registered pharmacy:
(a) diazepam 5 mg per ml emulsion for injection
(b) succinylated modified fluid gelatin 4 per cent intravenous infusion;

(c) medicines containing the substances ergometrine maleate 500mcg per ml with oxytocin 5iu per ml, but no other active ingredient;
(d) prescription-only medicines for parenteral administration containing one or more of the following substances but no other active ingredients:
Adrenaline acid tartrate
Amiodarone
Anhydrous glucose
Benzylpenicillin
Bretylium tosylate
Compound sodium lactate intravenous infusion (Hartmann's solution)
Ergometrine maleate
Frusemide
Glucose
Heparin sodium
Lignocaine (Lidocaine) hydrochloride
Metoclopramide
Morphine sulphate (injection to a maximum strength of 20mg)
Nalbuphine hydrochloride
Naloxone hydrochloride
Polygeline
Reteplase
Sodium bicarbonate
Sodium chloride
Streptokinase
Tenecteplase

The registered paramedic can only administer these medicinal products, under certain conditions. These conditions are:
(i) That the administration shall be only for the immediate, necessary treatment of sick or injured persons;
(ii) In the case of a prescription-only medicine containing heparin sodium shall be only for the purpose of cannula flushing.

A registered paramedic can also obtain morphine sulphate oral for the purpose of its administration for the immediate necessary treatment of sick or injured person.

These exemptions apply to both NHS paramedics and privately employed (including self-employed) paramedics.

A supply made by a registered pharmacy to a registered paramedic under these exemptions is a wholesale transaction. For the requirements concerned with wholesale transactions *see* Section 1.2.4.

Any pharmacist who is asked for advice or wishes to check on the legality of supplying any of the Controlled Drugs listed above, i.e., diazepam or morphine sulphate to a registered paramedic should contact the Society's Legal and Ethical Advisory Service for advice.

Her Majesty's armed forces

The wholesale of medicines to persons who are members of Her Majesty's armed forces from a registered pharmacy for the SUPPLY (BUT NOT SALE) to sick or injured persons or to prevent ill-health

Persons who are members of Her Majesty's armed forces may supply the following medicines. Therefore, they can obtain these medicines by wholesale from a registered pharmacy:
(a) all general sale list medicine;
(b) all pharmacy medicines;
(c) all prescription-only medicines.

Persons ("P") who are members of Her Majesty's armed forces can only supply these medicinal products, under certain conditions. These conditions are:

(i) In the case of general sale list medicines and pharmacy medicines the supply shall be only so far as is necessary for the treatment of a sick or injured person or the prevention of ill-health

(ii) In the case of a prescription-only medicine the supply shall be in the course of P undertaking any function as a member of Her Majesty's armed forces: and

(iii) That where P is satisfied that it is not practicable for another person who is legally entitled to supply a prescription only medicine to do so; and

(iv) That the supply shall only be in so far as is necessary for the treatment of a sick or injured person in a medical emergency; or

(v) That the supply shall only be in so far as is necessary to prevent ill-health where there is a risk that a person would suffer ill-health if the prescription only medicine is not supplied.

A supply made by a registered pharmacy to person who is a member of Her Majesty's armed forces under this exemption is a wholesale transaction. For the requirements concerned with wholesale transactions *see* Section 1.2.4.

The wholesale of medicines to persons who are members of Her Majesty's armed forces from a registered pharmacy for persons who are members of Her Majesty's armed forces to ADMINISTER to sick or injured persons or to prevent ill-health

Persons "(P)" who are members of Her Majesty's armed forces can administer the following parenteral medicines. Therefore, they can obtain these medicines by wholesale from a registered pharmacy.

(a) all general sale list medicines
(b) all pharmacy medicines
(c) all prescription-only medicines.

A person who is a member of Her Majesty's armed forces can only administer the above parenteral medicines under certain circumstances. These are:

(i) That the administration shall be in the course of P undertaking any function as a member of Her Majesty's armed forces: and

(ii) That where P is satisfied that it is not practicable for another person who is legally entitled to administer a prescription only medicine to do so; and

(iii) That the administration shall only be in so far as is necessary for the treatment of a sick or injured person in a medical emergency; or

(iv) That the administration shall only be in so far as is necessary to prevent ill-health where there is a risk that a person would suffer ill-health if the prescription only medicine is not administered.

A supply made by a registered pharmacy to person who is a member of Her Majesty's armed forces under this exemption is a wholesale transaction. For the requirements concerned with wholesale transactions *see* Section 1.2.4.

Other exempted persons and organisations

The following persons or organisations have exemptions from restrictions of the retail sale and/or supply of certain medicinal products in relation to certain specified purposes:

Dental schemes
Unorthodox practitioners
Marketing authorisation holders and holders of manufacturers' licences
Group authorities and licences
Persons selling or supplying to universities, institutions concerned with higher education or institutions concerned with research
Persons selling or supplying to public analysts / sampling officers / NHS drug testing / British Standards Institution
Prison officers
Health authorities or primary care trusts
Persons holding a certificate in first aid from the Mountain Rescue Council of England and Wales, or from the Northern Ireland Mountain Rescue Co-ordinating Committee
Persons carrying on the business of a school providing full-time education

A pharmacist who is approached to make a sale or supply to any of the above can check with the Society's Legal and Ethical Advisory Service if any doubts exist as to the extent of the purchasers' authority.

1.2.6 Labelling of medicinal products

This section outlines what must appear on the container of relevant medicinal products that are general sale list medicines, pharmacy medicines and prescription only medicines.

This section also details the information that must appear on the dispensing label when relevant medicinal products are dispensed.

The legislation that underpins the labelling of medicines is the Medicines for Human Use (Marketing Authorisations Etc.) Regulations 1994, the Medicines (Labelling) Regulations 1976 and European Directives. Those medicinal products that are Controlled Drugs must also be labelled in accordance with the Misuse of Drugs Regulations 2001.

For a definition of "relevant medicinal product" *see* p6. Effectively this refers to a licensed medicinal product.

Changes in the event of a pandemic See pp14-15 for changes to this legislation in the event of a pandemic.

1.2.6.1 Labelling of dispensed relevant medicinal products

A dispensed relevant medicinal product, so far as a pharmacist is concerned, is defined as a relevant medicinal product prepared or dispensed in accordance with a prescription given by a practitioner.

The following must appear on the label when relevant medicinal products are dispensed:

(a) the name of the person to whom the medicine is to be administered;

(b) the name and address of the person who sells or supplies the medicinal product;

(c) the date on which dispensed;

(d) where the medicinal product has been prescribed by a practitioner the following particulars as s/he may request;

(i) the name of the product or its common name,

(ii) directions for use, and

(iii) precautions relating to the use of the product.

If the professional opinion of the pharmacist is that any of those particulars (d (i), (ii), (iii)) are inappropriate and having taken necessary steps to consult with the practitioner, s/he is unable to do so, s/he may substitute other particulars of the same kind;

(e) the words "Keep out of the reach of children" or words of direction bearing a similar meaning.

If a pharmacist is dispensing an embrocation, liniment, lotion, liquid antiseptic or other liquid preparation or gel in a container other than in a manufacturers original pack (which will be fully labelled as described below) and is for external application, the words "For external use only."

NB: The Society would strongly advise that pharmacists place the phrase "Keep out of the reach and sight of children" on dispensing labels as good practice, to be in line with the requirements for manufacturers. This is a good practice requirement and not mandatory.

Where the container of a dispensed medicinal product is enclosed in a package immediately enclosing that container, the particulars required under (a), (b), (c) and (d) may be omitted from the label on the container if they appear on the label on the package.

Where several containers of medicinal products of the same description are supplied in a package, the particulars required under (d) need only appear on the label on the package containing all the products, or may appear on only one of the labels of the individual containers or packages. All the remaining containers must however, be labelled with all the other particulars.

Other information may be added if the pharmacist considers it to be necessary. For other/additional labelling requirements see below.

1.2.6.2 Labelling of dispensed non-relevant medicinal products

A non-relevant medicinal product is essentially an unlicensed medicine, for example a medicine extemporaneously prepared by a pharmacist under Section 10 of the Medicines Act 1968 against a prescription.

The requirements for the dispensing label for non-relevant medicinal products are the same as the requirements for the dispensing label of a relevant medicinal product (see Section 1.2.6.1). The only exemption to this is when a pharmacist extemporaneously prepares a product in accordance with a specification furnished by the person to whom the product will be sold or supplied, under Section 10(3)(a) of the Medicines Act 1968. In this case the "directions for use" may be omitted from the dispensing label.

1.2.6.3 Labelling of assembled (prepacked) medicines

Some pharmacists assemble medicines by breaking down bulk containers into quantities more appropriate for use against prescriptions. This, technically, falls within the definition of assembly, and all medicines should be properly labelled. Medicines repackaged in this way can only be sold or supplied from that pharmacy or from another pharmacy under the same ownership. Prepacking at the request of medical practitioners or for a separate legal entity is not permitted without an assembly licence.

The particulars which are required are:
(a) the name of the medicinal product;
(b) the appropriate quantitative particulars of the medicinal product (the ingredients);
(c) the quantity of the medicinal product in the container;
(d) any special requirements for the handling and storage of the medicinal product;
(e) the expiry date;
(f) the batch reference, preceded by the letters "BN" or "LOT" or other letters indicating a batch reference.

All medicines assembled in such a way must be relabelled before being supplied to a patient as a dispensed medicinal product.

1.2.6.4 Labelling of chemists' nostrums

The following requirements apply to medicinal products which are prepared in a registered pharmacy for retail sale from that pharmacy and which are not advertised (such products are familiarly known as "chemists' nostrums"). The preparation and the sale or supply must be carried out by or under the supervision of a pharmacist.

The label of the container of such a medicinal product and any package immediately enclosing it must show the following standard labelling particulars:
(a) name of the product;
(b) pharmaceutical form;
(c) appropriate quantitative particulars;
(d) quantity;
(e) directions for use;
(f) handling and storage requirements (if any);
(g) expiry date;
(h) the words "Keep out of the reach of children" or words of a similar meaning;
(i) where appropriate, the words "Warning. Do not exceed the stated dose," in a rectangle in which there is no other matter (this would be necessary where one or more of the ingredients are prescription-only medicines, incorporated in such a way as to exempt it from prescription-only control);
(j) the words "For external use only." if the product is an embrocation, liniment, lotion, liquid antiseptic or other liquid preparation or gel and is for external application;
(k) the name and address of the seller;
(l) the letter P in a rectangle.

1.2.6.5 Manufacturers' labelling requirements for relevant medicinal products

The regulations covering labelling and patient information leaflets are set out in Title V of Council Directive 2001/83/EC which was amended by Council Directive 2004/27/EC. The information below is from the updated regulation as amended by Council Directive 2004/27/EC. However, pharmacists should note that although the amendments made by Council Directive 2004/27/EC have been implemented into UK legislation and affect all new applications submitted to the MHRA from 30 October 2005, existing marketing authorisations have until 30 October 2010 to comply.

The following particulars must appear on the outer packaging of medicinal products or, where there is no outer packaging, on the immediate packaging.
(a) the name of the medicinal product followed by its strength and pharmaceutical form, and, if appropriate, whether it is intended for babies, children or adults; where the product contains up to three active substances, the international non-proprietary name (INN) shall be included, or, if one does not exist, the common name (this information must also be expressed in Braille format on the packaging);
(b) a statement of the active substances expressed qualitatively and quantitatively per dosage unit or according to the form of administration for a given volume or weight, using their common names;
(c) the pharmaceutical form and the contents by weight, by volume or by number of doses of the product;

(d) a list of those excipients known to have a recognized action or effect and included in the detailed guidance published pursuant to Article 65. However, if the product is injectable, or a topical or eye preparation, all excipients must be stated;

(e) the method of administration and, if necessary, the route of administration. Space shall be provided for the prescribed dose to be indicated;

(f) a special warning that the medicinal product must be stored out of the reach and sight of children;

(g) a special warning, if this is necessary for the medicinal product;

(h) the expiry date in clear terms (month/year);

(i) special storage precautions, if any;

(j) specific precautions relating to the disposal of unused medicinal products or waste derived from medicinal products, where appropriate, as well as reference to any appropriate collection system in place;

(k) the name and address of the marketing authorisation holder and, where applicable, the name of the representative appointed by the holder to represent him;

(l) the number of the authorisation for placing the medicinal product on the market;

(m) the manufacturer's batch number;

(n) in the case of non-prescription medicinal products, instructions for use.

All labelling of containers and packages of relevant medicinal products shall be:
(i) legible;
(ii) indelible;
(iii) clearly comprehensible; and
(iv) either in the English language only or in English and in one or more other languages provided that the same particulars appear in all languages used.

Containers and packages of relevant medicinal products may be labelled to show:
(1) a symbol or pictogram designed to clarify the above particulars;
(2) other information compatible with the summary of product characteristics which is useful for health education.

There must not be any labelling of a promotional nature.

The requirement for a container or package of a relevant medicinal product to be labelled to show its name is not met by the container or package being labelled to show an invented name which is liable to be confused with the common name.

1.2.6.6 Warnings and other special labelling requirements

For dispensed medicines *see* Sections 1.2.6.1 and 1.2.6.2 for the labelling of dispensed medicinal products. In addition to the labelling particulars shown for chemists' nostrums and relevant medicinal products above (1.2.6.5), there are certain other particulars, warnings and phrases which must be shown on the labels of containers and packages of certain medicinal products. Different requirements apply to general sale list products, pharmacy medicines and prescription-only medicines.

1.2.6.7 Manufacturers' labelling requirements for general sale list products

When a relevant medicinal product, on a general sale list is sold or supplied by retail (but not as a dispensed relevant medicinal product), in addition to the appropriate particulars listed in section 1.2.6.5 it must be also labelled to show the following:

(a) if the product contains aloxiprin, aspirin or paracetamol, the words "If symptoms persist consult your doctor" and, except where the product is for external use only, the recommended dosage;

(b) if the product contains aloxiprin, the words "Contains an aspirin derivative";

(c) if the product contains aspirin, except where the product is for external use only or where the name of the product includes the word "aspirin" and appears on the container or package, the words "Contains aspirin";

(d) if the product contains paracetamol, except where the name of the product includes the word "paracetamol" and appears on the container or package, the words "Contains paracetamol";

(e) if the product contains paracetamol, the words "Do not exceed the stated dose" (this should appear adjacent to the directions for use/recommended dosage where this appear on the container or package);

(f) if the product contains paracetamol, unless it is wholly or mainly intended for children who are twelve years old or younger, the words "Do not take with any other paracetamol-containing products", and

(i) if a package leaflet accompanying the product displays the words "Immediate medical advice should be sought in the event of an overdose, even if you feel well, because of the risk of delayed, serious liver damage", the words "Immediate medical advice should be sought in the event of an overdose, even if you feel well", or

(ii) if no package leaflet accompanies the product or the package leaflet does not display the words "Immediate medical advice should be sought in the event of an overdose, even if you feel well, because of the risk of delayed, serious liver damage", the words "Immediate medical advice should be sought in the event of an overdose, even if you feel well, because of the risk of delayed, serious liver damage";

(g) if the product contains paracetamol and is wholly or mainly intended for children who are twelve years old or younger, the words "Do not give with any other paracetamol-containing products"; and

(i) if a package leaflet accompanying the product displays the words "Immediate medical advice should be sought in the event of an overdose, even if the child seems well, because of the risk of delayed, serious liver damage", the words "Immediate medical advice should be sought in the [event] of an overdose, even if the child seems well", or

(ii) if no package leaflet accompanies the product or the package leaflet does not display the words "Immediate medical advice should be sought in the event of an overdose, even if the child seems well, because of the risk of delayed, serious liver damage", the words "Immediate medical advice should be sought in the event of an overdose, even if the child seems well, because of the risk of delayed, serious liver damage";

(h) if the product contains aspirin or aloxiprin, the words "Do not give to children aged under 16 years, unless on the advice of a doctor".

NB: Where the words set out in more than one of the paragraphs above (ie, [b], [c] and [d]) are required, there may be substituted for those words other words showing that the product contains more than one of the substances aloxiprin, aspirin and paracetamol and naming the substances so contained, except that in the case of aloxiprin the words "aspirin derivative" shall appear and the word "aloxiprin" need not appear.

Where the words set out in one or more of paragraphs (b), (c), (d), (f) or (g) above are required, such words must appear in a prominent position and be within a rectangle within which there is no other matter, except where words set out in more than one of those paragraphs appear on the container or package then any of them may appear together within a rectangle within which there must be no other matter of any kind.

1.2.6.8 Manufacturers' labelling requirements of products for pharmacy sale only

Medicinal products, including relevant medicinal products, for pharmacy sale only, when sold or supplied by retail in addition to appropriate particulars above (1.2.6.7), must be labelled as follows:

(1) With the capital letter "P" in a rectangle containing no other matter. (2) If exempt from prescription-only control by reason of the proportion or level in the product of the prescription-only substance, with the words "Warning. Do not exceed the stated dose." (This does not apply to products for external use or products containing any of the substances set out in 5 below.)

(3) If for the treatment of asthma or other conditions associated with bronchial spasm or if they contain ephedrine or any of its salts, with the words "Warning. Asthmatics should consult their doctor before using this product." (This does not apply to products for external use.)

(4) If the product contains an antihistamine or similar substances or any of their salts or molecular compounds with the words "Warning. May cause drowsiness. If affected do not drive or operate machinery. Avoid alcoholic drink." (This does not apply to products for external use or where the product is for external use only or where the marketing authorisation contains no warning relating to the sedating effect of the product in use.)

(5) If the product is an embrocation, liniment, lotion, liquid antiseptic or other liquid preparation or gel and is for external application, with the words "For external use only."

(6) If the product contains hexachlorophane, either with the words "Not to be used for babies" or a warning that the product is not to be administered to a child under two years except on medical advice.

The relevant warning phrase or phrases described under "Manufacturers' labelling requirements for general sale list products" and "Manufacturers' labelling requirements for products for pharmacy sale only" above must be in a rectangle within which there is no other matter. That does not apply to the phrases "Do not exceed the stated dose" or "If symptoms persist consult your doctor" on the labels of products required to be labelled because of their aspirin, aloxiprin or paracetamol content.

Where more than one of the phrases (1) to (6) in this section ("Manufacturers' labelling requirementsof products for pharmacy sale only") is applicable to a particular product, the phrases may be together within a rectangle although the wording must not be altered or combined except that the word "Warning" need only appear once.

1.2.6.9 Manufacturers' labelling requirements for-prescription-only medicines

In addition to appropriate particulars above, the container and package of every relevant medicinal product which is a prescription-only medicine must be labelled:

(a) to show the letters "POM" in capitals within a rectangle within which there shall be no other matter of any kind (except in the case of a dispensed medicine);

(b) if the product is an embrocation, liniment, lotion, liquid antiseptic, or other liquid preparation or gel and is for external application, with the words "For external use only;"

(c) if the product contains hexachlorophane, either with the words "Not to be used for babies" or a warning that the product is not to be administered to a child under two years except on medical advice.

The phrases described above must be within a rectangle within which there is no other matter of any kind.

1.2.7 Patient information leaflets

Each time a relevant medicinal product is supplied a patient information leaflet must also be supplied.

1.2.8 Use of fluted bottles

The Medicines (Fluted Bottles) Regulations 1978, as amended, require liquid medicinal products for external use to be sold or supplied in a bottle the outer surface of which is fluted vertically with ribs or grooves recognisable by touch if, and only if, the product contains any of the substances listed in the following Schedule:

Aconite; alkaloids of

Adrenaline; its salts

Amino-alcohols esterified with benzoic acid, phenylacetic acid, phenylpropionic acid, cinnamic acid or the derivatives of these acids; their salts

p-Aminobenzenesulphonamide; its salts; derivatives of p-aminobenzenesulphonamide having any of the hydrogen atoms of the p-amino group or of the sulphonamide group substituted by another radical; their salts

p-Aminobenzoic acid; esters of; their salts

Ammonia except in medicinal products containing less than 5% weight in weight of ammonia

Arsenical substances, the following: arsenic sulphides; arsenates; arsenites; halides of arsenic; oxides of arsenic; organic compounds of arsenic

Atropine; its salts

Cantharidin; cantharidates

Carbachol

Chloral; its addition and its condensation products other than alphachloralose; their molecular compounds

Chloroform except in medicinal products containing less than 1% volume in volume of chloroform

Cocaine; its salts

Creosote obtained from wood except in medicinal products containing less than 50% volume in volume of creosote obtained from wood

Croton, oil of

Demecarium bromide

Dyflos

Ecothiopate iodide

Ephedrine; its salts except in medicinal products containing less than the equivalent of 1% weight in volume of ephedrine

Ethylmorphine; its salts

Homatropine; its salts

Hydrofluoric acid; alkali metal bifluorides; potassium fluoride; sodium fluoride; sodium silicofluoride except in mouth washes containing not more than 0.05% weight in volume of sodium fluoride

Hyoscine; its salts

Hyoscyamine; its salts

Lead acetates except in medicinal products containing lead acetates equivalent to not more than 2.2% weight in volume of lead calculated as elemental lead

Mercury, oxides of; nitrates of mercury; mercuric ammonium chloride; mercuric chloride; mercuric iodide; potassium mercuric iodide; organic compounds of mercury; mercuric oxycyanide; mercuric thiocyanate except in medicinal products containing not more than 0.01% weight in volume of phenylmercuric salts or 0.01% weight in volume of sodium ethyl mercurithiosalicylate as a preservative

Nitric acid except in medicinal products containing less than 9% weight in weight of nitric acid

Opium

Phenols (any member of the series of phenols of which the first member is phenol and of which the molecular composition varies from member to member by one atom of carbon and two atoms of hydrogen); compounds of phenol with a metal except in:

(a) medicinal products containing one or more of the following:
   Butylated hydroxytoluene
   Carvacrol
   Creosote obtained from coal tar
   Essential oils in which phenols occur naturally
   Tar (coal or wood), crude or refined
   tert-Butylcresol
   p-tert-Butylphenol
   p-tert-Pentylphenol
   p-(1,1,3,3-tetramethylbutyl) phenol
   Thymol

(b) mouth washes containing less than 2.5% weight in volume of phenols;

(c) any liquid disinfectant or antiseptics not containing phenol and containing less than 2.5% weight in volume of other phenols;

(d) other medicinal products containing less than 1% weight in volume of phenols

Physostigmine; its salts

Picric acid except in medicinal products containing less than 5% weight in volume of picric acid

Pilocarpine; its salts except in medicinal products containing less than the equivalent of 0.025% weight in volume of pilocarpine

Podophyllum resin except in medicinal products containing not more than 1.5% weight in weight of podophyllum resin

Solanaceous alkaloids not otherwise included in this Schedule

Some exceptions to fluted bottle requirements

The fluted bottle requirements do not apply where:

(a) medicinal products are contained in bottles with a capacity greater than 1.14 litres;

(b) medicinal products are packed for export for use solely outside the UK;

(c) medicinal products are sold or supplied solely for the purpose of scientific education, research or analysis;

(d) eye or ear drops are sold or supplied in a plastic container;

(e) the product licence, marketing authorisation or any variation of any such licence or authorisation, enables medicinal products to be contained in a bottle otherwise than in accordance with the requirements;

(f) the clinical trial certificate otherwise provides;

(g) a substance listed above is contained in a medicinal product which is classified as being on prescription only, unless sold or supplied by retail sale or in accordance with a prescription given by a practitioner.

1.2.9 Medical devices

The Medical Devices Regulations 2002, as amended, have implemented international law, European Devices Directives which provide for mandatory CE Marking of all medical devices covered by them. This includes some dressings, blood pressure monitors, contact lens care products, glucose meters, test kits e.g. cholesterol and screening tests.

The CE Marking means that a manufacturer claims that his device is safe within a benefit risk analysis, performs as claimed and is fit for its intended purpose. For all except the simplest devices, this CE Marking is checked by a certification organisation known as a notified body, of which there are over 80 across Europe, each designated by their national competent authority.

Nowadays many medical devices are being used or sold by pharmacists. There are a number of considerations that all pharmacists and pharmacists staff should know about such devices when deciding to recommend, sell, stock, or employ within a supplied pharmacy service. Principals of appropriate procurement, safe use, maintenance and repair and guidance on reporting device related adverse events are set out as a series of practical check lists in 'Devices in Practice' available from the Medicines and Healthcare products Regulatory Agency website (_www.mhra.gov.uk_).

Emphasis is placed on post market surveillance which includes the mandatory reporting of all serious adverse events by the manufacturer. Voluntary reporting of all adverse events by Healthcare Professionals including Pharmacists is also promoted in order that adverse events can be investigated promptly and addressed as soon as possible. Further information can be obtained from the Society's Legal and Ethical Advisory Service or directly from the Medicines and Healthcare and products Regulatory Agency (_www.mhra.gov.uk_).

1.2.10 Restrictions on the sale of plano (zero powered) cosmetic contact lenses

Pharmacists are advised that they must not sell plano (zero powered) cosmetic contact lenses unless they are sold under the supervision of a registered optician, dispensing optician or doctor.

Pharmacists wishing to sell zero powered contact lenses must do so in accordance with the relevant legal requirements contained within The Opticians Act 1989, and the subsequent Rules and Regulations. Failure to do so could result in action being taken for breach of the legislation. For further information on these legal requirements, the General Optical Council should be consulted on 020 7580 3898 (_www.optical.org_; e-mail: goc@optical.org).

1.2.11 Chloroform: sale and supply

The Medicines (Chloroform Prohibition) Order 1979, as amended, prohibits the sale or supply of any medicinal product consisting of or containing chloroform, which is for human use, except in the following circumstances.

A sale or supply may be made:

(1) (a) by a doctor or dentist to a patient of his, where the medicinal product has been specially prepared by that doctor or dentist for administration to that particular patient, or

(b) by a doctor or dentist who has specially prepared the medicinal product at the request of another doctor or dentist for administration to a particular patient of that other doctor or dentist, or

(c) from a registered pharmacy, hospital or by a doctor or dentist where the medicinal product has been specially prepared, in accordance with a prescription given by a doctor or dentist for a particular patient of his, in a registered pharmacy, hospital or by a doctor or dentist

(2) (a) to a hospital, doctor or dentist either solely for use as an anaesthetic or solely for use as an ingredient in the preparation of a substance to be used as an anaesthetic, or both

(b) to a person who buys or obtains it for the purpose of selling or supplying it to a hospital, doctor or dentist either solely for use as an anaesthetic or solely for use as an ingredient in the preparation of a substance or article to be used as an anaesthetic, or both, or

(3) (a) where the medicinal product contains chloroform in a proportion of not more than 0.5% (w/w) or (v/v), or

(b) where the medicinal product is solely for use in dental surgery, or

(c) where the medicinal product is solely for use by being applied to the external surface of the body which for the purpose of this Order does not include any part of the mouth, teeth or mucous membranes, or

(4) where the medicinal product is for export, or

(5) where the medicinal product is sold for use as an ingredient in the preparation of a substance or article in a registered pharmacy, a hospital or by a doctor or dentist.

See also "Substances restricted to professional users" (p92).

1.2.12 Advertising and promotion of medicines: Accepting gifts and inducements to prescribe or supply

The Medicines (Advertising) Regulations 1994 govern the supply, offer or promise of gifts to healthcare professionals, including pharmacists, by drug manufacturers and distributors. Pharmacists accepting items such as gift vouchers, bonus points, discount holidays, sports equipment, etc, would be in breach of Regulation 21. Pharmacists are, therefore, advised not to participate in such offers.

1.2.13 Handling of waste medicines

England and Wales

Following the Environment Agency's review of waste exemptions, a pharmacy no longer needs to register an exemption to receive waste medicines from households and individuals under the Non-Waste Framework Directive (NWFD) exemptions. Providing that the conditions and limits below are met, a pharmacy can now accept back waste medicines and sharps from any source including other healthcare professionals (doctors, dentists, veterinarians, midwives or nurses) and nursing homes. With regard to accepting Controlled Drugs as waste back into the pharmacy, please refer to p42 for further guidance.

This exemption allows the temporary storage of waste medicines (other than any substances that have a flash point of less than 21 C) and waste sharps, at a pharmacy for the purposes of recovering or disposing of the waste elsewhere. No more than 5 cubic metres of waste may be stored at any one time. Waste can only be stored temporarily, as a general rule, wastes should not be stored for longer than three months. All wastes must be stored in secure containers. A pharmacy does not need to register an exemption to collect waste sharps.

It should be noted that the carriage of waste requires a licence from the Environment Agency (08708 506506). The removal of individual tablets or capsules from a blister strip or the decanting of liquids from bottles should be avoided as this falls within the definition of waste treatment, which is a licensable activity. The Environment Agency has confirmed that the removal of a blister strip from other inert packaging, so that the blister strip can be placed in the waste container and the outer packaging can be recycled, would not be regulated as a licensable waste treatment.

Scotland

In Scotland, the Waste Management Licensing Amendment (Scotland) Regulations 2006 allow registered pharmacies to accept patient returned medication from patients or individuals. The Regulations have enabled certain waste to be returned to pharmacies from care services, including all care homes (irrespective of whether or not they employ nurses). "Care services" for the purposes on the above Regulations has the same meaning as in Section 2 of the Regulation of Care (Scotland) Act 2001. By way of clarification the care services defined as those from which pharmacies in Scotland may accept returned waste include the following:

(a) a support service

(b) a care home service

(c) a school care accommodation service

(d) an independent health care service

(e) a nurse agency

(f) a child care agency

(g) a secure accommodation service

(h) an offender accommodation service

(i) an adoption service

(j) a fostering service

(k) an adult placement service

(l) child minding

(m) day care of children; and

(n) a housing support service.

The Scottish Environment Protection Agency can be contacted on 01786 457700.

Deblistering is allowed only in the case of Controlled Drugs where it is necessary to remove the solid dosage form from the blister strip or tablet bottle in order to denature the drug and render it irretrievable. (*See* pp42-45 for further information on the denaturing of Controlled Drugs.)

1.2.14 Controlled Drugs

The Misuse of Drugs Act 1971 controls "dangerous or otherwise harmful drugs" which are designated as "Controlled Drugs." The primary purpose of the Misuse of Drugs Act is to prevent the misuse of Controlled Drugs. It does that by imposing a total prohibition on the possession, supply, manufacture, import or export of Controlled Drugs except as allowed by regulations or by licence from the Secretary of State. The use of Controlled Drugs in medicine is permitted by the Misuse of Drugs Regulations 2001, as amended. Other regulations deal with the safe custody of Controlled Drugs and with the notification of and supply of drugs to misusers.

The classes to the Act are of no practical importance to pharmacists and practitioners. In the Misuse of Drugs Regulations, the drugs are classified in five schedules according to different levels of control. It is those classifications that are described in the following paragraphs. In the main alphabetical list of medicines for human use in this book they are marked CD Lic, CD POM, CD No Register POM, CD Benz POM, CD Anab POM, or CD Inv. P or POM, according to the controls (detailed below) which apply to each drug.

Schedule 1 drugs (CD Lic)

Schedule 1 includes the hallucinogenic drugs (for example LSD), the ecstasy-type substances and cannabis, which have virtually no therapeutic use. Production, possession and supply of drugs in this Schedule are limited, in the public interest, to purposes of research or other special purposes. A licence from the Home Office is needed for any of these purposes, and, apart from licence holders, the class of persons who may lawfully possess them is very limited. It does not include practitioners and pharmacists except under licence. There is an exception to the prohibition on the possession of a Schedule 1 Controlled Drug under certain conditions for specific purposes in the case of a fungus that contains psilocin or an ester of psilocin.

Some pharmacists, particularly those working within hospital, may be asked to deal with substances removed from patients on admission, which may be Schedule 1 products (for example cannabis). As a licence is required to possess Schedule 1 products, the pharmacist cannot take possession of the product other than in the two cases where exemptions are granted. The first exemption, is where a person takes possession of a Controlled Drug for the purpose of destruction, and the second, for the purpose of handing over to a police officer. Guidance should be sought from the Home Office regarding destruction of Schedule 1 Controlled Drugs.

The patient's confidentiality should normally be maintained, and the police should be called in on the understanding that there will be no identification of the source. If, however, the quantity is so large that the drug could not be purely for personal use, the pharmacist may decide that the greater interests of the public require identification of the source. Such a decision should not be taken without first discussing with the other health professionals involved in the patient's care, and the hospital's legal adviser.

In theory, the patient should give authority for the removal and destruction of the drug. If the patient refuses, then the hospital may feel that it has no alternative other than to call in the police. Under no circumstances can a Schedule 1 drug be handed back to a patient at discharge, as the person doing so could be guilty of an offence of unlawful supply of a Controlled Drug. The penalties for this type of offence are high, and often involve a custodial sentence.

Schedule 2 drugs (CD POM)

Schedule 2 includes the opiates (such as diamorphine, morphine and methadone), the major stimulants (such as the amphetamines) and quinalbarbitone. A licence is needed to import or export drugs in this Schedule, but they may be manufactured or compounded by a licence holder, a practitioner, a pharmacist, or a person lawfully conducting a retail pharmacy business acting in his capacity as such. A pharmacist may supply them to a patient only on the authority of a prescription in the required form (*see* below) issued by an appropriate practitioner.

The drugs may be administered to a patient by a doctor or dentist, a nurse independent prescriber (who may administer certain Controlled Drugs under certain circumstances, *see* p40), a supplementary prescriber in accordance with a clinical management plan, or by any person acting in accordance with the directions of a doctor, dentist, nurse independent prescriber or a supplementary prescriber in accordance with a clinical management plan.

Requirements for safe custody in pharmacies apply to all Schedule 2 Controlled Drugs except quinalbarbitone. The requirement for safe custody of Schedule 2 drugs also applies to patient returned Schedule 2 drugs, until such time as they are denatured for disposal. **NB. *See* p42 for further information on denaturing of Controlled Drugs and Controlled Drug waste.** Restrictions concerning the destruction of stock (requiring an authorised witness to be present) applies to these drugs, and the provisions relating to the marking of containers and the keeping of records must also be observed.

Schedule 3 drugs (CD No Register POM)

Schedule 3 includes a small number of minor stimulant drugs such as benzphetamine, and other drugs (such as buprenorphine, midazolam, phenobarbitone and temazepam) which are not thought so likely to be misused as the drugs in Schedule 2, nor to be so harmful if misused. The controls which apply to Schedule 2 also apply to drugs in this schedule, except:
(a) there is a difference in the classes of persons who may possess and supply them;
(b) the requirements for an authorised witness to attend during the destruction of date expired stock does not apply in retail pharmacy, (unless the pharmacist is a "producer" of Schedule 3 Controlled Drugs, ie, they manufacture or compound these items);
(c) records in the register of Controlled Drugs need not be kept in respect of these drugs, (unless the pharmacist is a "producer" of these items, as above);
(d) while safe custody requirements apply, currently most drugs in this Schedule are exempted. Currently, the four Schedule 3 Controlled Drugs that do require safe custody are temazepam, diethylpropion, buprenorphine and flunitrazepam. Neither phenobarbitone nor midazolam require safe custody. The requirement for safe custody of the four Schedule 3 drugs listed above, also applies to these drugs when they are returned by patients for disposal, until such time as they are denatured. Any drugs added to Schedule 3 require safe custody, unless specifically exempted. Invoices need to be retained by retail dealers.

Schedule 4 drugs (CD Benz POM or CD Anab POM)

Schedule 4 is split into two parts. Part I (CD Benz POM) contains most of the benzodiazepines. Part II (CD Anab POM) contains most of the anabolic and androgenic steroids, together with clenbuterol (adrenoceptor stimulant) and growth hormones (5 polypeptide hormones). The restrictions applicable to Schedule 3 drugs apply to them with the following relaxations:

(a) if the substance from Part II (CD Anab POM) is in the form of a medicinal product and is for administration by a person to himself a Home Office import or export licence is not required for the importation and exportation of this substance (a Home Office import or export licence would still be required for the importation and exportation of substances in Part I [CD Benz POM] and Part II [CD Anab POM] of Schedule 4 not falling under the above exemption);

(b) there is no restriction on the possession of any Schedule 4 Part II (CD Anab POM) when contained in a medicinal product;

(c) the labelling requirements of the Misuse of Drugs Regulations 2001, as amended, do not apply. However, the labelling requirements falling under the controls of the Medicines Act 1968 would still apply;

(d) prescription requirements under the Misuse of Drugs Regulations 2001, as amended, do not apply, except for the validity of a prescription being limited to 28 days; prescription requirements falling under the controls of the Medicines Act 1968 continue to apply;

(e) Controlled Drug register entries need not be kept by retailers;

(f) the requirement for an authorised witness for the destruction of Schedule 4 CDs applies only to importers, exporters and manufacturers;

(g) there are no safe custody requirements.

Schedule 5 drugs (CD Inv. P or CD Inv. POM)

Schedule 5 contains preparations of certain Controlled Drugs, for example, codeine, pholcodine and morphine, which are exempt from full control when present in medicinal products of low strength. There is no restriction on the import, export, possession or administration of these preparations, and safe custody requirements do not apply. A practitioner or pharmacist acting in his capacity as such, or a person holding an appropriate licence, may manufacture or compound any of them.

No record in the register of Controlled Drugs need be made in respect of drugs obtained or supplied by a person lawfully conducting a retail pharmacy business unless that person is a "producer", ie, a manufacturer or compounder of such items. The invoices or copies of Schedule 5 Controlled Drugs obtained or supplied must be kept for two years. No authorised witness is required to witness the destruction of these drugs, and there are no special labelling requirements other than the labelling requirements of the Medicines Act 1968.

Possession and supply of Controlled Drugs

It is unlawful for any person to be in possession of Controlled Drugs in Schedules 2, 3 and 4 unless:

(a) that person holds an appropriate licence from the Home Office; or

(b) that person is a member of a class specified in the Regulations; or

(c) the Regulations provide that possession of that drug or group of drugs is not unlawful, for example there is no restriction on the possession of any Schedule 4 Part II (CD Anab POM) drug when contained in a medicinal product; or

(d) they have been lawfully prescribed for that person (or for that person's animal).

In any case, possession or supply is not lawful unless the person concerned is acting in his capacity as a member of his class, or in accordance with the terms of his licence or group authority.

Practitioners and pharmacists when acting in their capacity as such are amongst those who have a general authority to possess, supply and procure all Controlled Drugs except those in Schedule 1.

Certain other persons, including wholesalers, importers and exporters, must obtain licences from the Secretary of State. "Wholesale dealer" in this context means a person who carries on the business of selling drugs to persons who buy to sell again.

Any person who is lawfully in possession of a Controlled Drug may supply that drug to the person from whom he lawfully obtained it.

Secretary of State prohibitions

The Home Secretary also has the power, under the Misuse of Drugs Act 1971, to make a direction against a practitioner prohibiting him from having in his possession, prescribing, administering, manufacturing, compounding and supplying, and from authorising the administration and supply of those Controlled Drugs specified in the direction. In order to confirm whether or not a practitioner has had a direction made against him under the Misuse of Drugs Act 1971, prohibiting him from dealing with Controlled Drugs as indicated above, pharmacists are advised to contact the Home Office directly on 020 7035 4848.

Safe custody of Controlled Drugs

The regulations relating to safe custody apply to all Controlled Drugs included in Schedules 1, 2 (except quinalbarbitone [secobarbital]) and 3 (except any 5,5 disubstituted barbituric acid, cathine, ethchlorvynol, ethinamate, mazindol, meprobamate, methylphenobarbitone, methprylone, midazolam, pentazocine, phentermine or any stereoisomeric form of the above, or any salts of the above). Phenobarbitone (Phenobarbital) is a 5,5 disubstituted barbituric acid and therefore does not require safe custody.

Any liquid preparations designed for administration otherwise than by injection which contain any of the following substances and products are exempt from safe custody requirements:

(a) amphetamine
(b) benzphetamine
(c) chlorphentermine
(d) fenethylline
(e) mephentermine
(f) methaqualone
(g) methylamphetamine
(h) methylphenidate
(i) phendimetrazine
(j) phenmetrazine
(k) pipradrol
(l) any stereoisomeric form of a substance specified in (a) to (k) or any salt of a substance specified in (a) to (l).

However, pharmacists may wish to keep these drugs in the Controlled Drug cupboard.

Retail dealers and care homes must comply with the requirements for safe custody where they apply and must ensure that the relevant Controlled Drugs are kept in a locked safe, cabinet or room which is so constructed and maintained in accordance with the Misuse of Drugs (Safe Custody) Regulations 1973, as amended. This requirement does not apply in respect of any Controlled Drug which is for the time being constantly under the direct personal supervision of a pharmacist, for example, when dispensing a prescription.

The specifications with which safes, cabinets and rooms must comply are given in great detail in the Regulations (obtainable from The Stationery Office, _www.tso.co.uk_.) The owner of a pharmacy may, however, elect to apply, as an alternative, to the police for a certificate that his safes, cabinets or rooms provide an adequate degree of security. Applications must be made in writing. The certificate may specify conditions to be observed.

The requirement for safe custody for certain Controlled Drugs applies equally to patient returned and out-of-date Controlled Drugs, which until such time that they can be denatured and be rendered irretrievable, must be kept in the Controlled Drug cabinet. NB. _See_ **p42 for further information on denaturing of Controlled Drugs and Controlled Drug waste.** Patient returned Controlled Drugs must be kept segregated from stock Controlled Drugs, and clearly marked as such to minimise the risk of errors and inadvertent supply.

Requisitions for Schedules 1, 2 and 3 Controlled Drugs

A requisition in writing must be obtained by a supplier before he delivers any Schedule 2 or 3 Controlled Drug. The requisition does not have to be in the recipient's handwriting but must:

(a) be signed by the recipient;
(b) state the recipient's name;
(c) state the recipient's address;
(d) state the recipient's profession or occupation;
(e) specify the total quantity of the drug;
(f) specify the purpose for which it is required.

The supplier must be reasonably satisfied that the signature is that of the person purporting to sign the requisition and that he is engaged in the occupation stated.

The requisition must be obtained prior to supply to any of the following:

(a) a practitioner (a practitioner urgently requiring a drug and unable to supply a written requisition before delivery may be supplied on his giving an undertaking to furnish a requisition within the next 24 hours; failure to furnish the requisition within 24 hours is an offence on the part of the practitioner);
(b) the person or acting person in charge of a hospital or care home (a requisition from the person in charge of a hospital or care home must be signed by a doctor or dentist employed or engaged there);
(c) a person who is in charge of a laboratory the recognised activities of which consist in or include the conduct of scientific education or research and in relation to Schedule 2 Controlled Drugs, which is attached to a university, university college or such a hospital as aforesaid or to any other institution approved for such a purpose by the Secretary of State;

(d) the owner of a ship or the master of a ship which does not carry a doctor among the seamen employed on board;
(e) the installation manager of an offshore installation;
(f) the master of a foreign ship in a port in Great Britain (a requisition from the master of a foreign ship must contain a statement from the proper officer of the port health authority, or, in Scotland, the medical officer designated under section 14 of the National Health Service (Scotland) Act 1978 by the Health Board, within whose jurisdiction the ship is, that the quantity of drug is necessary for the equipment of the ship);
(g) a supplementary prescriber;
(h) a senior registered nurse or acting senior registered nurse for the time being in charge of any ward, theatre or other department of a hospital or care home who obtains a supply of a Controlled Drug from the person responsible for dispensing and supplying medicines at that hospital or care home must furnish a requisition in writing signed by the recipient which specifies the total quantity of the drug required. The recipient must retain a copy or note of the requisition. The person responsible for the dispensing and supply of the Controlled Drug must mark the requisition in such a manner as to show that it has been complied with and must retain the requisition in the dispensary;
(i) an operating department practitioner (ODP) can order Schedule 2, 3, 4 and 5 Controlled Drugs from a hospital pharmacy and the hospital pharmacy, in which the ODP is practising, can supply the ODP with these drugs. Currently, when ordering Controlled Drugs from a hospital pharmacy, the ODP is under no legal obligation to provide a written requisition. However, pharmacists are advised as a matter of good practice and/or to comply with local standard operating procedures, supplies should be made on the receipt of a requisition signed by the ODP. The legislation is due to be changed to make the provision of a written requisition a legal requirement. (There is no provision to allow an ODP to obtain Controlled Drugs from a community pharmacy.)

Supply of Controlled Drugs stock from the community

Standardised requisition forms have been produced for use in England (FP10CDF), Scotland (CDRF) and Wales (WP10CDF). There is no legal requirement to use these standardised requisition forms, however, they should be used wherever possible as a matter of good practice. The standardised requisition forms can be obtained from the local Primary Care Organisation.

It is still lawful for a community pharmacist to supply against a requisition form written in a format other than on the newly introduced standardised forms as long as all the legal requirements for a requisition are complied with. When one community pharmacy supplies another community pharmacy, as a matter of good practice a written requisition should be obtained, and ideally this should be the standardised form.

In Scotland the arrangements for the requisition form used to obtain NHS stock remain unchanged. GP10A stock order forms should be used for NHS purposes. A duplicate GP10A will be required to be kept at the pharmacy. It should be noted that separate GP10A forms should be used for Schedule 1, 2 and 3 Controlled Drugs. Prescribers in Scotland who wish to obtain stocks of Schedule 1, 2 and 3 Controlled Drugs privately from a community pharmacy should use the standardised requisition form (CDRF). Those wishing to obtain a supply of CDRF forms must contact the local NHS Board to register as a private prescriber (if they are not already registered) and to order the forms.

On receipt of a requisition for a Schedule 1, 2 or 3 Controlled Drug by a pharmacist in a community setting (not a care home or a hospital), the pharmacist must:

(i) mark on the requisition (in ink or otherwise indelibly) the supplier's name and address. The Home Office has confirmed that a pharmacy stamp can be used to mark these details on the requisition if the address details appear in full and the information is clear and legible;

(ii) preserve and retain a copy of the requisition for two years from the date of supply;

(iii) send all original requisitions to the relevant National Health Service agency in accordance with arrangements specified by that agency.

The requirements to mark and send the requisition to the relevant NHS agency do not apply where the supplier is:

(a) a person responsible for the dispensing and supply of medicines at a hospital or care home. The original requisition must be kept for two years;

(b) a pharmaceutical manufacturer or pharmaceutical wholesaler;

(c) a person responsible for the supply of Controlled Drugs within a prison setting.

The requirements to mark and send the requisition to the relevant NHS agency do not apply to:

(a) midwives' supply orders. The arrangements for midwives' supply orders remain unchanged.

(b) veterinary requisitions. A "veterinary requisition" is a requisition which states that the recipient is a veterinary surgeon or veterinary practitioner. The requirements for a requisition, as described above, state that the requisition must specify "the recipient's profession or occupation". The original requisition must be kept for five years.

Where non-standardised Controlled Drug requisition forms have been used, these must also be marked on receipt, copied and sent to the relevant NHS agency, as above.

Collection by messenger (of stock)

A messenger sent by a purchaser (recipient) to collect Controlled Drug stock in response to a written requisition on the recipient's behalf may only be supplied with the Controlled Drug if he produces to the supplier a statement in writing given by the recipient to the effect that the messenger is empowered to receive the drugs on his behalf. The supplier must be reasonably satisfied that the document is genuine and must retain it for two years. The requirement for the written statement does not apply to a person carrying on a business as a carrier engaged by the supplier.

Controlled Drugs in hospitals

In hospitals additional requirements relating to administration and supply, prescriptions, requisitions and registers for Controlled Drugs include:

(a) A senior registered nurse or acting senior registered nurse, for the time being in charge of a ward, theatre, or other department, may not supply any drug otherwise than for administration to a patient in the ward, theatre or department in accordance with the directions of a doctor, dentist, supplementary prescriber acting under and in accordance with the terms of a clinical management plan, or of a nurse independent prescriber subject to the limited list of Controlled Drugs which they may prescribe which includes a specific purpose for which the drug may be prescribed (see pp40-41)*.

(b) The senior registered nurse or acting senior registered nurse, for the time being in charge of a ward, theatre or other department is not required by the Misuse of Drugs Regulations 2001, as amended, to keep any register. However, Department of Health guidance and good practice should be followed, which may require such a register to be kept. It follows that ward stocks of Controlled Drugs may legally be destroyed without the attendance of an "authorised person." However, Department of Health guidance must again be taken into account.

(c) An operating department practitioner is authorised to order Schedule 2, 3, 4 and 5 Controlled Drugs from the hospital pharmacy, in which the ODP is practising. That hospital pharmacy would be able to supply an ODP with those drugs. ODPs are able to possess and supply Schedule 2 to 5 Controlled Drugs for the purposes of administration to a patient in a ward, theatre or other department, at the hospital in which they are practising, in accordance with the directions of a doctor, dentist, supplementary prescriber acting under and in accordance with the terms of a clinical management plan, or of a nurse independent prescriber. The directions given by a nurse prescriber relate only to the limited list of Controlled Drugs which they may prescribe, and are subject to restrictions on the purpose for which they may be prescribed.†

(d) The person in charge or acting person in charge of a hospital or care home having a pharmacist responsible for the dispensing and supply of medicines may not supply or offer to supply any drug.

(e) A prescription issued for the treatment of a patient in a hospital or care home may be written on the patient's bed-card or casesheet. Where a bed-card or casesheet is used as an authorisation to administer a Controlled Drug, it would not need to comply with the full prescription requirements for a Controlled Drug. However, where a bed-card or casesheet is used as an authorisation to supply a Controlled Drug to a patient it would need to fully comply with the prescription requirements of a Controlled Drug (see below).

(f) Private prescriptions for Schedule 2 or 3 Controlled Drugs issued from within that hospital or from within its legal entities that are to be supplied by a pharmacist in that hospital, do not need to be on a standardised private prescription form provided by the primary care organisa-

---

* When legislation changes, it is anticipated that pharmacist independent prescribers and nurse independent prescribers will be able to prescribe any Controlled Drug for any condition

† When legislation changes, it is anticipated that this would also include supply in accordance with the directions of a pharmacist independent prescriber and the full range of Controlled Drugs by a nurse independent prescriber

tion and do not need to specify the prescriber identification number.

(g) In order for a hospital pharmacy to lawfully supply a Schedule 2 or 3 Controlled Drug against a private prescription issued outside that hospital (i.e. outside its legal entity), the private prescription must be issued on a standardised private prescription form.

(h) Requisitions for Schedule 2 or 3 Controlled Drugs that are to be supplied by a pharmacist in a hospital do not need to be sent to a National Health Service agency and do not need to be marked with the name and address of the supplying pharmacy.

Prescriptions for Controlled Drugs

No prescription is required under the Misuse of Drugs Regulations for the supply by a pharmacist of a Schedule 5 drug but, for preparations above certain strengths, a prescription is required under the Medicines Act 1968. Prescriptions are necessary for all other categories of Controlled Drugs which are always prescription-only medicines. The requirements of both the Misuse of Drugs Act 1971 and the Medicines Act 1968 must be satisfied. In the case of a prescription for an animal, *see* Section 1.8.1 (p97).

It is unlawful for a practitioner to issue a prescription containing a Schedule 2 or 3 Controlled Drug (except temazepam) or for a pharmacist to dispense it, unless it complies with the following requirements:

The prescription must:

(a) be signed by the person issuing it with his usual signature;

(b) be dated;

(c) be written so as to be indelible;

(d) except in the case of an NHS or local health authority prescription, specify the address of the person issuing it. NB: The Medicines Act requires that all prescriptions for prescription-only medicines contain the prescriber's address;

(e) in the case of a private prescription (including one for temazepam and midazolam) be on a standardised form, when dispensed in a community pharmacy or GP practice. The forms issued in England, Scotland or Wales, are called FP10PCD, PPCD(1) and WP10PCD respectively. NB: The requirement to use standardised prescription forms when prescribing Schedule 2 and 3 Controlled Drugs does not apply to veterinary prescriptions, but does apply to private prescriptions issued by doctors, dentists and non-medical prescribers (eg, nurse and pharmacist prescribers);

(f) in the case of a private prescription for human use (including temazepam and midazolam), contain the private prescriber's identification number on the prescription.

(g) specify the dose to be taken (NB: The Home Office has expressed the view that a dose of "as directed" or "when required" is not acceptable, but "one to be taken as directed/when required" is acceptable); and:

(i) in the case of preparations, the form and, where appropriate, the strength of the preparation;

(ii) and either the total quantity (in both words and figures) of the preparation, or the number (in both words and figures) of dosage units, as appropriate, to be supplied; in any other case, the total quantity (in both words and figures) of the Controlled Drug to be supplied

(*see* Technical errors on Controlled Drug prescriptions, p37);

(h) have written on it, if issued by a dentist, the words "for dental treatment only";

(i) specify the name and address of the person for whose treatment it is issued;

(j) in the case of a prescription for a total quantity intended to be dispensed by instalments, contain a direction specifying the amount of the instalments which may be supplied and the intervals to be observed when supplying.

The Home Office has confirmed that an instalment prescription must have both a dose and an instalment amount on the prescription (ie, they both have to be specified separately.)

Prescriptions for Schedule 2 and 3 Controlled Drugs do not have to be written in the handwriting of the prescriber. Apart from the prescriber's signature, the entire prescription, including the date, may be computer generated.

The requirement for certain particulars to be on the prescription does not apply to prescriptions for temazepam (eg, total quantity in words and figures), or to prescriptions for Controlled Drugs in Schedule 4. For the purpose of prescription writing, temazepam can be written up as for any other prescription-only medicine (*see* Prescriptions for prescription-only medicines, p13)

A Schedule 2 or 3 Controlled Drug must not be supplied by any person on a prescription:

(a) unless the prescription complies with the provisions set out above (except temazepam);

(b) unless the prescriber's address on the prescription is within the United Kingdom;

(c) unless the supplier is either acquainted with the prescriber's signature and has no reason to suppose that it is not genuine, or has taken reasonably sufficient steps to satisfy himself that it is genuine;

(d) before the appropriate date on the prescription;

(e) in the case of an instalment prescription (FP10MDA or equivalent), unless the first instalment is dispensed within 28 days of the appropriate date. The remainder of the instalments can be dispensed in accordance with the instructions (even when this runs past the 28-day limit).

(f) later than 28 days after the appropriate date on the prescription. (This also applies to temazepam, midazolam and Schedule 4 Controlled Drugs.)

The "appropriate date" for the purposes of these Regulations is defined as "the later of the date on which it was signed by the person issuing it or the date indicated by him as being the date before which it shall not be supplied."

Where a prescriber wishes the 28-day period to start on a date other than the date of signing, he may specify a start date from which the period will begin. The start date specified can be more than 28 days from the date of signing / issue.

Owings of dispensed prescriptions for Schedule 2, 3 or 4 Controlled Drugs cannot be supplied more than 28 days after the appropriate date.

The date must be marked on the prescription at the time of supply of a Schedule 2 or 3 Controlled Drug.

Private Controlled Drug prescriptions

In order for a hospital pharmacy to lawfully supply a Schedule 2 or 3 Controlled Drug against a private prescription issued outside that hospital (i.e. outside its legal entity), the private prescription must be issued on a standardised private rescription form. Private prescriptions for Schedule 2 or 3 Controlled Drugs issued from within that hospital or from within its legal entities that are to be supplied by a pharmacist in that hospital, do not need to be on a standardised private prescription form provided by the primary care organisation and do not need to specify the prescriber identification number. In any other case the private prescription for a Schedule 2 and 3 Controlled Drug must:

(i) be on a standardised form (FP10PCD for England, PPCD(1) for Scotland and WP10PCD for Wales). Private Controlled Drug prescriptions which are not on the designated form must not be dispensed, and should not be accepted.

(ii) For Schedule 2 and 3 Controlled Drugs for human use, a private prescription that is to be dispensed in community must contain the private prescriber's identification number.

(iii) There is a requirement for pharmacists in England, Scotland and Wales to submit the original of Schedule 2 and 3 private prescription forms for human use to the relevant NHS agency. An identifying code, assigned to the pharmacy for this purpose, will be required to submit private Controlled Drug prescriptions to the PPD-NHSB-SA (or equivalent).

No other items should be prescribed on a private standardised form (FP10PCD, PPCD(1) or WP10PCD) other than Controlled Drugs, as the prescription has to be sent away and pharmacists would therefore be unable to comply with the requirement to keep the private prescription of a POM for two years.

These requirements (i), (ii) and (iii) do not apply to certain prison arrangements in England and Wales. Where a service level agreement exists between a community pharmacy and a primary care organisation to supply items to a prison, the local primary care organisation should be consulted to determine whether it would not be necessary to use the standardised private prescription form for such supplies. Whether or not standardised private prescription forms are required, a robust audit trail must be maintained. Where it is determined that this is a private (not an NHS) arrangement, prescribers would need to use a standardised private prescription form for Schedule 2 or 3 Controlled Drugs to be supplied in a community setting. Where the private standardised form is required, the prescriber's identification number would also need to appear on the form.

These requirements (i), (ii) and (iii) do not apply to veterinary prescriptions for Controlled Drugs. Veterinary prescriptions do not need to be sent to any NHS agency but must be retained for at least five years (*see* p97).

Sativex (a cannabis oro-mucosal spray) does not have to be prescribed on a standardised private prescription form when being dispensed in community.

Repeat prescriptions

Repeat prescriptions for Schedule 2 and 3 Controlled Drugs are not allowed. Instalment prescriptions allow Schedule 2 and 3 Controlled Drugs to be issued over a period of time.

With reference to Schedule 4 Controlled Drugs and repeats on prescriptions, after the first dispensing, legislation does not specify the time frame in which the repeat dispensing(s) of private prescriptions should be made. As long as the first dispensing of a repeat for a Schedule 4 Controlled Drug is within 28 days of the appropriate date, repeat dispensing of Schedule 4 Controlled Drugs can be made after 28 days. However, for the NHS repeat dispensing scheme in England and Wales, batch repeats are valid for a maximum of 12 months.

Prescribing for up to 30 days' clinical need

Although not a legal requirement, the Department of Health and the Scottish Executive have issued a strong recommendation that as good practice, the quantity of Schedule 2, 3 and 4 Controlled Drugs prescribed should not exceed 30 days' supply. Pharmacists may legally supply a quantity greater than 30 days' supply, if appropriate. Prescribers will need to be able to justify on the basis of clinical need, a supply of more than 30 days.

Technical errors on Controlled Drug prescriptions

Pharmacists may supply Schedule 2 or 3 Controlled Drugs (excluding temazepam) if the prescription contains a minor typographical error or spelling mistake. A supply can also be made if the total quantity of the preparation or the number of dosage units (as the case may be) is specified on the prescription in either words or figures, but not both. Pharmacists can make a supply against a prescription containing these technical errors provided that:

(a) having exercised all due diligence, the pharmacist is satisfied on reasonable grounds that the prescription is genuine;

(b) having exercised all due diligence, the pharmacist is satisfied on reasonable grounds that he or she is supplying the drug in accordance with the intention of the person issuing the prescription;

(c) the pharmacist amends the prescription in ink or otherwise indelibly to correct the minor typographical errors or spelling mistakes or so that the prescription complies with the requirement to contain the total quantity of the preparation or the number of dosage units in both words and figures; and

(d) the pharmacist marks the prescription so that the amendment he has made under (c) is attributable to him or her.

No other amendments, such as the date, the dose and the form can be made, or added if omitted, as minor typographical errors by the pharmacist.

Supply of Controlled Drugs to misusers

A person is regarded as being addicted to a drug if, and only if, he has as a result of repeated administration become so dependent on a drug that he has an overpowering desire for the administration of it to be continued.

No doctor may administer or authorise the supply of cocaine, diamorphine or dipipanone, or their salts, to an addicted person, except for the purpose of treating organic disease or injury, unless he is licensed to do so by the Secretary of State.

There is provision for misusers to receive daily supplies of cocaine or diamorphine on special prescriptions. This is an administrative arrangement under the National Health

Service and does not form part of the Misuse of Drugs legislation.

Instalment prescriptions

In the case of instalment prescriptions for Schedule 2, 3 and 4 Controlled Drugs, the first instalment must be dispensed within 28 days of the appropriate date, with the remainder of instalments dispensed in accordance with the instructions. The 28-day period of validity starts from the appropriate date on the prescription form. The appropriate date is the later of the date of signing or a date expressly specified by the prescriber as being the date before which the Controlled Drug should not be supplied. The start date specified can be more than 28 days from the date of signing/issue.

Although there is no legal requirement for a starting date to be specified, where one is given in the prescription, it must be complied with and the instalment directions run from that date. If no start date is specified then the date of first dispensing would need to take place within 28 days of the date of signing. The prescription must be marked with the date of each supply.

It is a legal requirement that the instalment amount and the dose are specified separately on the prescription. Prescriptions which contain a direction that specified instalments of the total amount may be dispensed at stated intervals must not be dispensed otherwise than in accordance with the directions.

However, the Home Office has confirmed that if specified, approved wording is included in the prescription, it will enable those supplying Controlled Drugs to issue the remainder of an instalment prescription when the person fails to collect the instalment on the specified day. If the prescription does not reflect such wording, the Regulations only permit the supply to be in accordance with the prescriber's instalment direction. The direction must be clear and unambiguous.

The Home Office approved wording does not appear in the Misuse of Drugs Regulations 2001, as amended, and a strict interpretation of the legislation allows no scope for dispensing a prescription for a Schedule 2 or 3 Controlled Drug outside of a prescriber's directions, ie each supply against an instalment prescription must be dispensed on the date specified on the prescription. However, the Home Office has approved wording in the past that, in their opinion, would cover a pharmacist supplying when instalments have been missed or supplies for days on which the pharmacy is closed (*see* below).

The approved wording is not included in legislation but the fact that the wording (*see* below) has been approved by the Home Office gives the dispensing pharmacist a degree of protection against the consequences of supplying against a strictly unlawful prescription. An instalment prescription that contains wording different from that approved by the Home Office would not provide the dispensing pharmacist the security conferred by a prescription containing Home Office approved wording.

If a pharmacist decides to supply against an instalment prescription that utilises wording that is not approved by the Home Office the pharmacist must be aware that they do not have the protection afforded by Home Office approved wording. Therefore, in this situation a pharmacist would be advised to get the prescription amended to reflect the Home Office approved wording. It should be noted that the Home Office no longer approve any new versions of approved wording that vary from those that already exist.

Home Office approved wording is in addition to the usual Controlled Drug prescription requirements (i.e. all the other prescription requirements apply).

Where Home Office approved wording is included on the prescription, allowing a reduced amount of Controlled Drug to be supplied on a day other than that specified on the prescription, the pharmacist must still use his or her professional judgment in deciding whether making the supply, less the days missed, would be appropriate.

The versions of Home Office approved wording for use when the day for an instalment to be collected is missed are as follows:

For supervised consumption: "Supervised consumption of daily dose on specified days; the remainder of supply to take home. If an instalment prescription covers more than one day and is not collected on the specified day, the total amount prescribed less the amount prescribed for the day(s) missed may be supplied."

For unsupervised consumption: "Instalment prescriptions covering more than one day should be collected on the specified day; if this collection is missed the remainder of the instalment (i.e., the instalment less the amount prescribed for the day(s) missed) may be supplied."

Or alternative wording permitted:

For unsupervised consumption: "If an instalment prescription covers more than one day and is not collected on the specified day, the total amount prescribed less the amount prescribed for the days missed may be supplied"

The Home Office approved wording to be used if the prescriber would like to ensure that the patient is not supplied with their dose if they have missed collecting their dose for three days is: "Instalment prescriptions covering more than one day should be collected on the specified day. If this collection is missed, the remainder of the instalment (i.e. the total amount less the instalments for the days missed) may continue to be supplied in the specified instalments at the stated intervals, provided no more than three days are missed."

Other Home Office approved wording to be used when the pharmacy is closed is given here. This approved wording will enable those supplying Controlled Drugs to issue instalments on the day immediately prior to closure should the pharmacy be closed on days when instalments are due. The wording approved by the Home Office is: "Instalments due on days when the pharmacy is closed should be dispensed on the day immediately prior to closure."

Where a third party collects a Controlled Drug for a patient being treated for drug addiction, although not a legal requirement it is good practice that a letter of authorisation from the patient is obtained on every occasion that the representative collects the medicine, and that the letter should be retained in the pharmacy for a period so that a comparison of signatures can be made.

National Health prescriptions for the treatment of misusers

In England, prescription form FP10(MDA) is used for instalment prescribing by both drug treatment centres and GPs. A maximum of 14 days' supply of any Schedule 2 Controlled Drug, buprenorphine and diazepam can be prescribed for the treatment of addiction using this form.

In Scotland, forms HBP(A) and HBP are issued from drug misuse centres and hospitals respectively and can be used to prescribe, in instalments, any drug used in the treatment of addiction. General practitioners may prescribe by instalment for the treatment of addiction on a GP10 of GP10-SS form. The doctor may specify that the drug should be dispensed in instalments and the prescription must comply with the Misuse of Drugs Regulations 2001, as amended.

In Wales, two types of prescription form are used for the treatment of misusers by instalment: WP10(MDA), issued by general practitioners, and WP10(HP)Ad, used principally by drug treatment centres. Up to 14 days' supply of drugs listed in Schedules 2 to 5 of the Misuse of Drugs Regulations 2001, as amended, will be reimbursed.

Cocaine, diamorphine and dipipanone can only be prescribed for the treatment of addiction by specially authorised doctors licensed by the Secretary of State..

Supplying drug paraphernalia

Legislation permits practitioners, pharmacists, persons employed or engaged in the lawful provision of drug treatment services and supplementary prescribers acting under and in accordance with the terms of a clinical management plan to supply specified drug paraphernalia to illicit drug users.

The items that a pharmacist can supply are:
swabs;
utensils for the preparation of Controlled Drugs;
citric acid;
ascorbic acid; and
filters.

Pharmacists employed or engaged in the lawful provision of a drug treatment service can supply only in the course of those services:
ampoules of sterile water for injection (on the condition that each ampoule does not contain more than 2ml).

A pharmacist who is not engaged or employed in such services, can only supply water for injection against a prescription or under a patient group direction.

Collection of Schedule 2 and 3 Controlled Drugs

Schedule 2 and 3 Controlled Drug prescriptions have a space on the reverse of the form for the person collecting to sign. There is no legal requirement for a signature on collection, but it is good practice to obtain one. The pharmacist must exercise their discretion as to whether or not to make a supply if the collector does not sign the back of the prescription.

Patients who collect their prescription in instalments via an FP10(MDA) or equivalent are not required to sign for each instalment, nor will a third party collecting the Controlled Drug on the patient's behalf. However, it would be good practice to have the back of the prescription signed on at least one occasion.

The patient may nominate a person to sign the back of the prescription on their behalf, who could be a delivery driver, or another representative. There should be a robust audit trail in place to show the successful delivery to the patient.

On collection of a Schedule 2 Controlled Drug, it is a legal requirement for the pharmacist asked to supply the drug on the prescription, to ascertain whether the person collecting is the patient, the patient's representative or a healthcare professional acting in their professional capacity on behalf of the patient.

Where a patient or their representative (other than a healthcare professional acting in their professional capacity) is collecting the Controlled Drug, the pharmacist may request evidence of that person's identity, and may refuse to make the supply if he is not satisfied as to the identity of that person.

Where a healthcare professional acting in their capacity as such is collecting the Controlled Drug on behalf of the patient, the pharmacist must obtain the healthcare professional's name and address, and unless acquainted with that professional, must request evidence of that professional's identity. The pharmacist may proceed with the supply even if he is not satisfied as to the healthcare professional's identity.

The Home Office has indicated that ID fields of the Controlled Drug Register (CDR) should be completed in the case of supplies made against requisitions as well as against prescriptions.

Details regarding the person collecting Schedule 2 Controlled Drugs must be recorded in the CDR. (*See* below and also table on p45 for further information.)

When a delivery driver is taking a dispensed Schedule 2 Controlled Drug to a patient, either at their own home or in a care home, his/her details should be entered in the Controlled Drug register. The delivery driver would be classed as the patient's representative. However, the pharmacy may wish to annotate the register to show that the person collecting was the delivery driver.

The requirements to check ID apply where Schedule 2 Controlled Drugs are supplied. In a hospital, the porter should be asked for ID unless they are already known by the pharmacist, but legislation does not require the porter's name and address to be recorded.

Controlled Drug registers

Records must be kept by pharmacists of all Schedule 1 (except Sativex) and 2 Controlled Drugs received or supplied. The headings under which information must be recorded in the Controlled Drug register are as follows:

For Controlled Drugs obtained, the following must be recorded:
(a) date supply received;
(b) name and address from whom received;
(c) quantity received.

For Controlled Drugs supplied, the following must be recorded:
(a) date supplied;
(b) name/address of person or firm supplied;
(c) details of authority to possess – prescriber or licence holder's details;
(d) quantity supplied;
(e) person collecting Schedule 2 Controlled Drug (patient/patient's representative/healthcare professional), and if a healthcare professional collecting a Schedule 2 Controlled Drug, their name and address;
(f) was proof of identity requested of patient / patient's representative (Yes/No);
(g) was proof of identity of person collecting provided (Yes/No).

These particulars are the minimum fields of information that must be recorded in the Controlled Drug register. The regulations allow additional related information to be recorded. The proof of identity and evidence seen requirements apply to all CDRs that are required by legislation (i.e. even to registered retail hospital pharmacy CDRs).

The following points must be complied with in relation to the keeping of Controlled Drug registers:

(a) Entries must be in chronological sequence.

(b) A separate register or separate part of the register must be used for each class of drugs. NB - Separate sections are required for amphetamines (which includes dexamphetamine) and methylamphetamine.

(c) In the separate register or separate part of the register used for each class of drug, a separate page shall be used for each strength and form of that drug.

(d) The class of the drug, its strength and form must be specified at the head of each page.

(e) Entries must be made on the day of the transaction or on the next day following.

(f) No cancellation, obliteration or alteration may be made; correction must be dated by marginal note or footnote.

(g) Entries must be in ink or otherwise indelible, or shall be in a computerised form.

(h) The computerised form must ensure every such entry is attributable and capable of being audited. Electronic Controlled Drug registers must comply with best practice guidance.

(i) The register must be kept at the premises to which it is related and a separate register must be kept for each premises of the business, but not more than one register can be kept at one time in respect to each class of drug. Where the register is in computerised form, it must be accessible from those premises.

(j) With Home Office approval, separate registers may be kept for each department of a business.

(k) Particulars of stocks, receipts and supplies must be furnished to any authorised person on request (this includes inspectors of the Royal Pharmaceutical Society and Controlled Drug liaison officers). Other documents and stocks of drugs must also be produced if required.

(l) Registers must be kept for two years from the last date of entry.

(m) Records must be kept in their original form or copied and kept in an approved computerised form.

(n) A copy of the register, in its computerised or other specified form may be requested to be sent to persons authorised by the Secretary of State (eg, the Society's Inspectors).

Entries made in respect of drugs obtained and drugs supplied may be made on the same page or on separate pages in the register.

The following is good practice in relation to the keeping of Controlled Drug registers:

(a) It is good practice that all Controlled Drug registers contain a running balance.

(b) Where an entry has been made in the Controlled Drug register no entry need be made in the prescription-only register under the Medicines Act 1968, but it is good practice to make such entries.

Electronic Controlled Drugs registers

As an alternative to a bound book, pharmacists may elect to keep their Controlled Drug register electronically. They must be capable of printing or displaying the name, form and strength of the drug in such a way that the details appear at the top of each display or printout to comply with the new Regulations. Electronic Controlled Drug registers must also comply with best practice guidance. Current best practice guidance states that:

(a) Registers may only be kept in computerised form if safeguards are incorporated into the software to ensure all of the following:
- the author of each entry is identifiable;
- entries cannot be altered at a later date;
- a log of all data entered is kept and can be recalled for audit purposes.

(b) Access control systems should be in place to minimise the risk of unauthorised or unnecessary access to the data in computerised registers.

(c) Adequate backups must be made of computerised registers.

(d) Arrangements should be made so that Inspectors can examine computerised registers during a visit with minimum disruption to the dispensing process.

The most up to date guidance can be found at the National Prescribing Centre website at _www.npc.co.uk_ or on the Society's website at _www.rpsgb.org.._.

Controlled Drugs and supplementary prescribing

A supplementary prescriber is permitted, when acting under and in accordance with the terms of a clinical management plan (CMP) to administer and/or supply or direct any person to administer Controlled Drugs in Schedules 2, 3, 4 and 5.

In England, supplementary prescribers use FP10MDA-SS or FP10MDA-SP prescription forms for drug misusers, and FP10SP and FP10SS prescription forms for general practice patients. In Wales, WP10SP, WP10SP-SS and WP10HSP prescription forms are issued by supplementary prescribers for general practice patients and hospital outpatients. In Scotland, GP10(N), GP10(N)SS and HBPN prescription forms are issued by nurse supplementary prescribers for general practice patients and hospital outpatients. In Scotland, GP10P and HBPP prescription forms are issued by pharmacist supplementary prescribers for general practice patients and hospital outpatients.

Controlled Drugs and nurse independent prescribers

Currently, nurse independent prescribers are permitted to prescribe, supply, administer or direct any other person to administer the following Controlled Drugs, solely for the medical conditions indicated:

(a) Diamorphine hydrochloride (orally or parenterally), morphine hydrochloride (rectally), morphine sulphate (orally, parenterally or rectally), or oxycodone hydrochloride (orally or parenterally) for use in palliative care;

(b) Buprenorphine (by transdermal route) or fentanyl (by transdermal route) in palliative care;

(c) Diamorphine hydrochloride (orally or parenterally), or morphine hydrochloride (rectally), morphine sulphate (orally, parenterally or rectally) for pain relief in respect of suspected myocardial infarction or for relief of acute or severe pain after trauma, including in either case postoperative pain relief;

(d) Chlordiazepoxide hydrochloride (orally) and diazepam (orally, parenterally or rectally) for treatment of initial or acute alcohol withdrawal symptoms;

(e) Codeine phosphate (orally), dihydrocodeine tartrate (orally) and co-phenotrope (orally) (no restriction on medical conditions).

(f) Diazepam (orally, parenterally or rectally), lorazepam (orally or parenterally) or midazolam (parenterally or via buccal route) for use in palliative care or treatment of tonic-clonic seizures.

This situation is currently being changed. Further guidance will be issued following the amendments to legislation.

In England, independent nurse prescribers use FP10P prescription forms for general practice patients and FP10SS for hospital outpatients. In Wales, independent nurse prescribers use WP10PN prescription forms for general practice patients, WP10IP by hospital independent prescribers, WP10CN by community nurses and WP10HP for hospital outpatients. In Scotland, independent nurse prescribers use GP10(N) prescription forms for general practice patients and HBPN for hospital outpatients.

Controlled Drugs and pharmacist independent prescribers

Pharmacist independent prescribers are not currently permitted to prescribe, administer in their own right or direct the administration of Controlled Drugs. The restriction applies to all Controlled Drugs including Schedule 5 Controlled Drugs (these may appear in pharmacy only preparations that are available for over the counter sale).

This situation is currently being changed. Further guidance will be issued following the amendments to legislation.

Controlled Drugs and midwives

A registered midwife may possess diamorphine, morphine, pethidine and pentazocine in her own right so far as is necessary for the practice of her profession (see p20). Supplies of diamorphine, morphine, pethidine and pentazocine may only be made to her on the authority of a midwife's supply order signed by the "appropriate medical officer" who is a doctor authorised in writing by the local supervising authority for the region or area, or the person appointed by the local supervising authority to exercise supervision over midwives within their area. The order must be in writing and must contain the following particulars:

(a) the name of the midwife;

(b) the occupation of the midwife;

(c) the purpose for which the Controlled Drug is required:

(d) the total quantity to be obtained;

(e) the signature of the "appropriate medical officer"

A midwife is required to keep a record of supplies of diamorphine, morphine and pethidine received and administered in a book used solely for that purpose. She must not destroy surplus stock but may surrender it to the "appropriate medical officer."

The pharmacist should retain the midwives supply order for two years. As diamorphine, morphine and pethidine are Schedule 2 Controlled Drugs, an appropriate entry is required in the Controlled Drug register. Pentazocine is a Schedule 3 Controlled Drug and therefore no entry is required in the Controlled Drug register, although an entry should be made in the prescription-only register.

Controlled Drugs and operating department practitioners

An operating department practitioner (ODP) may, when acting in their capacity as such, supply Controlled Drugs for administration to a patient in a ward, theatre or other department in accordance with the directions of a doctor, dentist, supplementary prescriber acting under and in accordance with the terms of a clinical management plan, or of a nurse independent prescriber. The Controlled Drugs to which this relates are those which have been supplied to the ODP by a person responsible for the dispensing and supply of medicines at that hospital.

The directions given by a nurse independent prescriber relate only to the limited list of Controlled Drugs which they may prescribe and are subject to restrictions on the purpose for which the drug may be prescribed (see above).

An ODP can order Schedule 2, 3, 4 and 5 Controlled Drugs from a hospital pharmacy. The hospital pharmacy in which the ODP is practising, can supply the ODP with these drugs. ODPs are able to possess and supply Schedule 2 to 5 Controlled Drugs for the purposes of administration to a patient in a ward, theatre or other department, at the hospital in which they are practising, in accordance with the directions of an appropriate practitioner for that particular drug.

Currently, when ordering Controlled Drugs from a hospital pharmacy, the ODP is under no legal obligation to provide a written requisition. However, pharmacists are advised as a matter of good practice and/or to comply with local standard operating procedures, supplies should be made on the receipt of a requisition signed by the ODP. The legislation is due to be changed to make the provision of a written requisition a legal requirement. There is no provision to allow an ODP to obtain Controlled Drugs from a community pharmacy.

Controlled Drugs and patient group directions

There are currently only three circumstances in which certain Controlled Drugs may be administered or supplied under a patient group direction (PGD). These are outlined below:

(a) A registered nurse may, when acting in her capacity as such, supply or administer diamorphine under a PGD for the treatment of cardiac pain to a person admitted as a patient to a coronary care unit or accident and emergency department of a hospital.

(b) A registered nurse, pharmacist or any of the other named healthcare professionals listed in Schedule 8 of the Misuse of Drugs Regulations 2001, as amended, may, when acting in their capacity as such, supply or administer any Schedule 5 Controlled Drug in accordance with a valid PGD.

(c) A registered nurse, pharmacist or any of the other named healthcare professionals listed in Schedule 8 of the Misuse of Drugs Regulations 2001, as amended, may, when acting in their capacity as such, supply or administer any Part 1 Schedule 4 Controlled Drug or midazolam in accordance with a valid PGD provided that it is not a drug in parenteral form for the treatment of addiction.

Midazolam is the only Schedule 3 Controlled Drug that can be included in a PGD. Under no other circumstances can a Controlled Drug be considered for inclusion in a PGD.

The list of Controlled Drugs that can be included in a PGD and the circumstances in which they can be supplied or administered is currently being reviewed and may be extended. Further guidance will be issued when changes in legislation have been made.

Standard operating procedures for Controlled Drugs

In England, Scotland and Wales, all healthcare providers who hold a stock of Controlled Drugs on their premises, including community pharmacies, must have up to date standard operating procedures (SOPs) in place that cover the following matters:
(a) who has access to the Controlled Drugs;
(b where the Controlled Drugs are stored;
(c) security in relation to the storage and transportation of Controlled Drugs as required by misuse of drugs legislation;
(d) disposal and destruction of Controlled Drugs;
(e) who is to be alerted if complications arise (which may include details of when and how the relevant accountable officer (*see* p3) (within a primary care organisation, trust or independent hospital) should be made aware of incidents); and
(f) record keeping, including:
 (i) maintaining relevant Controlled Drugs registers under misuse of drugs legislation, and
 (ii) maintaining a record of the Controlled Drugs specified in Schedule 2 to the Misuse of Drugs Regulations 2001, as amended, that have been returned by patients.

The Department of Health (in England) has issued guidance giving more detailed advice on the areas that may need to be covered by the SOP. The guidance is entitled the "Safer management of Controlled Drugs: guidance on standard operating procedures for Controlled Drugs" and is available on the Department of Health website at *www.dh.gov.uk*. The Scottish Executive Health Department has also issued more detailed advice in the document "Safer management of Controlled Drugs: standard operating procedures", which is available on *www.sehd.scot.nhs.uk*. The Department for Health and Social Services in Wales will issue guidance on what should be covered by SOPs in Wales in the near future.

Although the recording of patient returned Controlled Drugs is not a current legal requirement in relation to the Misuse of Drugs Regulations 2001, as amended, the Controlled Drugs (Supervision of Management and Use) Regulations 2006 and Controlled Drugs (Supervision of Management and Use) (Wales) Regulations 2008 as described in (f)(ii), above, require SOPs to be in place for maintaining a record of Schedule 2 Controlled Drugs that have been returned by patients. NB. *See* **p42 for further information on denaturing of Controlled Drugs and Controlled Drug waste.**

Pharmacists are therefore advised to keep a record of patient returned Schedule 2 Controlled Drugs, and their destruction, and to ensure that another member of staff, preferably a pharmacist or pharmacy technician if available, witnesses the destruction. The record of destruction should be made somewhere other than the Controlled Drug register, for example at the back of the private prescription register or in a separate book designated for that purpose.

It is recommended that the following details are recorded:
• the date of return of the Controlled Drugs;
• details of the Controlled Drugs:
 (i) name of the Controlled Drug
 (ii) quantity of the Controlled Drug;
 (iii) strength of the Controlled Drug; and
 (iv) form of the Controlled Drug;
• the role of the person who returned the Controlled Drugs (if known);
• the name and signature of the person who received the Controlled Drugs;
• the patient's name and address (if known);
• the names, positions and signatures of:
 (i) the person destroying the Controlled Drugs; and
 (ii) the person witnessing the destruction; and
• the date of destruction.

The recommendation is that these records be retained for a period of at least seven years.

Forms to record these details are available from the Society's website, *www.rpsgb.org*. Other bodies, organisations and suppliers may produce a record book specifically designed for this purpose.

Marking of containers for Controlled Drugs

A container in which a Controlled Drug other than a preparation is supplied must be plainly marked with the amount of drug contained in it.

If the drug is a preparation made up into tablets, capsules or other dosage units, the container must be marked with the amount of Controlled Drug(s) in each dosage unit and the number of dosage units in it. For any other kind of preparation, the container must be marked with the total amount of the preparation in it and the percentage of each of its components which are Controlled Drugs in the preparation.

These requirements do not apply to certain Schedule 3 Controlled Drugs, Schedule 4 and 5 Controlled Drugs, to poppy straw, to the supply of a Controlled Drug by or on the prescription of a practitioner or supplementary prescriber, to the supply of a Controlled Drug for administration in a clinical trial or a medicinal test on animals, or any exempt products.

Destruction of Controlled Drugs

England and Wales

The Environment Agency is in the process of reviewing its waste exemptions. We are currently seeking clarification from the Environment Agency in relation to the destruction of Controlled Drugs that have been returned to the pharmacy as waste. Further guidance will be published in a Law and Ethics Bulletin and via the pharmaceutical press.

Scotland

In Scotland, pharmacies should register an exemption under paragraph 39 of Schedule 3 to the Waste Management Licensing Regulations 1994 (as amended) with the Scottish Environment Protection Agency (SEPA). The exemption covers the secure storage of Controlled Drugs at a pharmacy prior to subsequent collection and disposal. SEPA has currently accepted that the denaturing of

Table B: Additional requirements for private prescriptions for Controlled Drugs

	Schedule 2	Schedule 3	Schedule 4, Part I	Schedule 4, Part II	Schedule 5
Private prescriber identification number required on private prescription (*see* Note B1)	Yes	Yes	No	No	No
Private CD prescriptions to be written only on standardised form (*see* Note B2)	Yes	Yes	No	No	No
Private CD prescription forms to be sent to relevant NHS agency (*see* Note B3)	Yes	Yes	No	No	No

Notes

B1. *Private prescriber identification number:* This number is required on private prescriptions for human use intended to be dispensed in community. Private prescriptions for temazepam must also contain the prescriber's identification number

B2. *Private prescription standardised forms:* Private prescriptions for human use intended to be dispensed outside the legal entity of a hospital or in community must be issued on the relevant standardised form. Private prescriptions for temazepam must also be on a standardised form.

B3. *Submission of private CD prescriptions:* The original of a Schedule 2 or 3 private CD prescription for human use must be sent to the relevant NHS agency in accordance with their arrangements for collection and analysis purposes (*see* p33)

Table C: Requirements for record keeping of Controlled Drugs

	Schedule 2	Schedule 3	Schedule 4, Part I	Schedule 4, Part II	Schedule 5
Records to be kept in CD register	Yes	No	No	No	No
Pharmacist must ascertain the identity of the person collecting CD (*see* Note C1)	Yes	No	No	No	No
Pharmacist must record in the CD register whether the person collecting is the patient, the patient's representative or a healthcare professional	Yes	No	No	No	No
Pharmacist must record in the CD register, where the person collecting is a healthcare professional, their name and address (*see* Note C2)	Yes	No	No	No	No
Pharmacist must record in the CD register whether proof of identity was requested of the patient or patient's representative	Yes	No	No	No	No
Pharmacist must record in the CD register whether proof of identity was provided by the person collecting	Yes	No	No	No	No

Notes

C1. *Identity of person collecting:* The pharmacist must ascertain the role of anyone collecting a Schedule 2 Controlled Drug. It must be ascertained whether the person is the patient, the patient's representative or a healthcare professional acting within their professional capacity as such. If a healthcare professional is collecting, their name and address (which may be their professional/work address) must be obtained and if they are not known to the pharmacist, ID must be requested (*see* p39)

C2. *Healthcare professional collecting:* The name and address of the healthcare professional collecting a Schedule 2 CD must be recorded in the CD register. The Home Office has confirmed that this may be their professional/work address.

native method of disposing of a large quantity of a liquid Controlled Drug is by adding and adsorbing it into an appropriate amount of cat litter, or similar product in accordance with Health and Safety regulations. The cat litter or similar product should be disposed of for incineration via the usual waste disposal methods for medicines.

<u>Fentanyl and buprenorphine patches</u> should have the backing removed and the patch folded over onto itself and placed in the waste disposal bin, or preferably a Controlled Drug denaturing kit.

<u>Ampoules</u> should be opened, the liquid poured into the Controlled Drug denaturing kit and the ampoule itself be put in the sharps bin. An ampoule that contains powder can have water added to it to dissolve the powder, and the resulting mixture can be poured into the Controlled Drug denaturing kit.

<u>Aerosol formulations</u> should be expelled into water (to prevent droplets of drug entering the air) and the resultant liquid disposed of as a liquid formulation.

For further information and advice on safe methods of destruction and precautions to be followed, *see* the guidance document "Guidance for Pharmacists on the safe destruction of Controlled Drugs, England, Scotland and Wales" on the Society's website *www.rpsgb.org*.

Summary of legal requirements for possession and supply of Controlled Drugs

The tables on pp44-45 summarise the legal requirements of the Regulations for Schedules 2 to 5 for the possession and supply of Controlled Drugs by pharmacists.

1.3: Alphabetical list of medicines for human use

This list of medicines for human use brings together medicines listed in the "Prescription Only Medicines" Order, the "General Sale List" Order and the Misuse of Drugs Regulations 2001. Generic medicines not specifically named in legislation are listed with the legal status granted under the marketing authorisation of the proprietary products in which they are contained.

However, changes to the reclassification procedure for medicines since 2003 mean that the legal status of a product now becomes part of its marketing authorisation rather than being determined by the active substance listed in secondary legislation.

Because a change of legal status will be conferred only on products that are the subject of an application for reclassification, users of this list should refer to the entry for the specific proprietary product and not rely on the entry for the active substance.

Since the POM Order remains in force, entries for active substances will remain in the list but will include cross references wherever proprietary products have been reclassified.

Further guidance or clarification on the status of individual products can be obtained from manufacturers or from the Medicines and Healthcare products Regulatory Agency (tel 020 7084 2000; e-mail info@mhra.gsi.gov.uk; website *www.mhra.gov.uk*).

The Royal Pharmaceutical Society's support service (RPS support) welcomes details of any errors or omissions in this list. RPS support can be contacted by email at support@rpsgb.org or by telephone 020 7572 2302.

KEY TO ANNOTATIONS

CD Lic: A substance controlled by the Misuse of Drugs Act 1971 to which the restrictions of the Regulations apply and, in addition, the production, possession and supply of which is limited in the public interest to purposes of research or other special purposes. A Home Office licence is required for such purposes. CD Lic substances are listed in Schedule 1 of the Misuse of Drugs Regulations 2001, as amended

CD POM: A substance controlled by the Misuse of Drugs Act 1971 to which the principal restrictions of the Misuse of Drugs Regulations 2001 apply. CD POM substances are listed in Schedule 2 of the Misuse of Drugs Regulations 2001, as amended

CD No Register POM: A substance controlled by the Misuse of Drugs Act 1971 to which the restrictions of the Regulations apply except that no entry in the Controlled Drugs Register is required and invoices must be retained for two years. CD No Register POM substances are listed in Schedule 3 of the Misuse of Drugs Regulations 2001, as amended

CD Benz POM: A substance controlled by the Misuse of Drugs Act 1971 to which the restrictions of the Regulations apply but with the following relaxation: prescription and labelling requirements do not apply (except those under the Medicines Act 1968), records in the CD register need not be kept by retailers, destruction requirements apply only to importers, exporters and manufacturers, there are no safe custody requirements. CD Benz POM substances are listed in Schedule 4, Part I of the Misuse of Drugs Regulations 2001, as amended

CD Anab POM: A substance controlled by the Misuse of Drugs Act 1971 to which the restrictions of the Regulations apply but with the following relaxation: prescription and labelling requirements do not apply (except those under the Medicines Act 1968), records in the CD register need not be kept by retailers, destruction requirements apply only to importers, exporters and manufacturers, there are no safe custody requirements. There is no restriction on possession when contained in a medicinal product. A Home Office import or export licence is required for the importation and exportation of these substances, unless they are imported or exported in the form of a medicinal product by a person for administration to himself. CD Anab POM substances are listed in Schedule 4, Part II of the Misuse of Drugs Regulations 2001, as amended

CD Inv. POM: A substance controlled by the Misuse of Drugs Act 1971 but which is exempt from all restrictions under the Regulations except that the invoice or a copy of it must be kept for two years. CD Inv. POM substances are listed in Schedule 5 of the Misuse of Drugs Regulations 2001, as amended

POM: A substance which, by virtue of an entry in the Prescription Only Medicines (Human Use) Order 1997, as amended, or by virtue of its marketing authorisation may be sold or supplied to the public only on a practitioner's prescription or in accordance with another legal authority, eg, patient group direction

P: A substance which is a pharmacy medicine by virtue of its marketing authorisation or a substance which is not subject to the prescription-only requirements of the Prescription Only Medicines (Human Use) Order 1997, as amended, and which is not included in the Medicines (Products Other Than Veterinary Drugs) (General Sale List) Order 1984, as amended

GSL: A substance which is licensed as a general sale list medicine or one which is described in the Medicines (Products Other Than Veterinary Drugs) (General Sale List) Order 1984, as amended, made under the Medicines Act 1968

PO: A substance which contains GSL ingredients but is licensed for sale through pharmacies only

md (maximum dose), ie, the maximum quantity of the substance contained in the amount of a medicinal product which is recommended to be taken or administered at any one time

mdd (maximum daily dose), ie, the maximum quantity of the substance that is contained in the amount of a medicinal product which is recommended to be taken or administered in any period of 24 hours

ms (maximum strength), ie, either or, if so specified, both of the following: (a) the maximum quantity of the substance by weight or volume that is contained in the dosage unit of a medicinal product; or (b) the maximum percentage of the substance contained in a medicinal product calculated in terms of w/w, w/v, v/w or v/v, as appropriate

External use means for application to the skin, teeth, mucosa of the mouth, throat, nose, eye, ear, vagina or anal canal when a local action only is necessary and extensive systemic absorption is unlikely to occur.
Note: The following are not regarded as for external use: throat sprays, throat pastilles, throat lozenges, throat tablets, nasal drops, nasal sprays, nasal inhalations or teething preparations

Parenteral administration means administration by breach of the skin or mucous membrane

A

A and P infant powders GSL
AAA mouth and throat spray P
Abacavir POM
Abciximab POM
Abelcet infusion POM
Abidec drops GSL
Abietis oil GSL
Abilify preparations POM
Abraxane POM
Abstral sublingual tablets CD POM
Abtrim P
AC Vax POM
Acamprosate tablets POM
Acarbose POM
Accolate tablets POM
Accupro tablets POM
Accuretic tablets POM
Accusite injectable gel POM
Acebutolol hydrochloride POM
Acea gel POM
Aceclofenac tablets POM
Acemetacin POM
Acenocoumarol/Nicoumalone POM
Acepril tablets POM
Acepromazine POM
Acepromazine maleate POM
Acerola GSL
Acetanilide POM
Acetarsol POM
Acetazolamide POM
Acetazolamide sodium POM
Acetic acid, if internal use maximum
  strength 7.5 per cent or external use
  maximum strength 15.0 per cent GSL
Acetohexamide POM
Acetone, external use only GSL
Acetorphine; its salts, esters and ethers
  CD POM
Acetylcholine chloride POM but if exter-
  nal use and maximum strength 0.2
  per cent, P
Acetylcysteine POM
Acetyldihydrocodeine CD POM
Acezide tablets POM
Achromycin ear/eye ointment POM
Achromycin preparations POM
Aci-Jel GSL
Aciclovir POM but if external for treat-
  ment of herpes simplex virus infec-
  tions of the lips and face (Herpes labi-
  alis) and maximum strength 5.0 per
  cent, and container or package con-
  tains not more than 2g of medicinal
  product, P or GSL. Please refer to pro-
  prietary names for the classification
  granted under the marketing authori-
  sation (See Zovirax products)
Acid-eze tablets P
Acidex GSL
Acipimox POM
Acitak tablets POM
Acitretin POM
Aclacin POM
Aclarubicin hydrochloride POM
Aclasta solution for infusion POM
Acnamino MR POM
Acnecide gel 10% P
Acnecide gel 5% P
Acnidazil cream P
Acnisal P
Acnocin tablets POM
Acoflam Retard tablets POM
Acoflam SR tablets POM
Acoflam tablets POM
Acomplia POM
Aconite POM but if external and maxi-
  mum strength 1.3 per cent, P
Acorvio P
Acorvio plus POM
Acriflex cream GSL
Acrivastine POM but if 24 mg (MDD)
  and container or package containing
  not more than 240mg of acrivastine,
  P; if for internal use for the sympto-
  matic relief of allergic rhinitis, includ-
  ing hayfever, and chronic idiopathic

urticaria in adults and children 12-65
  years with a maximum strength of
  8mg, 8mg (MD) 24mg (MDD) in a
  pack containing no more than 21
  doses (168mg acrivastine), GSL.
  Please refer to proprietary names for
  the classification granted under the
  marketing authorisation (see
  Benadryl Allergy Relief products)
Acrosoxacin POM
ACT-HIB POM
ACT-HIB DTP POM
Actal pastils PO
Actal tablets GSL
ACTH injection POM
Actidose Aqua Advance suspension P
Actidose Aqua suspension P
Actifed Chesty P
Actifed Linctus CD Inv P
Actifed syrup P
Actifed tablets P
Actilyse POM
Actinac POM
Actinomycin C POM
Actinomycin D POM
Actinomycin D inj POM
Actiq lozenges CD POM
Activated Attapulgite GSL
Activated dimeticone/dimethicone GSL
Actonel Combi preparations POM
Actonel Once a Week tablets POM
Actonel tablets POM
Actonorm gel P
Actonorm powder P
Actos tablets POM
Actrapid insulins POM
Acular ophthalmic solution POM
Acumed patch GSL
Acupan preparations POM
ACWY Vax vaccine POM
Adalat capsules POM
Adalat LA tablets POM
Adalat Retard tablets POM
Adalimumab POM
Adapalene gel POM
Adartrel tablets POM
Adcal chewable tablets P
Adcal D3 P
Adcortyl in Orabase POM
Adcortyl in Orabase for mouth ulcers (PL
  0034/0321) P
Adcortyl preparations POM
Adcortyl with Graneodin preparations
  POM
Addamel POM
Addiphos solution POM
Additrace solution POM
Adefovir Dipivoxil POM
Adenocor injection POM
Adenoscan vials POM
Adenosine POM
Adgyn Combi tablets POM
Adgyn Estro tablets POM
Adgyn Medro tablets POM
Adios P
Adipine MR POM
Adipine XL tablets POM
Adizem SR preps POM
Adizem XL capsules POM
Adizem XL Plus capsules POM
Adrenaline POM but if (1) by inhaler, (2)
  external (except ophthalmic), P
Adrenaline acid tartrate POM but if (1)
  by inhaler, (2) external, P
Adrenaline hydrochloride POM but if (1)
  by inhaler, (2) external, P
Adrenocortical extract POM
Adsorbed diphtheria and tetanus vaccine
  POM
Adsorbed diphtheria vaccine POM
Adsorbed diphtheria, tetanus and pertus-
  sis vaccine POM
Adsorbed tetanus vaccine POM
Advate solution for injection POM
Advil cold and sinus tablets P
Advil extra strength 400mg pack sizes
  24s P
Advil tablets 200mg pack sizes 12s GSL

Advil tablets pack sizes 24s P
Aerobec Autohaler POM
Aerobec Forte Autohaler POM
Aerocrom inhaler POM
Aerocrom Syncrone POM
Aerodiol nasal spray POM
Aerolin Autohaler POM
Aerrane POM
Aezodent P
Afinetor tablets POM
Afrazine nasal preparations GSL
After-bite GSL
Agalsidase alfa POM
Agalsidase Beta POM
Agarol P
Agenerase preparations POM
Aggrastat POM
Agnus castus (Chaste Tree) GSL
Agrimony GSL
Agrippal POM
Agropyron (triticum) GSL
Ailax Forte suspension POM
Ailax suspension POM
Air GSL
Airbron POM
Airomir autohaler POM
Airomir inhaler POM
Akineton preparations POM
Aklomide POM
Aknemin capsules POM
Aknemycin Plus POM
Albendazole POM
Albufilm GSL
Albumin Human (Immuno) POM
Albumin Human (Kabi) POM
Albumin Microspheres Human (3M)
  POM
Albuminar preps POM
Albutein preps POM
Alclofenac POM
Alclometasone dipropionate POM; but if
  cream for external use for the short-
  term treatment and control of patches
  of eczema and dermatitis including
  atopic eczema and primary irritant
  and allergic dermatitis in adults and
  children 12 years and over, maximum
  strength 0.05 per cent w/w, in a con-
  tainer or packaging containing not
  more than 15g of medicinal product P
Alcobon preparations POM
Alcoderm preparations P
Alcohol GSL
Alcon Isopto alkaline, eye drops P
Alcon Isopto atropine 1% eye drops
  POM
Alcon Isopto carbachol 3% eye drops
  POM
Alcon Isopto carpine 0.5%, 1%, 2%, 3%,
  4% POM
Alcon Isopto Frin, eye drops P
Alcon Isopto Plain, eye drops P
Alcon Maxidex eye drops POM
Alcon Maxitrol eye drops POM
Alcon Maxitrol oint POM
Alcon Mydriacyl 0.5% drops POM
Alcon Mydriacyl 1% drops POM
Alcon tears naturale eye drops P
Alcowipes GSL
Alcuronium chloride POM
Aldactide tablets POM
Aldactone tablets POM
Aldara cream POM
Aldesleukin POM
Aldioxa (aluminium dihydroxyallan-
  toinate), external use only GSL
Aldomet preparations POM
Aldosterone POM
Aldurazyme POM
ALEC vials POM
Alemtuzumab POM
Alendronic acid tablets POM
Alexitol sodium GSL
Alfa D capsules POM
Alfacalcidol POM
Alfentanil CD POM
Alfuzosin hydrochloride POM
Algesal cream P

Algicon tabs and suspension P
Alginic acid GSL
Algitec Chewtab POM
Algitec suspension POM
Algitec tablets POM
Alglucerase vials POM
Alimemazine/Trimeprazine POM
Alimemazine/Trimeprazine tartrate POM
Alimta POM
Alka Rapid crystals GSL
Alka-Seltzer GSL
Alka-Seltzer XS tablets GSL
Alkaline eye drops BPC P
Alkanna, external use only GSL
Alkeran preparations POM
n-Alkyl isoquinolinium bromide, exter-
  nal use only GSL
Allantoin, external use only GSL
Allegron preparations POM
Allens chesty cough GSL
Allens dry tickly cough GSL
Allens pine & honey balsam GSL
Aller-eze Plus preparations P
Aller-eze tablets P
Allergen Extracts POM
Allergy therapeutics POM
Allerief P
Allertek GSL
Allevyn Adhesive 17cm x 17cm GSL
Allevyn Lite GSL
Alli 60mg capsules P
Alloferin injection POM
Allopurinol POM
Allyloestrenol POM
Allylprodine CD POM
Almodan capsules POM
Almodan syrup POM
Almogran tablets POM
Almond oil GSL
Almotriptan POM
Aloes, Barbados, up to 50mg (MD) GSL
Aloes, Cape, up to 100mg (MD) GSL
Aloin, up to 20mg (MD) GSL
Alomide Allergy ophthalmic solution P
Alomide ophthalmic POM
Alophen pills P
Aloxi solution for injection POM
Aloxiprin POM but if non-effervescent
  tablets or capsules with ms 620mg
  supplied in a container not exceeding
  32 (unless the number of tablets, capsules or a combination of both supplied to a person at any one time
  exceeds 100) P; or if powders or granules maximum strength 800mg, or
  non-effervescent tablets or capsules
  with ms 400mg supplied in a container not exceeding 16 (unless the
  number of tablets, capsules or a combination of both supplied to a person
  at any one time exceeds 100), GSL
  (when combined with aspirin, the
  aspirin limits apply to the combina-
  tion of aspirin and aspirin equivalent)
Alpha Keri bath oil P
Alpha tocopheryl acid succinate GSL
Alpha-pinene, external use only GSL
Alphacetylmethadol; its salts CD POM
Alphaderm cream POM
Alphadolone acetate POM
Alphagan eye drops POM
Alphaglobin POM
Alphameprodine; its salts CD POM
Alphamethadol; its salts esters and
  ethers CD POM
Alphaparin POM
Alphaprodine; its salts CD POM
Alphavase tablets POM
Alphaxalone POM
Alphosyl 2 in 1 shampoo GSL
Alphosyl cream P
Alphosyl HC cream POM
Alphosyl lotion P
Alprazolam CD Benz POM
Alprenolol POM
Alprenolol hydrochloride POM
Alprostadil POM
Alseroxylon POM

Aspirin legal status

Product	Container size	Legal status	Where it can be sold	Maximum that can be sold to a person at any one time (*see* Note 2)
Aspirin tablets (non-effervescent) and capsules up to 325mg (including 75mg preparations)	Up to 16	GSL	Pharmacies and non-pharmacy retail outlets	Not more than 100 tablets or capsules
Aspirin tablets (non-effervescent) and capsules up to 325mg (including 75mg preparations)	Between 17 and 32	P (*see* Note 3)	Pharmacies only	Not more than 100 tablets or capsules
Aspirin enteric-coated tablets up to 75mg	Up to 28	GSL	Pharmacies and non-pharmacy retail outlets	Not more than 100 tablets or capsules
Aspirin tablets (non-effervescent) and capsules up to 75mg	Between 17 and 100	P (*see* Note 3)	Pharmacies only	Not more than 100 tablets or capsules
Aspirin tablets (non-effervescent) and capsules above 325mg and up to 500mg	Up to 32	P	Pharmacies only	Not more than 100 tablets or capsules
Aspirin tablets (non-effervescent) and capsules above 325mg and up to 500mg	Greater than 32	POM	Pharmacies only	To be sold or supplied only in accordance with a prescription
Aspirin tablets (effervescent) up to 325mg (*see* Note 1)	Up to 30	GSL	Pharmacies and non-pharmacy retail outlets	No legal limit
Aspirin tablets (effervescent) up to 325mg (*see* Note 1)	Greater than 30	P (*see* Note 3)	Pharmacies only	No legal limit
Aspirin tablets (effervescent) above 325mg and up to 500mg (*see* Note 1)	Up to 20	GSL	Pharmacies and non-pharmacy retail outlets	No legal limit
Aspirin tablets (effervescent) above 325mg and up to 500mg (*see* Note 1)	Greater than 20	P (*see* Note 3)	Pharmacies only	No legal limit
Aspirin powders up to 650mg	Up to 10	GSL	Pharmacies and non-pharmacy retail outlets	No legal limit
Aspirin powders up to 650mg	Greater than 10	P (*see* Note 3)	Pharmacies only	No legal limit

Note 1: Effervescent preparations in relation to a tablet, means containing not less than 75 per cent, by weight of the tablet, of ingredients included wholly or mainly for the purpose of releasing carbon dioxide when the tablets is dissolved or dispersed in water

Note 2: While several products have no legal limit for the amount that may be sold or supplied, pharmacists are expected to exercise professional control to limit the amount of aspirin which may be stored in a patient's home

Note 3: Strictly speaking, aspirin is a POM or GSL product, but limited to sale through pharmacies under certain conditions and exemptions. Products would be pharmacy medicines unless specifically licensed otherwise

Note 4: When aspirin is in combination with a pharmacy medicine (eg, low-strength codeine) or a prescription-only medicine (eg, dextropropoxyphene), the more stringent legal category applies

Altacite Plus suspension 500ml P
Altacite Plus suspension 100ml GSL
Altacite suspension P
Altargo POM
Alteplase inj POM
Altretamine capsules POM
Alu-Cap P
Aludrox liquid GSL
Alum BP, external use only GSL
Aluminium carbonate (Basic) GSL
Aluminium glycinate GSL
Aluminium hydroxide GSL
Aluminium oxide GSL
Aluminium sulphate, external use only GSL

Alupent aerosol inhalation POM
Alupent syrup POM
Alupent tablets POM
Alvedon suppositories P
Alvercol granules P
Alverine P
Alvesco POM
Amantadine hydrochloride POM
Amaranth GSL
Amaryl tablets POM
Ambenonium chloride POM
Amber oil, external use only GSL
Ambisome injection POM
Ambutonium bromide POM
Amcinonide POM

Ametazole hydrochloride POM
Amethocaine see Tetracaine
Ametop gel P
Amfetamine/Amphetamine; its salts CD POM
Amfiper preparations POM
Amias tablets POM
Amidone see Methadone
Amidopyrine POM
Amidox tablets POM
Amifostine infusion POM
Amikacin sulphate POM
Amikin injections POM
Amil-Co tablets POM
Amilamont solution POM

Amilmaxco 5/50 tablets POM
Amiloride hydrochloride POM
Amilospare tablets POM
Aminacrine see Aminoacridine
Aminoacetic acid (Glycine) GSL
Aminoacridine/aminacrine hydrochloride, external use only GSL
Aminobenzoic acid, if internal 30mg (MD) or external GSL
Aminocaproic acid POM
Aminoglutethimide POM
Aminogran food supplement P
Aminogran mineral mixture P
2-amino-1-phenyl-1-propanon structurally derived compounds (not being

bupropion, diethylpropion, pyrovalerone or a compound for the time being specified in sub-paragraph 1(a) of Schedule 1 of the Misuse of Drugs Regulations 2001) by modification in any of the following ways, that is to say: (i) by substitution in the phenyl ring to any extent with alkyl, alkoxy, alkylenedioxy, haloalkyl or halide substituents, whether or not further substituted in the phenyl ring by one or more other univalent substituents; (ii) by substitution at the 3-position with an alkyl substituent; (iii) by substitution at the nitrogen atom with alkyl or dialkyl groups, or by inclusion of the nitrogen atom in a cyclic structure CD Lic

Aminophylline injection BP POM
Aminoplex preparations POM
Aminopterin sodium POM
Aminorex CD Benz POM
Amiodarone hydrochloride POM
Amiphenazole hydrochloride POM
Amisulpride tablets POM
Amitriptyline POM
Amitriptyline embonate POM
Amitriptyline hydrochloride POM
Amix preps POM
Amlodipine besylate POM
Amlodipine maleate POM
Amlostin POM
Ammonaps POM
Ammonia, solutions of, up to maximum strength 5.0 per cent of NH3 (ammonia) in all preparations except smelling salts or 15.0 per cent of NH3 (ammonia) in smelling salts GSL
Ammonium acetate solution strong GSL
Ammonium bicarbonate GSL
Ammonium bromide POM
Ammonium carbonate GSL
Ammonium chloride GSL
Amnivent 225-SR tablets P
Amobarbital sodium/Amylobarbitone sodium CD No Register POM
Amobarbital/Amylobarbitone CD No Register POM
Amodiaquine hydrochloride POM
Amoram preps POM
Amorolfine hydrochloride POM; but in the form of a nail lacquer for the treatment of mild cases of distal and lateral subungual onychomycoses caused by dermatophytes, yeasts and moulds; treatment is limited to 2 nails, max strength 5% amorolfine (as the base), max pack 3ml of product, P
Amoxapine POM
Amoxicillin/Amoxycillin POM
Amoxicillin/Amoxycillin sodium POM
Amoxicillin/Amoxycillin trihydrate POM
Amoxil preparations POM
Amoxycillin see Amoxicillin
Amphetamine see Amfetamine
Amphocil infusion POM
Amphomycin calcium POM
Amphotericin POM
Ampicillin POM
Ampicillin sodium POM
Ampicillin trihydrate POM
Ampitrin preps POM
Amprenavir POM
Amsacrine POM
Amsidine preparations POM
Amyben POM
Amygdalin POM
Amyl nitrite POM but if sold or supplied by pharmacists to persons to whom cyanide salts may be sold by virtue of Section 3 (regulation of poisons) or Section 4 (exclusion of sales by wholesale and certain other sales) of the Poisons Act 1972 or by virtue of article 5 and the sale or supply shall only be so far as is necessary to enable an antidote to be available to persons at risk of cyanide poisoning P

Amylmetacresol, if internal 0.6mg (MD), or external except mouthwash maximum strength 0.5 per cent, or mouthwash maximum strength 0.001 per cent final concentration GSL
Amylobarbitone see Amobarbital
Amylobarbitone sodium see Amobarbital sodium
Amylocaine hydrochloride POM but if non-ophthalmic use P
Amyloglycosidase Concentrate GSL
Amytal tablets CD No Register POM
Ana-Kit POM
Anabact gel POM
Anacal preparations P
Anadin capsules, Maximum Strength P
Anadin Cold Control preparations GSL
Anadin Extra soluble tablets pack sizes 8s, 16s GSL
Anadin Extra tablets pack sizes 8s, 12s, 16s GSL; 32s P
Anadin Ibuprofen tablets pack sizes 16s GSL
Anadin Paracetamol tablets pack sizes 8s, 16s GSL; 32s P
Anadin tablets pack sizes 6s, 12s, 16s GSL; 32s P
Anadin Ultra capsules pack sizes 8s, 16s GSL; 32s P
Anadin Ultra Double Strength P
Anaflex cream P
Anafranil preparations POM
Anafranil SR tablets POM
Anagrelide POM
Anaguard POM
Anakinra POM
Anapen POM
Anapen Junior POM
Anastrazole tablets POM
Anbesol Adult Strength gel GSL
Anbesol liquid P
Anbesol teething gel P
Ancotil POM
Ancrod POM
Andrews Antacid tablets GSL
Andrews Liver Salts GSL
Andrews Plus GSL
Androcur tablets POM
Andropatch CD Anab POM
5a-Androstane-3,17-diol CD Anab POM
Androst-4-ene-3,17-diol CD Anab POM
1-Androstenediol CD Anab POM
1-Androstenedione CD Anab POM
5-Androstenedione CD Anab POM
4-Androstene-3,17-dione CD Anab POM
5-Androstene-3,17-diol CD Anab POM
Androsterone POM
Anectine injection POM
Anethaine cream P
Anethole GSL
Anexate injection POM
Angelica GSL
Angeliq tablets POM
Angettes tablets P
Angettes-75 tablets P
Angeze SR capsules POM
Angeze tablets P
Angilol tablets POM
Angiopine 40 LA tablets POM
Angiopine capsules POM
Angiopine LA tablets POM
Angiopine MR tablets POM
Angiotensin amide POM
Angiox POM
Angiozem CR tablets POM
Angiozem tablets POM
Angitak spray P
Angitil SR capsules POM
Angitil XL capsules POM
Anhydrol Forte P
Anileridine; its salts CD POM
Animalintex GSL
Anise Oil GSL
Aniseed (Anise) GSL
Anistreplase POM
Anodesyn preparations GSL
Anquil tablets POM
Antabuse tablets POM

Antepsin suspension POM
Antepsin tablets POM
Anterior Pituitary Extract POM
Anthisan Bite & Sting cream GSL
Anthisan cream P
Anthisan Plus spray GSL
Anthrax vaccine (Bacillus Anthracis) POM
Anti-D (Rh:) Immuno globulin inj POM
Antihepatitis B Immunoglobulin inj POM
Antimony barium tartrate POM
Antimony dimercaptosuccinate POM
Antimony lithium thiomalate POM
Antimony pentasulphide POM
Antimony potassium tartrate POM
Antimony sodium tartrate POM
Antimony sodium thioglycollate POM
Antimony sulphate POM
Antimony trichloride POM
Antimony trioxide POM
Antimony trisulphide POM
Antipeol GSL
Antipressan tablets POM
Antirabies Immunoglobulin inj POM
Antirobe capsules POM
Antistreplase inj POM
Antitetanus Immunoglobulin inj POM
Antivaricella-zoster Immunoglobulin inj POM
Anturan tablets POM
Anugesic-HC preparations POM
Anusol Plus HC ointment (0018/0223) P
Anusol Plus HC suppositories (0018/0224) P
Anusol preparations GSL
Anusol-HC preparations POM
Anzemet preparations POM
Apidra preparations POM
Apiol POM
APO-go pen injector POM
Apomorphine POM
Apomorphine hydrochloride POM
APP stomach powder and tablets POM
Apraclonidine ophthalmic solution 0.5%; 1% POM
Apramycin POM
Aprepitant POM
Apresoline preparations POM
Aprinox tablets POM
Aprotinin POM
Aprovel tablets POM
Apsin preparations POM
Apsolol tablets POM
Apstil tablets POM
Aptivus capsules POM
APV Acellular Pertussis Vaccine POM
Aquaban tablets GSL
Aquaban Herbal GSL
Aquadrate cream P
Aquaform GSL
Aqualette tablets GSL
Aquasept skin cleanser GSL
Aquasol sachets P
Aqueous cream BP GSL
Arachis oil GSL
Aramine injection POM
Aranesp injection POM
Arava tablets POM
Arbralene tablets POM
Arcoxia tablets POM
Arecoline hydrobromide POM
Aredia Dry Powder inj POM
Aredia vials POM
Arelix capsules POM
Argipressin POM
Aricept tablets POM
Aricept Evess POM
Aridil tablets POM
Arilvax yellow fever vaccine POM
Arimidex tablets POM
Aripiprazole POM
Aristolochia POM
Aristolochia Clematitis POM
Aristolochia Contorta POM
Aristolochia Debelis POM
Aristolochia Fang-chi POM
Aristolochia Manshuriensis POM

Aristolochia Serpentaria POM
Arixtra injection POM
Arlevert POM
Arnica, external use only GSL
Aromasin tablets POM
Arpicolin syrup POM
Arpimycin suspension POM
Arret capsules P
Arrowroot GSL
Arsenic POM
Arsenic triiodide POM
Arsenic trioxide POM
Arsphenamine POM
Artelac eye-drops P
Artesunate POM
Arthrocin tablets POM
Arthrofen tablets POM
Arthrotec 50 tablets POM
Arthrotec 75 tablets POM
Arthroxen tablets POM
Artichoke GSL
Artilan tablets POM
Arythmol tablets POM
Asacol foam enema POM
Asacol suppositories POM
Asacol MR tablets POM
Asafetida GSL
Asasantin Retard POM
Ascabiol P
Ascorbic acid GSL
Asendis tablets POM
Aserbine cream P
Aserbine solution P
Ashbourne emollient GSL
Ashton and Parsons infants powders GSL
Asilone Heartburn GSL
Asilone liquid GSL
Asilone suspension GSL
Asilone tablets GSL
Asilone Windcheaters GSL
Askit preparations GSL
Asmabec Clickhaler POM
Asmabec Spacehaler POM
Asmal tablets POM
Asmanex Twisthaler POM
Asmasal Clickhaler POM
Asmasal Spacehaler POM
Asmaven Inhaler POM
Asmaven tablets POM
Aspav tablets CD Inv POM
Aspergum P
Aspirin (see table p49) POM but if (1) non-effervescent tablets and capsules above 325mg up to maximum strength 500mg, and the quantity sold or supplied in one container or package does not exceed 32, and the quantity sold or supplied to a person at any one time does not exceed 100 P; or (2) non effervescent tablets and capsules maximum strength 75mg, and the quantity sold or supplied in one container or package does not exceed 100, and the quantity sold or supplied to a person at any one time does not exceed 100 GSL (Note there is a pack size limit in non- pharmacy premises); (3) in the case of non-effervescent tablets where they are enteric coated, maximum strength 75mg and not more than 28 tablets, GSL; (4) non-effervescent tablets and capsules maximum strength 325mg (and the quantity sold or supplied at any one time does not exceed 100), powder or granules maximum strength 650mg or effervescent tablets maximum strength 500mg GSL (Note there is a pack size limit in non-pharmacy premises)
Aspirin (dispersible) and papaveretum tablets (Cox) CD Inv POM
Aspro Clear maximum strength GSL
Aspro Clear pack sizes 18s, 30s GSL
Astemizole POM
AT 10 P
Atamestane CD Anab POM
Atazanavir POM

Atarax preparations POM
Atenix tablets POM
AtenixCo 100 POM
AtenixCo 50 POM
Atenolol POM
Athranol 2.0% POM
Atimos Modulite inhaler POM
Ativan preparations CD Benz POM
Atomoxetine POM
Atorvastatin tablets POM
Atosiban POM
Atovaquone suspension POM
Atracurium POM
Atracurium besylate POM
Atriance POM
Atro arnica pain relief gel GSL
Atromid-S capsules POM
Atropine POM but if (1) in inhalers P; or
(2) in preparations for internal use
(other than inhalers) with md
300mcg and mdd 1mg P; or (3) in
preparations for external use (except
preparations for local ophthalmic use
POM) P
Atropine methobromide POM but if (1)
in inhalers P; or (2) in preparations
for internal use (other than inhalers)
with md 400mcg and mdd 1.3mg P;
or (3) in preparations for external use
(except preparations for local ophthalmic use POM) P
Atropine methonitrate POM but if (1)
internal by inhaler P; or (2) in preparations for internal use (other than
inhalers) with md 400mcg and mdd
1.3mg P
Atropine oxide hydrochloride POM but
if (1) in inhalers P; (2) in preparations
for internal use (other than inhalers)
with md 360mcg and mdd 1.2mg P;
or (3) in preparations for external use
(except preparations for local ophthalmic use POM) P
Atropine sulphate POM but if (1) in
inhalers P; (2) in preparations for
internal use (other than inhalers)
with md 360mcg and mdd 1.2mg P;
or (3) in preparations for external use
(except preparations for local oph-
thalmic use POM) P
Atrovent Aerocaps POM
Atrovent Autohalers POM
Atrovent CFC-free inhaler POM
Atrovent Forte inhaler POM
Atrovent inhaler POM
Atrovent Nebuliser solution POM
Audax ear drops P
Audicort ear drops POM
Augmentin Duo suspension POM
Augmentin preparations POM
Auralgan ear drops P
Auranofin POM
Aureocort preparations POM
Aureomycin eye ointment POM
Aureomycin preparations POM
Aurothiomalate sodium inj POM
Avamys spray POM
Avandamet tablets POM
Avandia tablets POM
Avastin concentrate for solution for
infusion POM
Avaxim vaccine POM
Avelox preparations POM
Avena (oats) GSL
Aviral cream P
Avloclor tablets POM but for prophylaxis
of malaria P
AVOCA P
Avodart capsules POM
Avomine tablets P
Avonex injection POM
Axid capsules POM
Axid injection POM
Axorid capsules POM
Axsain cream POM
Ayrton preparations GSL
Azactam injection POM
Azamune tablets POM

Azapropazone POM
Azarga eye drops suspension POM
Azatadine preps P
Azathioprine POM
Azathioprine sodium POM
Azelaic Acid POM
Azelastine hydrochloride POM but if for
nasal administration, for the treatment of seasonal allergic rhinitis or
perennial allergic rhinitis for use in
adults and children not less than five
years, as a non-aerosol, aqueous form
140mcg per nostril (MD), 280mcg per
nostril (MDD) and container or package contains not more than
5,040mcg of azelastine hydrochloride, P
Azidocillin potassium POM
Azidothymidine POM
Azilect tablets POM
Azithromycin POM but if for the treatment of confirmed aysmptomatic
Chlamydia trachomatis genital infection in individuals aged 16 years and
over, and for the epidemiological
treatment of their sexual partners, 1g
(MD), 1g (MDD) in a maximum pack
size of 1g, P
Azlocillin sodium POM
Azopt eye-drops POM
Aztreonam POM

B

Baby Meltus cough syrup GSL
Babyhaler GSL
Bacampicillin hydrochloride POM
Bach flower remedies GSL
Bach rescue cream GSL
Bach rescue remedy GSL
Bach spray GSL
Bacillus Calmette-Guerin vaccine POM
Bacillus Calmette-Guerin Vaccine,
Isoniazid-Resistant POM
Bacillus Calmette-Guerin Vaccine,
Percutaneous POM
Bacitracin POM
Bacitracin methylene disalicylate POM
Bacitracin zinc POM
Baclofen POM
Baclospas tablets POM
Bacticlor MR POM
Bactigras P
Bactroban cream POM
Bactroban nasal POM
Bactroban ointment POM
Balance Active RX vaginal gel POM
Balanced Salt Solution POM
Balgifen tablets POM
Balm GSL
Balm of Gilead GSL
Balmosa cream GSL
Balneum preparations GSL
Balneum Plus preparations GSL
Balsalazide capsules POM
Balto foot balm GSL
Bambec tablets POM
Bambuterol hydrochloride POM
Bansor mouth antiseptic GSL
Baraclude POM
Baratol tablets POM
Barberry Bark GSL
Barbitone CD No Register POM
Barbitone sodium CD No Register POM
Baritop 100 P
Baritop Plus powder P
Barium carbonate POM
Barium chloride POM
Barium sulphide POM
Basiliximab injection (powder for recon-
stitution) POM
Baxan preparations POM
Bay oil, external use only GSL
Bayberry GSL
Baycaron tablets POM
Bazetham MR capsules POM
Bazuka gel P
Becaplermin POM

Beclamide POM
Beclazone Easi-Breathe POM
Beclazone inhaler POM
Beclo-Aqua nasal spray POM
Becloforte Diskhaler POM
Becloforte Easi-Breathe POM
Becloforte inhaler POM
Becloforte Integra Inhaler POM
Beclometasone/Beclomethasone POM
Beclometasone/Beclomethasone dipropionate POM but if for nasal administration (non-aerosol), for the preven-
tion and treatment of allergic rhinitis
in persons aged 18 years and over,
100mcg per nostril (MD) 200mcg per
nostril (MDD) for a maximum period
of 3 months and container or pack-
age contains not more than
20,000mcg of beclometasone dipropi-
onate, please refer to proprietary
names for classification granted
under the marketing authorisation
(see Beconase products)
Beclomethasone see Beclometasone
Beclomist nasal spray P
Becodisks POM
Beconase Allergy nasal spray P
Beconase Hayfever nasal spray GSL
Beconase nasal spray (aqueous) POM
Becotide 50, 100, 200 inhaler POM
Becotide Easi-Breathe POM
Becotide Rotacaps POM
Bedol tablets POM
Bedranol SR capsules POM
Beechams All-in-One GSL
Beechams cold & flu GSL
Beechams decongestant plus with parac-
etamol capsules GSL
Beechams Flu Plus caplets pack sizes 16s
GSL; 24s P
Beechams Flu-Plus sachets GSL
Beechams for Natural Defence zinc and
vitamin C tablets GSL
Beechams hydrocortisone ointment (PL
0079/0203) P
Beechams powders capsules GSL
Beechams powders pack sizes 10s GSL;
20s P
Beechams sore throat relief max strength
lozenges GSL
Beechams Tablets lemon GSL
Beechams Throat-Plus lozenges GSL
Beeswax GSL
Begrivac vaccine POM
Belladonna herb POM but if internal
and 1 mg of the alkaloids (MDD), or
external, P
Belladonna root POM but if internal and
1 mg of the alkaloids (MDD), or
external, P
Bemegride POM
Bemegride sodium POM
Bemiparin POM
Benactyzine hydrochloride POM
Benadryl Allergy Relief capsules 12s P;
12s GSL; 24s P
Benadryl allergy relief solution 70ml
GSL; 100ml P
Benadryl for Children Allergy Solution
GSL
Benadryl cream and lotion P
Benadryl One A Day tablets GSL
Benadryl Plus capsules P
Benadryl Skin Allergy Relief preparations
P
Benapryzine hydrochloride POM
Bencard skin testing solutions POM
Bendrofluazide see Bendroflumethiazide
Bendroflumethiazide/Bendrofluazide
POM
Benefix recombinant factor IX POM
Benemid tablets POM
Benerva tablets GSL
Benethamine Penicillin POM
Benoral granules P
Benoral suspension P
Benoral tablets P
Benoxaprofen POM

Benoxyl 10 lotion P
Benoxyl 5 cream P
Benoxyl 5 lotion P
Benperidol POM
Benquil POM
Benserazide hydrochloride POM
Bentiromide POM
Benuryl POM
Benylin 4-Flu liquid and tablets P
Benylin Active Response oral solution
GSL
Benylin Day and Night cold treatment P
Benylin chesty cough (drowsy) P
Benylin for Chesty Coughs (non-drowsy
formulation) 125ml, 300ml GSL
Benylin childrens chesty cough GSL
Benylin childrens chesty cough sachets
GSL
Benylin for Children's Coughs and Colds
P
Benylin childrens dry cough P
Benylin for Children's Night Coughs P
Benylin childrens tickly cough GSL
Benylin cold & flu max strength cap-
sules GSL
Benylin cold & flu max strength hot
drink sachets GSL
Benylin cough and congestion P
Benylin dry cough (drowsy and non-
drowsy) P
Benylin Fortified linctus P
Benylin Mentholated linctus P
Benylin Paediatric P
Benylin sachets GSL
Benylin Sore Throat lozenges GSL
Benylin tickly cough (non-drowsy) GSL
Benylin with codeine CD Inv P
Benzalkonium chloride, if external use,
or internal (pastilles, lozenges, throat
tablets) max strength 600mcg GSL
Benzamycin gel POM
Benzathine penicillin POM
Benzatropine/Benztropine mesylate POM
Benzbromarone POM
Benzethidine; its salts CD POM
Benzethonium chloride, external use
only GSL
Benzfetamine/Benzphetamine; its salts
CD No Register POM
Benzhexol see Trihexyphenidyl
Benzilonium bromide POM
Benzocaine POM but any use except
ophthalmic use P, except preparations with maximum strength 3% for
use in adults and in children aged 12
years and over GSL; in spray form for
use in adults and children aged 2
years and over with maximum
strength 1% and maximum pack size
22g of product GSL; as a dental gel
for the temporary relief of toothache
pain associated with open carious
lesions and for use in adults and children aged 12 years and over with a
maximum strength of 10% and maximum pack size 5.3g of product GSL;
benzocaine throat spray delivering
1mg per spray for the symptomatic
relief of sore throat pain in adults
and children aged 6 years and over,
maximum dose 3mg, maximum daily
dose 24mg, maximum pack size
106.5mg of benzocaine GSL; in combination with mepyramine maleate,
for the treatment of insect bites and
stings, nettle stings and jellyfish
stings in adults and children aged 2
years and over, maximum pack size
22g of the product GSL, please refer
to proprietary names for the classification granted under the marketing
authorisation (See Waspeze preparations and Orajel Dental Gel)
Benzocaine 10% mouth gel for temporary relief from the pain and tender-
ness associated with mouth ulcers
and from wearing dentures GSL
Benzoctamine hydrochloride POM

Benzoic acid, if internal maximum strength 0.2 per cent or external maximum strength 5.0 per cent GSL

Benzoin Tincture, Compound BP, if external use or internal (pastilles maximum strength 0.8 per cent or vapour inhalations) GSL

Benzoyl peroxide POM but if external maximum strength 10.0 per cent P; or for the treatment of spots or pimples on the face maximum strength 2.5 per cent GSL

N-Benzoyl sulphanilamide POM

Benzphetamine see Benzfetamine

Benzquinamide POM

Benzquinamide hydrochloride POM

Benzthiazide POM

Benztropine see Benzatropine

Benzydamine P

Benzyl alcohol, if external use or internal (pastilles, lozenges, throat tablets maximum strength 4mg) GSL

Benzyl benzoate, external use only GSL

Benzyl cinnamate, external use only GSL

Benzyl nicotinate, external use only GSL

Benzylmorphine (3-benzylmorphine) CD POM

Benzylpenicillin calcium POM

Benzylpenicillin potassium POM

Benzylpenicillin sodium POM

1-Benzylpiperazinene or any compound (not being a compound for the time being specified in Schedule 4) structurally derived from 1-benzylpiperazine by modification in any of the following ways - (i) by substitution at the second nitrogen atom of the piperazine ring with alkyl, benzyl, haloalkyl or phenyl groups; (ii) by substitution in the aromatic ring to any extent with alkyl, alkoxy, alkylenedioxy, halide or haloalkyl groups CD Lic

Bepro Cough syrup CD Inv P

Beractant POM

Beractant suspension POM

Berberis P but if equivalent to 500mcg berberine (MD) (Bitter, Stomachic), GSL

Berkatens tablets POM

Berkmycen preparations POM

Berkolol tablets POM

Berkozide tablets POM

Berocca Vit B effervescent tablets GSL

Berotec inhaler POM

Beta-Adalat capsules POM

Beta-aminoisopropylbenzene see Amfetamine

Beta-Cardone preparations POM

Beta-Prograne capsules POM

Betacap scalp application POM

Betacarotene, up to 6mg (MD) GSL

Betacetylmethadol; its salts CD POM

Betadine alcoholic solution P

Betadine antiseptic paint GSL

Betadine cream P

Betadine dry powder spray GSL

Betadine gargle and mouthwash P

Betadine ointment GSL

Betadine scalp and skin cleanser GSL

Betadine shampoo GSL

Betadine skin cleanser GSL

Betadine spare parts pump dispenser GSL

Betadine Standardised antiseptic Solution P

Betadine surgical scrub P

Betadine vaginal gel P

Betadine vaginal pessaries P

Betadine VC Kit P

Betaferon injection POM

Betagan POM

Betahistine hydrochloride POM

Betaine Hcl P

Betaloc injection POM

Betaloc SA tablets POM

Betaloc tablets POM

Betameprodine; its salts CD POM

Betamethadol; its salts, esters and ethers CD POM

Betamethasone POM

Betamethasone adamantoate POM

Betamethasone benzoate POM

Betamethasone dipropionate POM

Betamethasone sodium phosphate POM

Betamethasone valerate POM

Betaprodine CD POM

Betaxolol hydrochloride POM

Bethanechol chloride POM

Bethanidine sulphate POM

Betim tablets POM

Betinex tablets POM

Betnelan tablets POM

Betnesol preparations POM

Betnesol-N eye, ear and nose drops POM

Betnovate preparations POM

Betnovate RD preparations POM

Betnovate-C preparations POM

Betnovate-N preparations POM

Betoptic eye drops POM

Bettamousse POM

Bevacizumab POM

Bexarotene POM

Bextra tablets POM

Bezafibrate POM

Bezalip tablets POM

Bezalip-Mono tablets POM

Bezitramide; its salts CD POM

Bicalutamide tablets POM

Bi-Carzem SR POM

Bi-Carzem XL POM

Bicillin injection POM

BiCNU injection POM

Bifonazole P but if for external use for the treatment of athlete's foot, in a cream with a maximum strength of 1 per cent and a maximum pack size of 30g of product, GSL

Bimatoprost POM

Binocrit prefilled syringes POM

Binovum tablets POM

Biolax tablets pack sizes 10s GSL; 30s P

Biolon syringe P

Bioplex granules for mouthwash POM

Bioral gel P

Biorphen oral solution POM

Biostrath elixir GSL

Bio-strath natural herb remedies GSL

Biotene dry mouth sensitive toothpaste GSL

Biotene oralbalance dry mouth moisturising liquid GSL

Biotin GSL

Biovital liquid P

Biovital tablets P

Biperiden hydrochloride POM

Biperiden lactate POM

Bipranix POM

Bisacodyl, if internal tablets (other than for use by children under 10 years of age) with a maximum strength of 5mg, 10mg (MD), not more than 40 tablets GSL

Bismuth aluminate, up to 6mg (MD), calculated as bismuth oxide GSL

Bismuth carbonate GSL

Bismuth citrate GSL

Bismuth glycollylarsanilate POM

Bismuth oxide GSL

Bismuth subgallate, external use only GSL

Bismuth subnitrate GSL

Bisodol Extra GSL

Bisodol Heartburn GSL

Bisodol tablets and powders GSL

Bisodol tablets extra strong mint GSL

Bisodol tablets flip top GSL

Bisodol wind relief tablets GSL

Bisoprolol fumarate POM

Bitrex GSL

Bivalirudin POM

Black Bryony, external use only GSL

Black Catechu GSL

Black Currant GSL

Black Haw GSL

Black Root GSL

Blackberry GSL

Bladderwrack (Fucus) GSL

Blemix tablets POM

Bleo-Kyowa POM

Bleomycin POM

Bleomycin sulphate POM

Blistex relief cream GSL

Blisteze cream GSL

Blocadren tablets POM

Blue Cohosh (Caulophyllum), up to 265mg (MD) GSL

Blue Flag, up to 600mg (MD) GSL

Bocasan P

Bolandiol CD Anab POM

Bolasterone CD Anab POM

Bolazine CD Anab POM

Boldenone CD Anab POM

Boldione CD Anab POM

Boldo, up to 1.5g (MD) GSL

Bolenol CD Anab POM

Bolmantalate CD Anab POM

Bondronat preparations POM

Bonefos preparations POM

Boneset (Eupatorium perfoliatum) GSL

Bonjela gel GSL

Bonviva solution for injection POM

Bonviva tablets POM

Borax (sodium borate), if maximum strength 5.0% in all preparations except ophthalmic lotions; or maximum strength 0.7% in ophthalmic lotions (external use only) GSL

Boric acid, maximum strength 2.5% (external use only) GSL

Bornyl acetate, external use only GSL

Bortezomib POM

Bosentan POM

Botox injection POM

Botox powder for solution for injection POM

Botulinium A toxin-Haemagglutinin complex injection POM

Botulinum B toxin POM

Botulism antitoxin POM

Bradosol lozenges GSL

Bradosol Plus lozenges P

Braggs Charcoal tablets GSL

Bran GSL

Brasivol 1 Fine GSL

Brasivol 2 Medium GSL

Bretylate injection POM

Bretylium tosylate POM

Brevibloc POM

Brevinor tablets POM

Brevoxyl cream P

Brexidol tablets POM

Bricanyl preparations POM

Bricanyl SA tablets POM

Bridion POM

Brietal sodium injections POM

Brimonidine tartrate POM

Brinzolamide POM

Britaject pens POM

Britaject preparations POM

BritLofex POM

Brochlor P

Broflex syrup POM

Brolene eye drops P

Brolene eye ointment P

Bromazepam CD Benz POM

Bromhexine hydrochloride POM

Bromocriptine mesylate POM

4-Bromo-2,5-dimethoxy-a-methylphenethylamine CD Lic

Bromperidol POM

Bromvaletone POM

Bronalin Decongestant P

Bronalin Dry Cough P

Bronalin Expectorant P

Bronalin Junior P

Bronchodil POM

Brotizolam CD Benz POM

Brovon asthma inhalant POM

Brufen preparations POM

Brufen Retard POM

Bruiseze P

Brulidine cream GSL

Buccastem M tablets P

Buccastem tablets POM

Buchu GSL

Buckthorn GSL

Budenofalk capsules POM

Budesonide POM but for nasal administration, for the prevention or treatment of seasonal allergic rhinitis in persons aged 18 years and over as a non-aerosol, aqueous form, 200mcg per nostril (MD) 200mcg per nostril (MDD), for a maximum period of 3 months and container or package contains not more than 10mg of budesonide, P

Budoneside Easyhaler POM

Bufexamac POM

Bufotenine; its salts, esters and ethers CD Lic

Bugleweed GSL

Bumetanide POM

Buphenine hydrochloride POM but if 6mg (MD) 18mg (MDD), P

Bupivacaine POM but any use except ophthalmic use P

Bupivacaine hydrochloride POM but any use except ophthalmic use, P

Buprenorphine CD No Register POM

Bupropion POM

Burgundy Pitch, external use only GSL

Burinex A tablets POM

Burinex K tablets POM

Burinex preparations POM

Burneze P

Buscopan ampoules POM

Buscopan Cramps tablets P

Buscopan IBS Relief GSL

Buscopan tablets, pack sizes 56s POM

Buserelin acetate POM

Buserelin nasal spray POM

Busilvex concentrate for solution for infusion POM

Buspar tablets POM

Buspirone hydrochloride POM

Busulfan/busulphan POM

Busulphan see Busulfan

Butacaine sulphate POM but any use except ophthalmic use, P

Butacote tablets POM

Butalbital CD No Register POM

Butobarbital/Butobarbitone CD No Register POM

Butobarbital/Butobarbitone sodium CD No Register POM

Butobarbitone see Butobarbital

Butorphanol tartrate POM

BuTrans CD No Reg POM

Butriptyline hydrochloride POM

Buttercup infant cough syrup GSL

Buttercup medicated sweets GSL

Buttercup syrup GSL

Butternut (White Walnut) GSL

Byetta POM

C

C-View GSL

Cabaser tablets POM

Cabdrivers Adult cough linctus P

Cabergoline POM

Cacit D3 granules P

Cacit tablets P

Cade oil, external use only GSL

Caelyx for infusion POM

Cafergot suppositories POM

Cafergot tablets POM

Caffeine GSL

Caffeine citrate GSL

Caffeine injection POM

Cajuput oil GSL

Calaband GSL

Calabren tablets POM

Caladryl cream P

Caladryl lotion P

Calamine, external use only GSL

Calamus (Sweet Flag) GSL

Calanif capsules POM

Calazem tablets POM

Calceos tablets P

Calchan MR POM
Calcicard CR tablets POM
Calcichew Forte tablets P
Calcichew tablets P
Calcichew-D3 Forte tablets P
Calcichew-D3 tablets P
Calcidrink sachets P
Calciferol injection POM
Calciferol tablets P
Calcijex injection POM
Calcimax syrup P
Calciparine injection POM
Calci-plus GSL
Calcipotriol POM
Calcisorb P
Calcitare POM
Calcitonin POM
Calcitonin (salmon)/Salcatonin POM
Calcitonin (salmon)/Salcatonin acetate
    POM
Calcitriol POM
Calcium alginate, external use only GSL
Calcium amphomycin POM
Calcium ascorbate GSL
Calcium benzamidosalicylate POM
Calcium bromide POM
Calcium bromidolactobionate POM
Calcium carbimide POM
Calcium carbonate GSL
Calcium chloride GSL
Calcium chloride injection POM
Calcium folinate POM
Calcium gluconate GSL
Calcium gluconate injection POM
Calcium glycerophosphate GSL
Calcium heptagluconate GSL
Calcium hydrogen phosphate GSL
Calcium lactate GSL
Calcium leucovorin preparations POM
Calcium metrizoate POM
Calcium pantothenate GSL
Calcium phosphate GSL
Calcium resonium P
Calcium sulphaloxate POM
Calcium undecylenate, external use only
    GSL
Calcium with vitamin D tablets BPC P
Calcium-Sandoz syrup P
Calcort tablets POM
Calendula (Marigold), external use only
    GSL
Calfovit D3 POM
Calgel GSL
Califig GSL
Califig, Junior GSL
Calimal P
Callanish Nutritional preparations GSL
Calmurid cream P
Calmurid HC cream POM
Calpol Fast melts 6+ tablets 12 GSL; 24 P
Calpol infant sachets sugar-free GSL
Calpol Infant suspension 70ml P; 100ml
    GSL; 140ml P; 200ml P
Calpol infant suspension sugar-free
    100ml GSL; 140ml P; 200ml P
Calpol Paediatric suspension P
Calpol sachets GSL
Calpol 6+ sugar-free sachets GSL
Calpol Six Plus suspension P
Calprofen paediatric suspension POM
Calprofen sachets GSL
Calprofen suspension 100ml P; 100ml
    GSL
Calsalettes P
Calsynar POM
Caltrate tablets GSL
Calumba GSL
Calusterone CD Anab POM
CAM P
Camazepam CD Benz POM
Camcolit tablets POM
Camphor oil, external use only GSL
Camphor up to 20mg (MD), 50mg
    (MDD) GSL
Camphorated opium tincture BP CD Inv
    POM
Campral EC tablets POM
Campto infusion POM

Cancidas POM
Candesartan cilexitil POM
Candicidin POM
Candida Yeast Extract GSL
Candiden preparations P
Canesten 1 vaginal Tablet P
Canesten 10% VC POM
Canesten 2% vaginal cream POM
Canesten AF GSL
Canesten AF Once Daily P
Canesten Cream Combi GSL
Canesten Combi GSL and POM
Canesten Complete P
Canesten cream P
Canesten dermatological spray P
Canesten Duo P
Canesten Duopack POM
Canesten HC cream 30g POM
Canesten hydrocortisone 15g P
Canesten Internal P
Canesten Oasis GSL
Canesten Once P
Canesten Oral P
Canesten pessary 500mg P and POM
Canesten powder P
Canesten solution P
Canesten thrush cream P
Canesten vaginal cream P
Canesten vaginal tablets P
Cannabinol CD Lic
Cannabinol derivatives not being dron-
    abinol or its stereoisomers CD Lic
Cannabis and cannabis resin CD Lic
Canrenoic Acid POM
Cantharidin POM but if external maxi-
    mum strength 0.01 per cent, P
Canusal injection POM
Capasal P
Capastat injection POM
Capecitabine POM
Caplenal tablets POM
Capoten tablets POM
Capozide LS tablets POM
Capozide tablets POM
Capreomycin sulphate POM
Caprin 75mg tablets P
Caprin 300mg tablets POM
Capsaicin POM
Capsicum GSL
Capsicum oleoresin (water soluble),
    external use only GSL
Capsicum oleoresin BPC 1923 GSL
Capsicum oleoresin BPC 1973, if inter-
    nal 1.2mg (MD) and 1.8mg (MDD) or
    external maximum strength 2.5 GSL
Capsicum oleoresin, external use only
    GSL
Capsuvac capsules POM
Capto-co POM
Captopril POM
Carace 10 Plus tablets POM
Carace 20 Plus tablets POM
Carace tablets POM
Caralpha tablets POM
Caramet CR POM
Caraway GSL
Caraway oil GSL
Carbachol POM
Carbadox POM
Carbagen CR tablets POM
Carbaglu POM
Carbalax suppositories GSL
Carbamazepine POM
Carbaryl POM
Carbasalate calcium POM
Carbellon tablets P
Carbenicillin sodium POM
Carbenoxolone sodium POM but if (1)
    Pellet 5mg (MD) 25mg (MDD); (2)
    Gel maximum strength 2.0 per cent;
    (3) Granules for mouthwash in adults
    and children not less than 12 years,
    20mg (MD) 80mg (MDD) and maxi-
    mum strength 1.0 percent and con-
    tainer or package containing not
    more than 560mg of carbenoxolone
    sodium, P
Carbetocin POM

Carbex P
Carbidopa POM
Carbidopa monohydrate POM
Carbimazole POM
Carbo-Cort cream POM
Carbo-Dome cream GSL
Carbocisteine POM
Carbomix P
Carbon Black GSL
Carbon tetrachloride POM
Carboplatin POM
Carboprost Trometamol POM
Carbromal POM
Carbuterol hydrochloride POM
Cardamom GSL
Cardamom Oil GSL
Cardene capsules POM
Cardene SR capsules POM
Cardicor tablets POM
Cardilate MR tablets POM
Cardinol tablets POM
Cardioplen XL tablets POM
Cardura tablets POM
Cardura XL tablets POM
Care ammonia & ipecacuanha mixture
    GSL
Care antiseptic first aid cream GSL
Care antiseptic mouthwash GSL
Care aqueous cream GSL
Care arnica tincture GSL
Care aspirin dispersible 75mg P
Care calamine aqueous cream GSL
Care calamine lotion GSL
Care castor oil GSL
Care Cetirizine Hayfever Relief tablets P
Care chlorhexidine antiseptic mouth-
    wash GSL
Care clotrimazole cream P
Care clove oil GSL
Care codeine oral solution CD Inv P
Care codeine linctus CD Inv P
Care Cystitis Relief Sachets GSL
Care ephedrine nasal drops P
Care epsom salts GSL
Care eucalyptus oil GSL
Care flu-strength liquid all-in-one P
Care fluconazole capsules P
Care friars balsam GSL
Care fullers earth cream GSL
Care gees linctus CD Inv P
Care glycerin GSL
Care glycerin suppositories GSL
Care glycerin, lemon & honey GSL
Care glycerin, lemon, honey &
    ipecacuanha GSL
Care haemorrhoid relief ointment GSL
Care hay fever relief nasal spray P
Care Heartburn & Indigestion liquid PO
Care Heartburn Relief tablets P
Care hydrogen peroxide GSL
Care ibuprofen gel 5% GSL
Care ibuprofen gel 10% P
Care ibuprofen suspension P
Care ibuprofen tablets P
Care indian brandee GSL
Care iodine tincture GSL
Care ipecacuanha & morphine mixture
    CD Inv P
Care kaolin & morphine mixture CD Inv
    P
Care kaolin mixture GSL
Care kaolin paediatric mixture GSL
Care loperamide capsules GSL
Care magnesium sulphate paste GSL
Care magnesium trisilicate mixture GSL
Care menthol & eucalyptus inhalation
    GSL
Care paracetamol junior suspension P
Care paraffin liquid P
Care pholcodine oral solution sugar-free
    CD Inv P
Care pholcodine linctus CD Inv P
Care potassium citrate mixture P
Care senna tablets GSL
Care simple linctus GSL
Care simple paediatric linctus GSL
Care sleep aid tablets P
Care sodium bicarbonate GSL

Care surgical spirit GSL
Care terpin with codeine linctus CD Inv P
Care white embrocation GSL
Care witch hazel GSL
Care zinc & castor oil cream GSL
Careline products GSL
Carfecillin sodium POM
Carfentanil; its stereoisomers, salts,
    esters and ethers CD POM
Carglumic acid POM
Carindacillin sodium POM
Carisoma tablets POM
Carisoprodol POM
Carmellose sodium GSL
Carmil XL P
Carmustine POM
Carnation Callous caps GSL
Carnation Corn caps GSL
Carnation Verruca treatment GSL
Carnitine POM
Carnitor preparations POM
Carperidine POM
Carrot GSL
Carteolol hydrochloride POM
Carvedilol POM
Carylderm lotion POM
Carylderm shampoo POM
Cascara GSL
Cascor POM
Casodex tablets POM
Caspofungin infusion POM
Cassia Oil GSL
Castor Oil GSL
Catapres preparations POM
Catarrh-Eeze tablets GSL
Catechu GSL
Cathine its salts, stereoisomers (other
    than phenylpropanolamine), their
    salts CD No Register POM
Cathinone; its salts, stereoisomers, esters
    and ethers CD Lic
Caverject injection POM
Cayston POM
CCNU POM
Ceanel concentrate P
Cedar wood oil, external use only GSL
Cedax capsules POM
Cedax suspension POM
Cedocard Retard tablets POM
Cefaclor POM
Cefaclor MR tablets POM
Cefadroxil POM
Cefalexin/Cephalexin POM
Cefalexin/Cephalexin sodium POM
Cefamandole nafate/Cephamandole
    nafate POM
Cefazedone sodium POM
Cefazolin/Cephazolin sodium POM
Cefdinir POM
Cefixime POM
Cefizox injection POM
Cefodizime sodium POM
Cefotaxime sodium POM
Cefoxitin sodium POM
Cefpirome POM
Cefpodoxime proxetil POM
Cefprozil POM
Cefradine/Cephradine POM
Cefrom vials POM
Cefsulodin sodium POM
Ceftazidime POM
Ceftizoxime sodium POM
Ceftriaxone sodium POM
Cefuroxime axetil POM
Cefuroxime sodium POM
Cefzil preparations POM
Celance tablets POM
Celebrex capsules POM
Celecoxib POM
Celectol tablets POM
Celery oil GSL
Celery seed GSL
Celevac tablets GSL
Celiprolol hydrochloride POM
Cellcept capsules POM
Cellcept powder for infusion POM
Cellcept powder for oral suspension
    POM

Cellcept tablets POM
Cellulose GSL
Celluvisc P
Centaury GSL
Centella, external use only GSL
Centrapryl tablets POM
Centyl K tablets POM
Cephalexin see Cefalexin
Cephaloridine POM
Cephalothin sodium POM
Cephamandole nafate
    see Cefamandole nafate
Cephazolin see Cefazolin
Cephradine see Cefradine
Ceplac GSL
Ceporex preparations POM
Ceprotin injection POM
Cepton Medicated cleansing lotion GSL
Cepton Medicated skinwash GSL
Cerazette POM
Cerebrovase tablets POM
Ceredase Concentrate POM
Cerezyme powder for reconstitution
    POM
Cerium oxalate POM
Cerivastatin POM
Cerivastatin sodium POM
Cernevit POM
Cerubidin powder for reconstitution
    POM
Ceruletide diethylamine POM
Cerumol ear drops P
Cetalkonium chloride, if external use or
    internal (teething gel maximum
    strength 0.01 per cent) GSL
Cetanorm cream GSL
Cetavlex cream GSL
Cetec GSL
Cetirizine hydrochloride POM but if
    10mg (MDD) P; or if maximum
    strength 10mg, in tablet form for the
    symptomatic relief of perennial rhini-
    tis, seasonal allergic rhinitis and idio-
    pathic chronic urticaria in adults and
    children aged 6 years and over, 10mg
    (MDD), in an individual container or
    package containing not more than 14
    tablets, GSL. If liquid preparations
    with a maximum strength of 1mg/ml
    for the symptomatic relief of perenni-
    al rhinitis, seasonal allergic rhinitis
    and idiopathic chronic urticaria in
    adults and children aged 6 years and
    over with a maximum pack size of no
    more than 70ml, GSL. Please refer to
    the proprietary names for classifica-
    tion granted under the marketing
    authorisation (see Galpharm Hayfever
    and Allergy Relief syrup)
Cetomacrogol, external use only GSL
Cetostearyl alcohol, external use only
    GSL
Cetraben Emollient bath additive GSL
Cetraben Emollient cream GSL
Cetrimide, external use only GSL
Cetrorelix POM
Cetrotide injection POM
Cetuximab POM
Cetylpyridinium chloride, all prepara-
    tions other than liquid preparations
    for oral administration 3mg (MD)
    and liquid preparations for oral
    administration 5mg (MD) GSL
Chalk GSL
Chamomile GSL
Chamomile oil, external use only GSL
Champix POM
Charas see Cannabis
Charcoal tabs GSL
Charcoal, medicinal GSL
Charcodote suspension P
Check-Mate pregnancy testing strips GSL
Chemotrim preparations POM
Chemydur 60XL tablets POM
Chenodeoxycholic acid POM
Chickenpox vaccine POM
Chickweed GSL
Chimax tablets POM

Chirocaine POM
Chloractil tablets POM
Chloral betaine see Cloral betaine
Chloral hydrate POM but if external, P
Chlorambucil POM
Chloramphenicol POM
Chloramphenicol cinnamate POM
Chloramphenicol ear drops POM
Chloramphenical eye drops POM, but
    containing 0.5% chloramphenicol,
    for the treatment of acute bacterial
    conjunctivitis in adults and children
    aged 2 years and over, maximum
    length of treatment 5 days, and pack
    size 10ml; Please refer to proprietary
    names for the classification granted
    under the marketing authorisation
Chloramphenicol eye/ear ointment POM
Chloramphenicol 1% eye ointment
    POM, but containing 1% chloram-
    phenicol, for the treatment of acute
    bacterial conjunctivitis in adults and
    children aged 2 years and over, maxi-
    mum length of treatment 5 days, and
    pack size 4g; please refer to propri-
    etary names for the classification
    granted under the marketing authori-
    sation
Chloramphenicol palmitate POM
Chloramphenicol sodium succinate
    POM
Chlorbutol see Chlorobutanol
Chlordiazepoxide CD Benz POM
Chlorhexadol POM
Chlorhexidine acetate, external use only
    GSL
Chlorhexidine gluconate, external use
    only GSL
Chlorhexidine hydrochloride, if external
    use or internal (pastilles, lozenges,
    throat tablets maximum strength
    5mg) GSL
Chlormadinone acetate POM
Chlormerodrin POM
Chlormethiazole see Clomethiazole
Chlormethine/Mustine hydrochloride
    POM
Chlormezanone POM
Chlorobutanol/chlorbutol, if internal
    (solid preparations 150mg (MD) or liq-
    uid preparations maximum strength
    0.5 per cent), or external (except
    toothache gel) maximum strength 2.5
    per cent, or external (toothache gel)
    maximum strength 7.0 per cent GSL
Chlorocresol, if maximum strength 0.2
    per cent (external use only) GSL
Chlorodyne BPC CD Inv POM
Chloroform POM but if (1) internal
    maximum strength 5.0 per cent, P;
    (2) internal maximum strength 0.5
    per cent, GSL, (3) external GSL
4-Chloromethandienone CD Anab POM
Chloromycetin preparations POM
Chlorophene, if maximum strength 1.25
    per cent (external use only) GSL
Chlorophenols, if internal maximum
    strength 1mg or external maximum
    strength 0.6 per cent GSL
1-(3-chlorophenyl)-4-(3-
    chloropropyl)piperazine CD Benz
    POM
1-(3-chlorophenyl)piperazine CD Benz
    POM
Chloroquine phosphate POM but for
    prophylaxis of malaria, P
Chloroquine sulphate POM but for pro-
    phylaxis of malaria, P
Chlorothiazide POM
Chlorotrianisene POM
Chloroxylenol, if internal maximum
    strength 0.5 per cent or external max-
    imum strength 5.0 per cent GSL
Chlorphenamine/Chlorpheniramine P
Chlorphenesin, external use only GSL
Chlorpheniramine see Chlorphenamine
Chlorphenoxamine hydrochloride POM
Chlorphentermine; its salts CD No

Register POM
Chlorpromazine POM
Chlorpromazine embonate POM
Chlorpromazine hydrochloride POM
Chlorpropamide POM
Chlorprothixene POM
Chlorprothixene hydrochloride POM
Chlortalidone/Chlorthalidone POM
Chlortetracycline POM
Chlortetracycline calcium POM
Chlortetracycline hydrochloride POM
Chlorthalidone see Chlortalidone
Chlorzoxazone POM
Cholera vaccine POM
Cholestyramine see Colestyramine
Choline salicylate, if external use or
    internal (teething gel maximum
    strength 9.0 per cent) GSL
Chondrus GSL
Choragon injection CD Anab POM
Chorionic Gonadotrophin (HCG) CD
    Anab POM
Christy caplets P
Chymol emollient balm GSL
Cialis tablets POM
Cialis Once-A-Day tablets POM
Cibral tablets POM
Cibral XL tablets POM
Cicafem POM
Cicatrin preparations POM
Ciclacillin POM
Ciclesonide POM
Ciclobendazole POM
Ciclosporin/Cyclosporin POM
Cidofovir POM
Cidomycin preparations POM
Cilastatin sodium POM
Cilazapril POM
Cilest POM
Cilostazol POM
Ciloxan eye drops POM
Cimetidine POM but if (1) For the
    short-term symptomatic relief of
    heartburn, dyspepsia, indigestion,
    acid indigestion and hyperacidity
    and for the prophylaxis of meal-
    induced heartburn 200mg (MD)
    800mg (MDD) for a maximum period
    of 14 days; or (2) For the prophylac-
    tic management of nocturnal heart-
    burn by a single dose taken at night
    100mg (MD) to be taken as a single
    dose at night, for a maximum period
    of 14 days, P
Cimetidine hydrochloride POM
Cimicifuga (Black Cohosh), up to 200mg
    (MD) GSL
Cimzia solution for injection in prefilled
    syringe POM
Cinacalcet POM
Cinaziere 15 tablets P
Cinchocaine POM but if non-oph-
    thalmic use maximum strength 3.0
    per cent, P
Cinchocaine hydrochloride POM but if
    non-ophthalmic use maximum
    strength equivalent of 3.0 per cent of
    cinchocaine, P
Cinchophen POM
Cinnamic acid, if external use or inter-
    nal (pastilles, lozenges, throat tablets
    maximum strength 500 GSL
Cinnamon GSL
Cinnamon oil GSL
Cinnarizine P
Cinobac capsules POM
Cinoxacin POM
Cipralex oral drops POM
Cipralex tablets POM
Cipramil preparations POM
Ciprofibrate POM
Ciprofloxacin POM
Ciprofloxacin hydrochloride POM
Ciproxin preparations POM
Circadin prolonged-release tablets POM
Cisatracurium besylate POM
Cisapride POM
Cisplatin POM

Citalopram POM
Citanest preparations POM
Citramag P
Citric acid GSL
Citronella oil, external use only GSL
Cladribine POM
Claforan injection POM
Clairette 2000/35 POM
Clarelux cutaneous foam POM
Clariteyes eye drops P
Clarithromycin POM
Clarityn preparations P; except Clarityn
    Allergy tablets pack size 7s GSL
Clarosip POM
Clarosip granules for suspension POM
Clavulanic acid POM
Clear complexion tablets GSL
Clear Ear GSL
Clearasil Max 10 P
Clearsore cream P
Clemastine P
Clenbuterol CD Anab POM
Clenil Modulite POM
Clexane injection POM
Clidinium bromide POM
Climagest POM
Climanor tablets POM
Climaval tablets POM
Climesse tablets POM
Clindamycin POM
Clindamycin hydrochloride POM
Clindamycin palmitate hydrochloride
    POM
Clindamycin phosphate POM
Clinitar preparations P
Clinorette tablets POM
Clinoril tablets POM
Clioquinol POM but if (1) external
    (other than treatment of mouth
    ulcers); (2) treatment of mouth ulcers
    350mg (MDD) and maximum
    strength 35mg, P
Clivarine injection POM
Clivers GSL
Clobazam CD Benz POM
Clobetasol propionate POM
Clobetasone butyrate POM but if cream
    for external use for the short term
    symptomatic treatment and control
    of patches of eczema and dermatitis
    (excluding seborrhoeic dermatitis) in
    adults and children 12 years and
    over, maximum strength 0.05 per
    cent, in a container or packaging
    containing not more than 15g of
    medicinal product P
Clofarabine POM
Clofazimine POM
Clofibrate POM
Clomethiazole/Chlormethiazole POM
Clomethiazole/Chlormethiazole edisy-
    late POM
Clomid tablets POM
Clomifene/Clomiphene citrate POM
Clomiphene see Clomifene
Clomipramine POM
Clomipramine hydrochloride POM
Clomocycline POM
Clomocycline sodium POM
Clonazepam CD Benz POM
Clonidine POM
Clonidine hydrochloride POM
Clonitazene; its salts CD POM
Clopamide POM
Clopenthixol decanoate POM
Clopenthixol hydrochloride POM
Clopidogrel hydrogen sulphate POM
Clopixol Acuphase injection POM
Clopixol injection POM
Clopixol tablets POM
Cloprostenol sodium POM
Cloral betaine/Chloral betaine POM
Clorazepic acid CD Benz POM
Clorexolone POM
Clostebol CD Anab POM
Clostet vaccine POM
Clotam Rapid tablets POM

Clotiazepam CD Benz POM
Clotrimazole POM but if external and in
the case of vaginal use only external
use for the treatment of vaginal candidiasis, P; if in a combination pack
containing a maximum of one
500mg pessary (for the treatment of
candidal vaginitis) and 2% cream
with a maximum of 200mg of clotrimazole per pack (for the treatment of
candidal vulvitis and as an adjunct to
treatment of candidal vaginitis), GSL;
please refer to proprietary names for
classification granted under the marketing authorisation (see Canesten
Combi); if maximum strength 1.0%
for the external treatment of tinea
pedis (athlete's foot) only, powders
for the prevention of, or as an
adjunct to the treatment of tinea
pedis, and all preparations other than
powders, for the treatment of tinea
pedis and tinea cruris, in a pack con-
taining no more than 500mg of
clotrimazole with a maximum
strength 1%, GSL
Clove GSL
Clove Oil GSL
Clover (Red Clover) GSL
Cloxacillin benzathine POM
Cloxacillin sodium POM
Cloxazolam CD Benz POM
Clozapine POM
Clozaril tablets POM
Co-amilofruse POM
Co-amilozide POM
Co-amoxiclav POM
Co-Aprovel tablets POM
Co-beneldopa POM
Co-Betaloc SA tablets POM
Co-Betaloc tablets POM
Co-careldopa POM
Co-codamol 30/500 preparations
CD Inv POM
Co-codamol 8/500 effervescent
CD Inv P
Co-codamol 8/500 pack sizes 32s CD Inv
P; greater than 32s CD Inv POM
Co-codaprin eff CD Inv P
Co-codaprin pack sizes 32s CD Inv P;
sizes greater than 32s CD Inv POM
Co-cyprindiol tablets POM
Co-danthramer POM
Co-danthrusate POM
Co-dergocrine mesylate POM
Co-diovan tablets POM
Co-dydramol CD Inv POM
Co-fluampicil POM
Co-flumactone POM
Co-phenotrope CD Inv POM
Co-prenozide POM
Co-proxamol CD Inv POM
Co-tenidone POM
Co-tetroxazine POM
Co-triamterzide POM
Co-trimoxazole POM
Co-zidacapt POM
Coal tar, external use only GSL
Cobadex cream POM
Cobalin-H injection POM
Cobalt sulphate, if MDD equivalent to
0.25mg elemental cobalt GSL
Coca alkaloids see Cocaine
Coca leaf CD Lic
Cocaine; its salts CD POM
Cocculus Indicus POM
Cocillana GSL
Cocois scalp application GSL
Cod liver oil as for Vitamin A and
Vitamin D GSL
Codafen Continus tablets CD Inv POM
Codalax Forte suspension POM
Codalax suspension POM
Codeine; its salts CD POM but if for
non-parenteral use and (a) in undi-
vided preparations with ms 2.5% (cal-
culated as base) CD Inv POM; or (b)
in single dose preparations with ms

per dosage unit 100mg (calculated as
base) CD Inv POM; or (c) in unit
preparations diluted to at least one
part in a million (6X) in response to a
specific request, CD Inv P; or (d) in
unit preparations diluted to at least
one part in a million million (6C),
CD Inv P
Codipar Caplets CD Inv POM
Codis 500 soluble tablets CD Inv P
Cogentin preparations POM
Colaspase POM
Colazide capsules POM
Colchicine POM
Colestid preparations POM
Colestipol hydrochloride POM
Colestyramine/Cholestyramine POM
Colfosceril palmitate POM
Colgate Chlorohex 1200 oral rinse GSL
Colgate Chlorohex 2000 oral rinse P
Colgate dental cream tartar control 50ml
GSL
Colgate dental cream ultra cavity protec-
tion 25ml GSL
Colgate dental cream ultra cavity protec-
tion 50ml GSL
Colgate Fluorigard alcohol-free daily
rinse GSL
Colgate Fluorigard daily drops P
Colgate Fluorigard daily rinse GSL
Colgate Fluorigard Gelkam gel P
Colgate Fluorigard tablets P
Colgate sensitive products GSL
Colgate Total products GSL
Colgate Total + whitening GSL
Colgate Total fresh stripe GSL
Colgate triple cool stripe gel GSL
Colgate ultra cavity protection GSL
Colifoam aerosol POM
Colistimethate sodium/Colistin
sulphomethate sodium POM
Colistin sulphate POM
Colistin sulphomethate POM
Colistin sulphomethate sodium see
Colistimethate sodium
Collins elixir P
Collis Browne's mixture, J. CD Inv P
Collis Browne's tablets, J. CD Inv P
Colloidal sulphur, external use only GSL
Colofac 100 tablets P
Colofac IBS tablets P
Colofac liquid POM
Colofac MR capsules POM
Colofac tablets POM
Colomycin preparations POM
Colophony, external use only GSL
Colpermin capsules GSL
Colsor cream GSL
Colsor lotion GSL
Combivent aerosol POM
Combigan eye-drops POM
Combivent UDV POM
Combivir tablets POM
Combodart capsules POM
Comfrey root, external use only GSL
Comixco Suspension POM
Competact POM
Compound W P
Comtess tablets POM
Concavit preparations P
Concentrate of poppy-straw CD Lic
Concerta XL tablets CD POM
Concordin tablets POM
Condrotec POM
Condyline liquid POM
Congescor POM
Coniine POM
Conium leaf POM but if external maxi-
mum strength 7.0 per cent, P
Conotrane cream GSL
Conray POM
Contac capsules P
Contiflo XL POM
Contigen POM
Contimin tablets POM
Contraflam capsules POM
Contraflam tablets POM
Convulex capsules POM

Copaxone injection POM
Copegus tablets POM
Copper carbonate, if MDD equivalent to
1mg elemental copper GSL
Copper sulphate, if internal equivalent
to 4mg elemental copper (MDD) or
external maximum strength 1.0 per
cent GSL
Coracten SR capsules POM
Coracten XL capsules POM
Cordarone X preparations POM
Cordilox preparations POM
Corgard tablets POM
Corgaretic tablets POM
Coriander GSL
Coriander oil GSL
Corlan Pellets (PL 0039/0397) P
Coro-Nitro spray P
Coroday MR POM
Corsodyl dental gel P
Corsodyl mouthwash GSL
Corsodyl spray P
Corticotrophin see Corticotropin
Corticotropin/Corticotrophin POM
Cortisone POM
Cortisone acetate POM
Cortisyl tablets POM
Corwin tablets POM
Cosalgesic tablets CD Inv POM
Cosmegen, Lyovac POM
Cosmofer POM
Cosopt eye-drops POM
Cosuric tablets POM
Cough Nurse Night Time liquid P
Coversyl Plus tablets POM
Coversyl tablets POM
Covonia Bronchial balsam original P
Covonia catarrh relief formula GSL
Covonia cold & flu formula P
Covonia menthol cough mixture expec-
torant GSL
Covonia night time formula P
Covonia throat spray P
Covonia vapour drops GSL
Cozaar tablets POM
Cozaar-Comp tablets POM
Crampex tablets P
Cranesbill (Geranium) GSL
Cranesbill tabs GSL
Cremalgin GSL
Creon 10,000 P
Creon 25,000 capsules POM
Creon 40,000 POM
Creon granules P
Creon Micro granules P
Creosote, if internal 0.125ml (MD) or
external maximum strength 0.5 per
cent GSL
Crestor tablets POM
Crinone gel POM
Crisantaspase POM
Crixivan capsules POM
Cromogen preps POM
Cromolux eye drops POM
Cromolux hayfever P
Cropropamide POM
Crotamiton, external use only GSL
Crotethamide POM
Croton oil POM
Croton seed POM
Crystacide cream P
Crystapen injections POM
Cubicin injection POM
Cuplex gel P
Cuprofen preparations P
Curanail nail lacquer P
Curare POM
Curatoderm ointment POM
Curosurf POM
Cutipen GSL
Cutivate cream POM
Cutivate ointment POM
Cuxson Gerrard belladonna plasters BPC
white cloth P
CX powder P
Cyanocobalamin, up to 10mcg (MDD)
GSL
4-Cyano-2-dimethylamino-4,4-

diphenylbutane CD POM
4-Cyano-1-methyl-4-phenylpiperidine
CD POM
Cyclimorph injections CD POM
Cyclizine hydrochloride tablets P
Cyclizine hydrochloride injection POM
Cyclo-Progynova tablets POM
Cyclobarbitone CD No Register POM
Cyclobarbitone calcium CD No Register
POM
Cyclodox Caps POM
Cyclofenil POM
Cyclogest suppositories POM
Cyclomin tabs POM
Cyclopenthiazide POM
Cyclopentolate hydrochloride POM
Cyclophosphamide POM
Cycloserine POM
Cyclosporin see Ciclosporin
Cyclothiazide POM
Cyklokapron preparations POM
Cymalon GSL
Cymbalta capsules POM
Cymevene capsules POM
Cymevene vials POM
Cymex GSL
Cymex Ultra cream GSL
Cypripedium GSL
Cyproheptadine P
Cyprostat tablets POM
Cyproterone acetate POM
Cystagon caps POM
Cystemme cystitis sachets 6 PO
Cystocalm sachets GSL
Cystofem sachets PO
Cystopurin granules GSL
Cystrin tablets POM
Cytacon liquid P
Cytacon tablets P
Cytamen injection POM
Cytarabine POM
Cytarabine hydrochloride POM
Cytosar injection POM
Cytotec tablets POM

D

Dacarbazine POM
Dactinomycin POM
Daclizumab POM
Daktacort cream POM
Daktacort HC cream P
Daktacort ointment POM
Daktarin (Janssen-Cilag) cream 2% P
Daktarin (Janssen-Cilag) oral gel POM
Daktarin cream 2% 15g P
Daktarin dual action cream 2% 15g GSL;
30g GSL
Daktarin dual action powder 2% 20g
GSL
Daktarin spray powder 2% 100g GSL
Daktarin oral gel 15g P
Daktarin powder 2% P
Daktarin Aktiv cream, powder and spray
powder GSL
Daktarin Gold P
Dalacin C preparations POM
Dalacin cream 2% POM
Dalacin T preps POM
Dalfopristin POM
Dalivit drops GSL
Dalmane caps CD Benz POM
Dalteparin sodium POM
Damiana GSL
Danaparoid sodium POM
Danazol CD Anab POM
Dandelion GSL
Dandrazol Antidandruff shampoo P
Dandrazol Dandruff Shampoo GSL
Dandrazol shampoo POM
Danlax syrup POM
Danol capsules POM
Danthron see Dantron
Dantrium preparations POM
Dantrolene sodium POM
Dantron/Danthron POM
Daonil tablets POM
Dapsone POM

Dapsone ethane ortho sulphonate POM
Daptomycin POM
Daraprim tablets POM
Darbopoetin alfa POM
Darifenacin POM
Dasatinib POM
Daunorubicin hydrochloride POM
Daunoxome injection POM
Davenol linctus CD Inv P
Day and Night Nurse capsules P
Day Nurse preparations CD Inv P
Dayleve cream P
DDAVP Melt POM
DDAVP preps POM
DDD preps GSL
De Witts analgesic pills pack sizes 16s GSL; 32s P
De Witts antacid powder GSL
De Witts antacid tablets GSL
De Witts antibiotic throat lozenges P
De Witts Kidney and Bladder pills GSL
De Witts Placidex syrup P
De Witts Secron catarrh syrup for children P
De Witts Secron susp P
De Witts worm syrup P
De-capeptyl SR vial POM
De-Nol P
De-Noltab tablets P
Deanol bitartrate POM but if 26mg (MDD) P
Debrisan P
Debrisoquine sulphate POM
Deca-Durabolin injection CD Anab POM
Decadron preparations POM
Decan POM
Decapeptyl SR injection POM
Decubal cream GSL
Deep Freeze cold gel GSL
Deep Freeze pain relief spray GSL
Deep Heat Liniment, rub, spray GSL
Deep Relief pack sizes 15g GSL; 30g GSL; 50g GSL; 100g P
Defanac POM
Defanac Retard POM
Deferasirox POM
Deferiprone POM
Deflazacort POM
Delfen foam GSL
Delorazepam CD Benz POM
Delta-9-tetrahydrocannabinol see Dronabinol
Deltacortril Enteric tablets POM
Deltacortril Gastro-resistant tablets POM
Deltaprim tablets POM
Deltastab injection POM
Delvas tablets POM
Demecarium bromide POM
Demeclocycline POM
Demeclocycline calcium POM
Demeclocycline hydrochloride POM
Demix caps POM
Demser capsules POM
Dencyl capsules P
Denes medicine products GSL
Denorex shampoo 125ml PO
Denorex shampoo with conditioner 125ml PO
Dentinox Infant Colic drops GSL
Dentinox shampoo GSL
Dentinox teething gel GSL
Dentogen gel GSL
Dentogen liquid GSL
Dentomycin gel POM
Denzapine tablets POM
Deoxycoformycin POM
Deoxycortone acetate POM
Deoxycortone pivalate POM
Depakote tablets POM
Depixol preparations POM
DepoCyte POM
Depodur suspension for injection CD POM
Depo-Medrone injection POM
Depo-Medrone with lidocaine POM
Depo-Provera injections POM
Deponit 10 P
Deponit 5 P

Depostat injection POM
Deptropine citrate POM
Dequa Spray P
Dequacaine lozenges P
Dequadin lozenges P
Dequalinium chloride POM but if (1) internal: throat lozenges or throat pastilles maximum strength 0.25mg, P; (2) external: paint maximum strength 1.0 percent, P; minor infections of the mouth and throat 0.25mg (MD) 2mg (MDD), GSL
Derbac M P
Dermabond GSL
Dermacort hydrocortisone cream (PL 8265/0002) P
Dermalo bath emollient GSL
Dermamist spray P
Dermax shampoo P
Dermestril transdermal patches POM
Dermestril-Septem transdermal patches POM
Dermidex P
Dermol P
Dermol 200 P
Dermol 500 lotion P
Dermol 600 bath emollient P
Dermovate preparations POM
Dermovate-NN skin preparations POM
Deseril tablets POM
Deserpidine POM
Desferal injection POM
Desferrioxamine mesylate POM
Desflurane POM
Desipramine hydrochloride POM
Deslanoside POM
Desloratadine POM
DesmoMelt POM
Desmopressin POM
Desmopressin acetate POM
Desmospray intranasal spray POM
Desmotabs POM
Desogestrel POM
Desomorphine; its salts, esters and ethers CD POM
Desonide POM
Desoximetasone/Desoxymethasone POM
Desoxymethasone see Desoximetasone
Desoxymethyltestosterone CD Anab POM
Destolit tablets POM
Deteclo preparations POM
Detrunorm POM
Detrunorm XL POM
Detrusitol tablets POM
Detrusitol XL capsules POM
Dettol anti-bacterial cleanser GSL
Dettol antiseptic cream GSL
Dettol antiseptic pain relief spray P
Dettol antiseptic wash GSL
Dettol disinfectant spray GSL
Dettol liquid GSL
Dexa-Rhinaspray Duo POM
Dexamethasone POM
Dexamethasone acetate POM
Dexamethasone isonicotinate POM
Dexamethasone phenylpropionate POM
Dexamethasone pivalate POM
Dexamethasone sodium metasulphobenzoate POM
Dexamethasone sodium phosphate POM
Dexamethasone troxundate POM
Dexamfetamine CD POM
Dexedrine preparations CD POM
Dexemel POM
Dexfenfluramine hydrochloride POM
Dexibuprofen POM
Deximine soft gel capsules POM
Dexketoprofen POM
Dexomon SR POM
Dexpanthenol GSL
Dexpanthenol (Panthenol, Pantothenol) GSL
Dexrazoxane POM
Dexsol POM
Dextran POM
Dextrodiphenopyrine see

Dextromoramide
Dextromethorphan hydrobromide POM but if internal (1) In the case of a prolonged release preparation: equivalent of 30mg of dextromethorphan (MD) equivalent of 75mg of dextromethorphan (MDD), P; (2) in any other case: equivalent of 15mg of dextromethorphan (MD) equivalent of 75mg of dextromethorphan (MDD), P
Dextromoramide; its salts CD POM
Dextropropoxyphene; its salts, esters and ethers CD POM but if in a preparation for oral use containing not more than 135mg of dextropropoxyphene (calculated as base) per dosage unit or with a total concentration of not more than 2.5% (calculated as base) CD Inv POM
Dextrose GSL
Dextrose injection POM
Dextrose monohydrate GSL
Dextrothyroxine sodium POM
DF 118 forte tabs CD Inv POM
DHC Continus tablets CD Inv POM
Diabact UBT POM
Diabetamide tabs POM
Diacetylmorphine see Diamorphine
Diagesil inj CD POM
Diaglyk tabs POM
Diah-Limit capsules GSL
Dialar POM
Diamicron MR tablets POM
Diamicron tablets POM
Diamorphine; its salts CD POM
Diamox preps POM
Diampromide; its salts CD POM
Dianette tablets POM
Diaquitte P
Diarrest liquid CD Inv POM
Diasorb capsules P
Diazemuls injection CD Benz POM
Diazepam CD Benz POM
Diazoxide POM
Dibenyline preparations POM
Dibenzepin hydrochloride POM
Dibromopropamidine see Dibrompropamidine
Dibrompropamidine/Dibrompropamidine isethionate, external use only GSL
Dichloralphenazone POM
Dichlorobenzyl alcohol, if external use or internal (pastilles, lozenges, throat tablets maximum strength 2mg) GSL
Dichlorodifluoromethane (Propellant 12), external use only GSL
Dichlorodifluoromethane (Propellant 21), external use only GSL
Dichlorophen, if maximum strength 1.0 per cent (external use only) GSL
Dichlorotetrafluroethane, external use only GSL
Dichloroxylenol, if internal maximum strength 0.5 per cent or external maximum strength 5.0 per cent GSL
Dichlorphenamide POM
Diclofenac diethylammonium POM but if external for local symptomatic relief of pain and inflammation in trauma of the tendons, ligaments, muscles and joints, eg, due to sprains, strains and bruises; localised forms of soft tissue rheumatism, for use in adults and children aged 12 years and over, for a maximum period of 7 days, maximum strength 1.16 per cent and container or package containing not more than 50g of medicinal product, GSL. Please refer to proprietary names for the classification granted under the marketing authorisation (See Voltarol Pain-Eze Emulgel)
Diclofenac ethylammonium POM; but if for external use for local symptomatic relief of pain and inflammation in trauma of the tendons, ligaments, muscles and joints and in localised

forms of soft tissue rheumatism; for relief of pain of non-serious arthritic conditions, for use in adults and children not less than 12 years, for a maximum period of 7 days, maximum strength 1.16 per cent maximum pack size 50g P. Please refer to proprietary names for the classification granted under the marketing authorisation
Diclofenac potassium POM but if for the short term relief of headache, dental pain, period pain, rheumatic and muscular pain, backache and the symptoms of colds and flu, including fever, in adults and children aged 14 years and over, maximum strength 12.5mg, 25mg (MD), 75mg (MDD), for a maximum duration of 3 days' treatment and in a maximum pack size of 18 tablets, P
Diclofenac sodium POM; but for the local symptomatic relief of mild to moderate pain and inflammation following acute blunt trauma of small and medium-sized joints and periarticular structures, such as trauma of the tendons, ligaments, muscles and joints eg due to sprains and strains, maximum length of treatment without medical advice 7 days, maximum dose 40mg, maximum daily dose 120mg, maximum strength 4%, maximum pack size 25g of product, P, please refer to proprietary names for the classification granted under the marketing authorisation
Diclofex 75mg SR tablets POM
Dicloflex Retard tablets POM
Dicloflex tablets POM
Diclomax Retard capsules POM
Diclomax SR capsules POM
Diclotard tablets POM
Diclovol tablets POM
Diclovol Retard POM
Diclozip tabs POM
Dicobalt edetate POM
Diconal tablets CD POM
Dicyclomine see Dicycloverine
Dicycloverine/Dicyclomine hydrochloride POM but if 10mg (MD) 60mg (MDD), P
Dicynene preparations POM
Didanosine POM
Didronel preps POM
Dienestrol/Dienoestrol POM
Dienoestrol see Dienestrol
Diethanolamine fusidate POM
Diethyl phthalate, external use only GSL
Diethylamine salicylate, external use only GSL
Diethylpropion; its salts CD No Register POM
Diethylstilbestrol/Stilboestrol POM
Diethylstilbestrol/Stilboestrol dipropionate POM
Diethylthiambutene; its salts CD POM
N,N-Diethyltryptamine; its salts CD Lic
Difenoxin CD POM but if in preparations containing per dosage unit, not more than 0.5mg of difenoxin and a quantity of atropine sulphate equivalent to at least 5% of the dose of difenoxin CD Inv POM
Differin gel POM
Difflam cream P
Difflam oral rinse P
Difflam spray P
Diffundox MR POM
Diflucan capsules POM
Diflucan infusion POM
Diflucan One capsule P
Diflucan Oral suspension POM
Diflucortolone valerate POM
Diflunisal POM
Diftavax vaccine POM
Digenac XL tabs POM
Digibind POM

Digitalin POM
Digitaline Nativelle preparations POM
Digitalis leaf POM
Digitalis prepared POM
Digitoxin POM
Digoxin POM
Dihydralazine sulphate POM
Dihydrocodeine; its salts CD POM but if
for non-parenteral use and (a) in undi-
vided preparations with ms 2.5% (cal-
culated as base) CD Inv POM; or (b) in
single dose preparations with ms per
dosage unit 100mg (calculated as base)
CD Inv POM; or (c) in unit prepara-
tions diluted to at least one part in a
million (6X) in response to a specific
request, CD Inv P; or (d) in unit prepa-
rations diluted to at least one part in a
million million (6C), CD Inv P
Dihydrocodeineone O-carboxymethy-
loxime; its salts esters and ethers CD
POM
Dihydroergotamine mesylate POM
Dihydroetorphine CD POM
Dihydrohydroxycodeinone see
Oxycodone
Dihydrohydroxymorphinone see
Oxymorphone
[2,3-Dihydro-5-methyl-3-(4-mor-
pholinylmethyl)pyrrolo[1, 2, 3-ce]-
1,4- benzoxazin-6-yl]-1-naphthalenyl-
methanone CD Lic
Dihydromorphine; its salts, esters and
ethers CD POM
Dihydromorphinone see
Hydromorphone
Dihydrone see Oxycodone
Dihydrostreptomycin POM
Dihydrostreptomycin sulphate POM
Dihydroxyaluminium sodium carbonate
GSL
Dilcardia SR capsules POM
Dilcardia XL capsules POM
Dill Oil GSL
Diloxanide furoate POM
Diltiazem hydrochloride POM
Dilzem SR capsules POM
Dilzem XL capsules POM
Dimenhydrinate P
Dimenoxadole; its salts CD POM
Dimepheptanol; its salts, esters and
ethers CD POM
Dimercaprol POM
Dimethicone see Dimeticone
Dimethisoquin hydrochloride POM but
if non-ophthalmic use, P
Dimethisterone POM
Dimethothiazine mesylate POM
2,5-Dimethoxy-a,4-dimethylphenethy-
lamine; its salts CD Lic
Dimethyl sulfoxide/Dimethyl sulphox-
ide POM
Dimethyl sulphoxide see Dimethyl
sulfoxide
3-Dimethylheptyl-11-hydroxyhexahy-
drocannabinol CD Lic
Dimethylthiambutene; its salts CD POM
N,N-Dimethyltryptamine; its salts CD
Lic
Dimethyltubocurarine bromide POM
Dimethyltubocurarine chloride POM
Dimethyltubocurarine iodide POM
Dimeticone/Dimethicone GSL; external
use for the eradication of headlice
infestations in adults and children
(aged six months and above) maxi-
mum strength 4% maximum pack
size 100ml GSL
Dimetriose capsules POM
Dimorphone see Hydrocodone
Dimotane elixir P
Dimotane expectorant P
Dimotane LA tabs P
Dimotane Plus elixir P
Dimotane Plus Paediatric elixir P
Dimotane tablets P
Dimotane with Codeine CD Inv P
Dimotane with Codeine Paediatric CD

Inv P
Dimotapp elixir P
Dimotapp elixir Paediatric P
Dimotapp LA tablets P
Dindevan tablets POM
Dinnefords Teejel GSL
Dinoprost POM
Dinoprost Trometamol POM
Dinoprostone POM
Diocalm tablets CD Inv P
Diocalm Complete GSL
Diocalm Ultra pack sizes 6s GSL; 12s P
Diocaps POM
Dioctyl capsules P
Dioderm cream POM
Dioralyte pack sizes 6s GSL; 20s P
Dioralyte Relief pack sizes 6s GSL; 20s P
Diovan caps POM
Dioxaphetyl butyrate; its salts CD POM
Dipentum capsules POM
Dipeptiven POM
Diperodon hydrochloride, external use
only GSL
Diphenhydramine hydrochloride POM
but all preparations except liquid-
filled capsules, P
Diphenoxylate hydrochloride POM but
if maximum strength 2.5mg, in combination with atropine sulphate for
short term use as an adjunctive thera-
py to appropriate rehydration in
acute diarrhoea, for use in persons
aged 16 years and over, in tablet
form, with MDD 25mg, in a container or package containing not more
than 20 tablets, P
Diphenoxylate; its salts CD POM but if
in preparations with ms per dosage
unit 2.5mg of diphenoxylate (calculated as base), and a quantity of
atropine sulphate equivalent to at
least 1% of the dose of diphenoxylate
CD Inv POM
Diphtheria and tetanus vaccine POM
Diphtheria vaccine POM
Diphtheria, tetanus and pertussis vac-
cine POM
Diphtheria, tetanus and poliomyelitis
vaccine POM
Diphtheria, tetanus, pertussis and
poliomyelitis vaccine POM
Dipipanone; its salts CD POM
Dipivefrine POM
Dipotassium clorazepate/Potassium clo-
razepate CD Benz POM
Diprivan injection POM
Diprobase cream and ointment GSL
Diprobath P
Diprosalic ointment and scalp applica-
tion POM
Diprosone preparations POM
Dipyridamole POM
Dirythmin SA tablets POM
Disipal POM
Disney multivitamins & minerals GSL
Disney vitamin C GSL
Disodium edetate, external use only GSL
Disodium etidronate POM
Disodium pamidronate POM
Disogram SR POM
Disopyramide POM
Disopyramide phosphate POM
Dispello GSL
Disprin CV P
Disprin Direct tablets pack sizes 16s GSL
Disprin Extra tablets pack sizes 16s GSL
Disprin tablets pack sizes 8s, 16s GSL;
32s P
Disprol suspension sugar-free 100ml P
and GSL
Disprol soluble tablets pack sizes 16s
GSL
Disprol susp sachets pack sizes 12s GSL
Distaclor MR tablets POM
Distaclor preparations POM
Distalgesic tablets CD Inv POM
Distamine tablets POM
Distigmine bromide POM

Disulfiram POM
Ditemic Spansule P
Dithranol POM but if maximum
strength 1.0 per cent, P
Dithrocream 0.1%, 0.25%, 1% P
Dithrocream 2% POM
Dithrocream forte 0.5% P
Ditropan preparations POM
Diumide-K Continus tablets POM
Diurexan tablets POM
Diva tablets POM
Dixarit tablets POM
DMT see N,N-Dimethyltryptamine
Do-Do tablets P
Doans backache pills GSL
Dobutamine hydrochloride POM
Dobutrex ampoules POM
Docetaxel POM
Docosahexaenoic acid (DHA) GSL
Docusate sodium GSL
Docusol liquid P
Dolasetron mesilate POM
Dolenio tablets POM
Dolmatil tablets POM
Dolobid tablets POM
Doloxene capsules CD Inv POM
Dolvan tablets P
Domical tablets POM
Dominion Pharma hayfever eye-drops P
Domiphen bromide GSL
Domperamol tabs POM
Domperidone POM but if for the relief
of post-prandial symptoms of exces-
sive fullness, nausea, epigastric bloat-
ing and belching, occasionally
accompanied by epigastric discomfort
and heartburn, 10mg of domperidone
(MD), 40mg of domperidone(MDD)
in a container or package containing
not more than 200mg of domperidone P; for the relief of nausea and
vomiting of less than 48 hours duration, for use by persons over the age
of 16, for a maximum period of 48
hours, P
Domperidone maleate POM but if for
the relief of post-prandial symptoms
of excessive fullness, nausea, epigastric bloating and belching, occasionally accompanied by epigastric discomfort and heartburn, 10mg of
domperidone as domperidone
maleate (MD), 40mg of domperidone as domperidone maleate
(MDD) in a container or package
containing not more than 200mg of
domperidone as domperidone
maleate P; for the relief of nausea
and vomiting of less than 48 hours
duration, for use by persons over
the age of 16, for a maximum peri-
od of 48 hours, P
Donepezil HCl POM
Dopacard injection POM
Dopamine hydrochloride POM
Dopexamine hydrochloride POM
Dopram injection POM
Doralese tiltabs tablets POM
Doribax POM
Dormonoct tabs CD Benz POM
Dornase alfa POM
Dorzolamide POM
Dostinex tablets POM
Dosulepin/Dothiepin POM
Dosulepin/Dothiepin hydrochloride
POM
Dothapax preps POM
Dothiepin see Dosulepin
Doublebase gel P
Dovobet ointment POM
Dovonex preps POM
Doxadura POM
Doxadura XL POM
Doxapram hydrochloride POM
Doxazosin mesylate POM
Doxepin hydrochloride POM
Doxorubicin POM
Doxorubicin hydrochloride POM

Doxycycline POM
Doxycycline calcium chelate POM
Doxycycline hyclate/Doxycycline
hydrochloride POM
Doxycycline hydrochloride see
Doxycycline hyclate
Doxylar capsules POM
Dozic liquid POM
Dozol liquid P
Dr. Greenfingers bumps & bruises oint-
ment GSL
Dr. Greenfingers cough soother GSL
Dr. Greenfingers cuts and grazes oint-
ment GSL
Dramamine tablets P
Drapolene cream GSL
Dreemon P
Driclor roll-on P
Dried smallpox vaccine POM
Dristan decongestant tablets P
Drogenil tablets POM
Droleptan preparations POM
Dromadol POM
Dronabinol CD POM
Droperidol POM
Drostanolone; its salts CD Anab POM
Drotebanol; its salts, esters and ethers
CD POM
Dryptal tablets POM
DTIC- Dome vial POM
DTP vaccine (pre-filled) POM
Duac Once Daily Gel POM
Dubam spray relief/cream GSL
Dukoral oral vaccine POM
Dulcobalance P
Dulcoease GSL
Dulco-Lax children's suppositories P
Dulco-Lax liquid P
Dulco-Lax Perles pack sizes 20s GSL; 50s
P
Dulco-Lax suppositories P
Dulco-lax tablets pack sizes 10s GSL; 20s
GSL; 40s GSL; 60s P; 100s P
Duloxetine POM
Dumicoat denture lacquer POM
Duodopa intestinal gel POM
Duofilm P
DuoTrav eye drops POM
Duovent preparations POM
Duphalac Dry P
Duphalac syrup P
Duphaston HRT POM
Duphaston tablets POM
Duragel gel GSL
Duraphat 5000 toothpaste POM
Duraphat weekly rinse P
Duraphat 2800 POM
Durogesic patches CD POM
Durogesic DTrans patches CD POM
Duromine capsules CD No Register
POM
Dutasteride POM
Dutonin tablets POM
Dyazide tablets POM
Dydrogesterone POM
Dyflos POM
Dymotil tablets P
Dynamin tabs P
Dynastat injection POM
Dysman preps POM
Dyspamet POM
Dysport inj POM
Dytac capsules POM
Dytide capsules POM

E

E45 cream GSL
E45 Itch Relief GSL
Earcalm P
Earex ear drops GSL
Earex Plus P
Earex protector plugs GSL
Easyhaler preparations POM
Ebixa tablets and oral drops POM
Ebufac tablets POM
Ecalta powder for concentrate for solu-

tion for infusion POM
Eccoxolac capsules POM
Ecgonine; and any derivative of ecgonine which is convertible to ecgonine or to cocaine CD POM
Echinacea GSL
Echinacea tabs GSL
Econac preparations POM
Econacort cream POM
Econazole POM but if external, and in the case of vaginal use only external use for the treatment of vaginal candidiasis P
Econazole nitrate POM but if external, and in the case of vaginal use only external use for the treatment of vaginal candidiasis P
Ecopace tabs POM
Ecostatin cream P
Ecostatin pessaries POM
Ecostatin Twinpack POM
Ecostatin-1 pessaries POM
Ecothiopate iodide POM
Eczmol emollient GSL
Edecrin preparations POM
Edetic acid, external use only GSL
Edible Bone Flour (bonemeal) GSL
Ednyt POM
Edronax tablets POM
Edrophonium chloride POM
Efalex caps GSL
Efalith ointment POM
Efalizumab POM
Efamast capsules POM
Efavirenz POM
Efcortelan cream, ointment POM
Efcortesol inj POM
Efexor capsules POM
Efexor XL tablets POM
Effentora buccal tablets CD POM
Effercitrate sachets GSL
Effercitrate tablets GSL
Effico GSL
Efient tablets POM
Eflornithine hydrochloride POM
Eformoterol see Formoterol
Efudix cream POM
Eicosapentaenoic acid (EPA) GSL
Elantan 10 tablets P
Elantan 20 tablets P
Elantan 40 tablets P
Elantan LA 25 capsules P
Elantan LA 50 capsules P
Elaprase POM
Elavil tablets POM
Eldepryl syrup POM
Eldepryl tablets POM
Elder GSL
Eldisine vials POM
Elecampane GSL
Electrolade sachets GSL
Eletriptan POM
Elidel cream POM
ellaOne tablets POM
Elleste Duet POM
Elleste Duet Conti tablets POM
Elleste Solo MX40 patches POM
Elleste Solo MX80 patches POM
Elleste Solo tablets POM
Elliman's embrocation GSL
Elocon preparations POM
Elohaes IV inf POM
Eloxatin infusion POM
Elset rayon/elastic bandages GSL
Eltor vaccine POM
Eltroxin tablets POM
Eludril mouthwash GSL
Eludril spray P
Elyzol gel POM
Emadine eye drops POM
Emblon tabs POM
Embrel injection POM
Embutramide POM
Emcor LS tablets POM
Emcor tablets POM
Emedastine POM
Emend capsules POM
Emepronium bromide POM

Emeside preparations POM
Emetine POM but if maximum strength 1.0 per cent, P
Emetine bismuth iodide POM
Emetine hydrochloride POM but if maximum strength equivalent of 1.0 per cent of emetine, P
Emfib caps POM
Emflex capsules POM
Eminase injection POM
Emla cream P
Emmolate bath oil P
Emselex POM
Emtricitabine POM
Emtriva preparations POM
Emulsiderm P
Emulsifying ointment BP GSL
Emulsifying wax, external use only GSL
En-de-kay Fluodrops P
En-De-Kay Fluoride mouthrinse daily GSL
En-de-kay Fluorinse POM
En-de-kay Fluotabs 3-6 years tablets P
En-de-kay Fluotabs 6+ years tablets P
Enalapril maleate POM
Enbrel injection POM
Encephalitis Virus, Tick-borne, Cent Eur POM
Endoxana preparations POM
Enestebol CD Anab POM
Enfamil AR GSL
Enfuvirtide POM
Engerix B Paediatric vaccine POM
Engerix B vaccine POM
Enos powder GSL
Enoxacin POM
Enoxaparin sodium POM
Enoximone POM
Enprin tabs 28 P
Entacapone POM
Entecavir POM
Enterosan tablets CD Inv P
Entocort CR capsules POM
Entocort enemas POM
Entonox P
Entrocalm preparations GSL
Entrolax constipation relief tablets P
Entrolax laxative tablets GSL
Enzed tablets POM
Enzira POM
Epaderm emollient GSL
Epanutin preparations POM
Epaxal POM
Ephedrine POM but if (1) internal (other than nasal sprays or nasal drops) 30mg (MD) 60mg (MDD); (2) nasal sprays or nasal drops maximum strength 2.0 per cent; (3) external, P
Ephedrine hydrochloride POM but if (1) internal (other than nasal sprays or nasal drops) equivalent of 30mg of ephedrine (MD) equivalent of 60mg of ephedrine (MDD); (2) nasal sprays or nasal drops maximum strength equivalent of 2.0 per cent of ephedrine; (3) external, P
Ephedrine sulphate POM but if (1) internal (other than nasal sprays or nasal drops) equivalent of 30mg of ephedrine (MD) equivalent of 60mg of ephedrine (MDD); (2) nasal sprays or nasal drops maximum strength equivalent of 2.0 per cent of ephedrine; (3) external, P
Ephynal tablets GSL
Epicillin POM
Epilim preparations POM
Epimaz tablets POM
Epinastine POM
Epinephrine see Adrenaline
Epipen pens POM
Epirubicin POM
Epirubicin hydrochloride POM
Episenta POM
Epithiazide POM
Epitiostanol CD Anab POM
Epivir solution POM
Epivir tablets POM

Eplerenone POM
Epoetin Alfa POM
Epoetin Beta POM
Epogam capsules POM
Epoprostenol sodium POM
Eporatio for intravenous and subcutaneous use POM
Eposin POM
Eppy POM
Eprex injection POM
Eprosartan POM
Epsom salts BP GSL
Eptifibatide POM
Equagesic tablets CD No Register POM
Equanil tablets CD No Register POM
Equasym tablets CD POM
Equasym XL capsules CD POM
Equilon herbal caps GSL
Equilon tabs P
Equisetum GSL
Erbitux POM
Erdosteine POM
Erdotin POM
Erecnos injection POM
Ergometrine maleate POM
Ergometrine tartrate POM
Ergot, Prepared POM
Ergotamine tartrate POM
Erlotinib POM
Ertapenem POM
Ervevax vial POM
Erwinase inj POM
Eryacne gel POM
Erycen tabs POM
Erymax capsules POM
Erymin suspension POM
Erythrocin preparations POM
Erythromycin POM
Erythromycin estolate POM
Erythromycin ethyl succinate POM
Erythromycin ethylcarbonate POM
Erythromycin lactobionate POM
Erythromycin phosphate POM
Erythromycin stearate POM
Erythromycin thiocyanate POM
Erythroped A tablets POM
Erythroped preparations POM
Erythropoietin POM
Erythrosine E127 GSL
Escitalopram POM
Eskamel cream P
Eskazole tablets POM
Eskornade Spansule capsules P
Esmeron ampoules POM
Esmolol hydrochloride POM
Esomeprazole POM
Estazolam CD Benz POM
Estracombi POM
Estracyt capsules POM
Estraderm MX patches POM
Estraderm TTS POM
Estradiol implant POM
Estradiol/Oestradiol POM
Estradiol/Oestradiol benzoate POM
Estradiol/Oestradiol cypionate POM
Estradiol/Oestradiol dipropionate POM
Estradiol/Oestradiol diundecanoate POM
Estradiol/Oestradiol enanthate POM
Estradiol/Oestradiol phenylpropionate POM
Estradiol/Oestradiol undecanoate POM
Estradiol/Oestradiol valerate POM
Estradot POM
Estragest TTS POM
Estramustine phosphate POM
Estramustine sodium phosphate POM
Estrapak 50 POM
Estring POM
Estriol/Oestriol POM
Estriol/Oestriol succinate POM
Estrone/Oestrone POM
Estropipate POM
Etacrynic acid/Ethacrynic acid POM
Etafedrine hydrochloride POM
Etamsylate/Ethamsylate POM
Etanercept POM
Ethacrynic acid see Etacrynic acid
Ethambutol hydrochloride POM

Ethamivan POM
Ethamsylate see Etamsylate
Ethanolamine oleate POM
Ethchlorvynol CD No Register POM
Ether, up to 0.25ml (MD) GSL
Ethiazide POM
Ethimil tabs POM
Ethinamate CD No Register POM
Ethinyl androstenediol POM
Ethinylestradiol/Ethinyloestradiol POM
Ethinyloestradiol see Ethinylestradiol
Ethionamide POM
Ethisterone POM
Ethmozine tablets POM
Ethoglucid POM
Ethoheptazine citrate POM
Ethopropazine hydrochloride POM
Ethosuximide POM
Ethotoin POM
Ethyl biscoumacetate POM
Ethyl loflazepate CD Benz POM
Ethyl nicotinate, external use only GSL
Ethyl salicylate, external use only GSL
N-Ethylamfetamine; its salts; its stereoisomers; their salts CD Benz POM
Ethyleostrenol CD Anab POM
Ethylmethylthiambutene; its salts CD POM
Ethylmorphine (3-ethylmorphine); its salts CD POM but if for non-parenteral use and (a) in undivided preparations with ms 2.5% (calculated as base) CD Inv POM; or (b) in single dose preparations with ms per dosage unit 100mg (calculated as base) CD Inv POM; or (c) in unit preparations diluted to at least one part in a million (6X) in response to a specific request, CD Inv P; or (d) in unit preparations diluted to at least one part in a million million (6C), CD Inv P
Ethylmorphine hydrochloride see Ethylmorphine
Ethynodiol see Etynodiol
Ethyol infusion POM
Eticyclidine CD Lic
Etodolac POM
Etomidate POM
Etomidate hydrochloride POM
Etonitazene; its salts CD POM
Etonogestrel POM
Etopan XL POM
Etopophos injection POM
Etoposide POM
Etoposide for injection concentrate POM
Etoricoxib POM
Etorphine; its salts, esters and ethers CD POM
Etoxeridine; its salts, esters and ethers CD POM
Etretinate POM
Etryptamine CD Lic
Etynodiol/Ethynodiol diacetate POM
Eucalyptol GSL
Eucalyptus oil GSL
Eucardic tablets POM
Eucerin extremely dry skin cream GSL
Eucerin extremely dry skin lotion GSL
Eucreas tablets POM
Eudemine preparations POM
Euflexxa POM
Eugenol, external use only GSL
Euglucon tablets POM
Eugynon 30 tablets POM
Eumovate eczema and dermatitis cream P
Eumovate preparations POM
Euphorbia hirta (Euphorbia pilulifera, Pill-Bearing Spurge) GSL
Eurax cream GSL
Eurax HC cream (PL 0001/5010R) P
Eurax Hydrocortisone POM
Eurax lotion GSL
European Birch, external use only GSL
Evista tablets POM
Evoltra POM

Evorel Conti patches POM
Evorel Pak POM
Evorel patches POM
Evorel Sequi patches POM
Evotrox POM
Evra transdermal patches POM
Ex-Lax laxative chocolate GSL
Exelderm cream P
Exelon capsules POM
Exelon oral solution POM
Exemestane POM
Exforge POM
Exjade POM
Exocin eye drops POM
Exorex lotion GSL
Exosurf Neonatal POM
Expulin children's cough linctus P
Expulin decongestant linctus for babies
    and children P
Expulin Dry Cough CD Inv P
Expulin For Chesty Coughs GSL
Expulin Paediatric linctus CD Inv P
Extavia 250mcg/ml powder and solvent
    for solution for injection POM
Exterol ear drops P
Exubera tablets POM
Eye Dew eye drops P
Ezetimibe POM
Ezetrol tablets POM

F

Fabrazyme POM
Factor VIIA, VIII, IX POM
Factor XIII concentrate POM
Fam-Lax tablets POM
Famciclovir POM
Famel Original CD Inv P
Famotidine POM but if for the short-
    term symptomatic relief of heartburn,
    dyspepsia, indigestion, acid indiges-
    tion and hyperacidity, and preven-
    tion of these symptoms when associ-
    ated with food and drink, including
    nocturnal symptoms, 10mg (MD)
    20mg (MDD) for maximum period of
    14 days, P; in the case of a tablet,
    maximum strength 10mg, for the
    short term symptomatic relief of
    heartburn, indigestion, acid indiges-
    tion and hyperacidity, 10mg (MD),
    20mg (MDD) and not more than 12
    tablets GSL
Famvir tablets POM
Fansidar tablets POM
Fareston tablets POM
Farlutal preparations POM
Fasigyn preparations POM
Faslodex injection POM
Fast Green FCF GSL
Fasturtec infusion POM
Faverin tablets POM
Fazadinium bromide POM
Fectrim preparations POM
Fedril preps P
Fefol Spansule capsules P
Fefol Z Spansule capsules P
Fefol-Vit Spansule capsules P
Fefol-Vit Z Spansule capsules P
Feiba Immuno POM
Felbinac POM but if external for the
    relief of rheumatic pain, pain of non-
    serious arthritic conditions and soft
    tissue injuries such as sprains, strains
    and contusions for use in adults and
    children not less than 12 years, for
    maximum period of 7 days maximum
    strength 3.17 per cent and container
    or package containing not more than
    30g of medicinal product, P
Feldene P gel P
Feldene capsules POM
Feldene Dispersible tablets POM
Feldene gel POM
Feldene IM POM
Feldene Melt POM
Feldene suppositories POM
Felendil XL POM

Felicium capsules POM
Felodipine POM
Felogen XL POM
Felotens XL POM
Felypressin POM
Femapak 40 HRT POM
Femapak 80 HRT POM
Femara tablets POM
Fematrix patches POM
Femeron cream P
Femeron pessaries P
Femfresh powder GSL
Femigraine P
Feminax tablets CD Inv P
Feminax Ultra tablets P
Feminine Balance GSL
Femodene preps POM
Femodette tablets POM
Femoston tablets POM
Femoston-conti tablets POM
FemSeven Conti patches POM
FemSeven patches POM
FemSeven Sequi patches POM
FemTab POM
FemTab Continuous POM
FemTab Sequi POM
Femulen tablets POM
Fenactol POM
Fenactol Retard POM
Fenbid Forte gel pack size 100g POM
Fenbid Forte gel pack size 30g P
Fenbid gel pack sizes 30g, 50g GSL; 100g
    P
Fenbid spansules POM
Fenbufen POM
Fenbuzip preps POM
Fencamfamin; its salts, stereoisomers CD
    Benz POM
Fenclofenac POM
Fendrix hepatitis B (rDNA) vaccine POM
Fenethylline; its salts and stereoisomers
    CD POM
Fenfluramine hydrochloride POM
Fenistil P
Fennel GSL
Fennel Oil GSL
Fennings Children's Cooling powder
    pack sizes 10s GSL; 20s P
Fennings Little Healers GSL
Fenofibrate POM
Fenogal capsules POM
Fenoket 200mg caps POM
Fenoprofen POM
Fenoprofen calcium POM
Fenopron tablets POM
Fenoterol hydrobromide POM
Fenox nasal drops P
Fenox nasal spray P
Fenpaed oral suspension P
Fenpaed sachets GSL
Fenproporex; its salts and stereoisomers
    CD Benz POM
Fertamox tabs POM
Fentanyl; its salts CD POM
Fentazin preparations POM
Fenticonazole nitrate POM but external
    use (but in the case of vaginal use,
    only for the treatment of vaginal can-
    didiasis) P
Fenugreek GSL
Feospan Spansule capsules P
Feprapax POM
Feprazone POM
Ferfolic SV tablets POM
Feroglobin B12 caps GSL
Ferric ammonium citrate, if MD equiva-
    lent to 24 mg elemental iron GSL
Ferric chloride, if MD equivalent to
    24mg elemental iron GSL
Ferriprox oral solution POM
Ferriprox tablets POM
Ferrograd C tablets P
Ferrograd Folic tablets P
Ferrograd tabs P
Ferrous arsenate POM
Ferrous carbonate, if MD equivalent to
    24 mg elemental iron GSL
Ferrous fumarate, if MD equivalent to 24

mg elemental iron GSL
Ferrous gluconate, if MD equivalent to
    24 mg elemental iron GSL
Ferrous sulphate, if internal (except for
    use as cyanide antidote) equivalent to
    24 mg elemental iron (MD) or inter-
    nal (for use as cyanide antidote only)
    maximum strength 15.8 per cent
    (FeSO4 7H2O) GSL
Fersaday tablets P
Fersamal syrup P
Fersamal tablets P
Fertiral injection POM
Fesovit Z Spansule capsules P
Feverfen P
Fexofenadine POM
Fibre, Vegetable GSL
Fibro-vein POM
Fiery Jack preparations GSL
Fig GSL
Filair preparations POM
Filgrastim POM
Filnarine SR tablets CD POM
Finacea POM
Finasteride POM
Fir Oil, Siberian GSL
Firazir POM
Firmagon powder and solvent for injec-
    tion POM
Flagyl Compak POM
Flagyl injection POM
Flagyl suppositories POM
Flagyl tablets POM
Flagyl-S suspension POM
Flamatak preps POM
Flamatrol caps POM
Flamazine cream POM
Flamrase preps POM
Flavoxate hydrochloride POM
Flaxedil injection POM
Flecainide acetate POM
Fleet preps P
Fletchers' arachis oil retention enema P
Fletchers' enemette P
Fletchers' phosphate enema P
Fletchers' prednisolone retention enema
    (Predenema) POM
Flexi-melt tablets GSL
Flexin Continus tablets POM
Flexotard MR POM
Flexotard tablets POM
Flixonase Allergy nasal spray P
Flixonase aqueous spray POM
Flixonase nasules POM
Flixotide preps POM
Flolan POM
Flomax MR capsules POM
Flomaxtra XL tablets POM
Florinef tablets POM
Flosequinan POM
Floxapen preparations POM
Flu-amp caps POM
Fluanisone POM
Fluanxol tablets POM
Fluarix vaccine POM
Flubendazole POM
Fluclomix caps POM
Fluclorolone acetonide POM
Flucloxacillin magnesium POM
Flucloxacillin sodium POM
Flucloxin preps POM
Fluconazole POM but if for oral adminis-
    tration for the treatment of vaginal
    candidiasis or associated candidal bal-
    anitis in persons aged not less than
    16 but less than 60 years, 150mg
    (MD) and container or package con-
    taining not more than 150mg of flu-
    conazole, P
Flucytosine POM
Fludara POM
Fludara oral tablets POM
Fludarabine POM
Fludiazepam CD Benz POM
Fludrocortisone acetate POM
Fludroxycortide/Flurandrenolone POM
Flufenamic acid POM
Flumazenil POM

Flumetasone/Flumethasone POM
Flumetasone/Flumethasone pivalate
    POM
Flumethasone see Flumetasone
Flunisolide POM but if for the preven-
    tion and treatment of seasonal aller-
    gic rhinitis, including hay fever, in
    persons aged 18 years and over in the
    form of a non-pressurised nasal spray
    50mcg per nostril (MD) 100mcg per
    nostril (MDD) for a maximum period
    of 3 months, maximum strength
    0.025 per cent and container or pack-
    age containing not more than
    6,000mcg of flunisolide, P
Flunitrazepam CD No Register POM
Fluocinolone acetonide POM
Fluocinonide POM
Fluocortin butyl POM
Fluocortolone POM
Fluocortolone hexanoate POM
Fluocortolone pivalate POM
Fluor-A-Day tablets P
Fluorescein dilaurate POM
Fluorets P
Fluorigard Daily drops P
Fluorigard Daily rinse GSL
Fluorigard Gelkam gel P
Fluorigard tablets P
Fluorigard Weekly rinse P
Fluorometholone POM
Fluorouracil POM
Fluorouracil trometamol POM
Fluoxetine hydrochloride POM
Fluoxymesterone CD Anab POM
Flupenthixol see Flupentixol
Flupentixol/Flupenthixol decanoate
    POM
Flupentixol/Flupenthixol hydrochloride
    POM
Fluperolone acetate POM
Fluphenazine decanoate POM
Fluphenazine enanthate POM
Fluphenazine hydrochloride POM
Fluprednidene acetate POM
Fluprednisolone POM
Fluprostenol sodium POM
Flurandrenolone see Fludroxycortide
Flurazepam; its salts CD Benz POM
Flurbiprofen POM but if maximum
    strength 8.75mg, in the form of a
    throat lozenge, with a MDD 43.75mg
    and in a container or package con-
    taining not more than 140mg of flur-
    biprofen, P
Flurbiprofen sodium POM
Fluspirilene POM
Flutamide POM
Fluticasone propionate POM
Flutrimazole POM
Fluvastatin sodium POM
Fluvirin vaccine POM
Fluvoxamine maleate POM
Fluzone POM
FML Liquifilm ophthalmic suspension
    POM
FML-Neo eye drops POM
Folex-350 tablets P
Folic acid POM but if 500mcg (MDD),
    GSL
Folicare oral solution GSL
Follicle stimulating hormone POM
Follitropin alpha POM
Follitropin beta POM
Fomac tabs POM
Fondaparinux sodium POM
Foradil capsules (for inhalation) POM
Forceval capsules P
Forceval Junior P
Forceval-Protein P
Formaldehyde solution, if maximum
    strength 0.47% in a dentifrice or
    maximum strength 0.75% for exter-
    nal use other than as a dentifrice,
    GSL
Formebolone CD Anab POM
Formestane POM
Formocortal POM

Formoterol/Eformoterol fumarate POM
Forsteo POM
Fortagesic tablets CD No Register POM
Fortespan P
Fortipine LA 40 POM
Fortovase capsules POM
Fortum injection POM
Fosamax Once Weekly tablets POM
Fosamax tablets POM
Fosamprenavir POM
Fosavance tablets POM
Foscan POM
Foscarnet sodium POM
Foscavir infusion POM
Fosfestrol sodium POM
Fosfomycin trometamol POM
Fosinopril sodium POM
Fosphenytoin POM
Fosrenol POM
Fostimon POM
Frador GSL
Fragmin injection POM
Framycetin sulphate POM
Framyspray aerosol POM
Frangula GSL
Frangula bark GSL
Frangulin GSL
Franol Plus tablets P
Franol tablets P
Freederm gel P
Freezone P
Friars' balsam BP GSL
Fringe tree GSL
Frisium tabs CD Benz POM
Froben SR capsules POM
Froben suppositories POM
Froben tablets POM
Froop preps POM
Frovatriptan POM
Fru-Co tablets POM
Fructose injection POM
Frumil Forte tablets POM
Frumil LS tablets POM
Frumil tablets POM
Frusemide see Furosemide
Frusene tablets POM
Frusid tablets POM
Frusol oral solution POM
FSC waterfall caps GSL
FSME-Immun POM
Fucibet cream POM
Fucidin H preparations POM
Fucidin preparations POM
Fucithalmic drops POM
Fulcin preparations POM
Full Marks preps P
Fullers earth, external use only GSL
Fulsovin suspension POM
Fulvestrant POM
Fumitory, up to 160mg (MD) GSL
Fungederm cream P
Fungilin preparations POM
Fungizone injection POM
Furadantin preparations POM
Furamide tablets POM
Furazabol CD Anab POM
Furazolidone POM
Furethidine; its salts CD POM
Furosemide/Frusemide POM
Fusafungine POM
Fusidic acid POM
Fuzeon injection POM
Fybogel Mebeverine sachets pack sizes
    10s P, 60s POM
Fybogel sachets pack sizes 10s, 30s PO
Fybozest Orange granules P

G

Gabapentin POM
Gabitril tablets POM
Gadoteridol POM
Galake tabs POM
Galantamine POM
Galcodine Linctus CD Inv P
Galcodine Linctus Paediatric CD Inv P
Galenamet tabs POM
Galenamox caps POM

Galenphol Linctus CD Inv P
Galenphol Linctus Paediatric CD Inv P
Galenphol Linctus Strong CD Inv P
Galenphol Original CD Inv P
Galfer preps P
Galfloxin capsules POM
Gallamine triethiodide POM
Galloway's Cough syrup GSL
Galpamol sachets GSL
Galpharm 3-in-1 antacid tablets GSL
Galpharm allergy eye drops P
Galpharm cold sore cream GSL
Galpharm dual action diarrhoea relief
    GSL
Galpharm extra power pain reliever
    tablets GSL
Galpharm Flu relief caps GSL
Galpharm flu strength all-in-one liquid P
Galpharm Hayfever and Allergy Relief
    Syrup GSL
Galpharm Hayfever and Allergy Relief
    Tablets pack sizes 7s GSL; 30s P
Galpharm Hayfever and Allergy Relief
    tablets non drowsy pack sizes 7s GSL;
    30s P
Galpharm hot lemon powders flu
    strength GSL
Galpharm ibuprofen caplets 16s GSL; 24,
    48, 96 P
Galpharm ibuprofen gel GSL
Galpharm ibuprofen 200mg tablets pack
    sizes 16s GSL
Galpharm ibuprofen 400mg tablets pack
    sizes 16s GSL; 96s P
Galpharm ibuprofen tablets max
    strength P
Galpharm migraine relief GSL
Galpharm Medical antiseptic cream GSL
Galpharm mouth ulcer treatment GSL
Galpharm nasal decongestant spray GSL
Galpharm paediatric suspension pack
    sizes 100ml P; 10 x 5ml GSL
Galpharm paracetamol caplets and
    tablets GSL
Galpharm senncalax GSL
Galpharm thrush preparations P
Galprofen cold & flu tablets GSL
Galprofen long lasting capsules 200mg
    GSL
Galprofen long lasting capsules 300mg P
Galpseud preps P
Galpseud Plus P
Galsud decongestant nasal spray GSL
Galsud linctus and tablets P
Galvus tablets POM
Gamanil tablets POM
Gamma Globulin (Kabi) ampoules POM
Gammabulin injection POM
Gammaderm cream GSL
Gammagard S/D POM
Gammahydroxy-butyrate (GHB) CD
    Benz POM
Ganciclovir POM
Ganciclovir sodium POM
Ganda eye drops POM
Ganfort eye drops POM
Ganirelix POM
Garamycin preparations POM
Gardasil POM
Gardenal sodium preparations CD No
    Register POM Note: emergency sup-
    ply at request of patient not permit-
    ted except for use in the treatment of
    epilepsy
Garlic GSL
Garlic Oil GSL
Gastrobid Continus tablets POM
Gastrocote liquid P
Gastrocote tablets GSL
Gastroflux tabs POM
Gastromax capsules POM
Gastromiro POM
Gavilast pack sizes 6s GSL; 12s GSL; 48s
    P
Gavilast-P P
Gaviscon 250 tablets GSL
Gaviscon Advance PO
Gaviscon Cool preparations GSL

Gaviscon Double Action GSL
Gaviscon Extra Strength PO
Gaviscon infant sachets PO
Gaviscon liquid GSL
Gee's linctus BPC CD Inv P
Gelcosal P
Gelofusine POM
Gelsemine POM but if maximum
    strength 0.1 per cent, P
Gelsemium POM but if 25mg (MD)
    75mg (MDD), P
Geltears P
Gemcitabine POM
Gemeprost POM
Gemfibrozil POM
Gemzar injection POM
Genalat retard tabs POM
Gencardia POM
Genotropin preps CD Anab POM
Gentamicin POM
Gentamicin Redibags POM
Gentamicin sulphate POM
Gentian GSL
Genticin preparations POM
Gentisone HC ear drops POM
Gentran IV inf POM
George's American Liniment GSL
Geranium oil, external use only GSL
Gerard House catarrh-eeze tablets GSL
Gerard House echinacea and garlic
    tablets GSL
Gerard House ginkgo tablets GSL
Gerard House hayfever aid tablets GSL
Gerard House herbulax tablets GSL
Gerard House reumalex tablets GSL
Gerard House serenity tablets GSL
Gerard House skin tablets GSL
Gerard House somnus tablets GSL
Gerard House water relief tablets GSL
Geref 50 POM
Germolene preparations GSL
Germoloids preparations GSL
Gestodene POM
Gestone injections POM
Gestonorone/Gestronol POM
Gestonorone/Gestronol hexanoate POM
Gestrinone CD Anab POM
Gestronol see Gestonorone
Ginger GSL
Ginger tabs GSL
Ginseng GSL
Givitol capsules P
Glamin sol POM
Glatiramer acetate POM
Glau-opt eye drops POM
Glaucol eye drops POM
Gliadel POM
Glibenclamide POM
Glibenese tablets POM
Glibornuride POM
Gliclazide POM
Gliken tabs POM
Glimepiride POM
Glipizide POM
Gliquidone POM
Glisoxepide POM
Glivec preparations POM
Glucagen inj POM
Glucagon POM
Glucamet tabs POM
Glucobay tablets POM
Glucophage powder for oral solution in
    sachets POM
Glucophage SR POM
Glucophage tablets POM
Glucoplex preparations POM
Glucose, liquid GSL
Glurenorm tablets POM
Glutamic acid hydrochloride GSL
Glutaraldehyde P
Glutarol P
Glutethimide; its salts; its stereoisomers;
    their salts CD POM
Glycerin BP GSL
Glycerin suppositories BP GSL
Glycerin thymol compound BP GSL
Glycerol GSL
Glycerol and saline injection POM

Glycerophosphoric acid GSL
Glycol salicylate, external use only GSL
Glyconon tablets POM
Glycophos POM
Glycopyrronium bromide POM but if
    1mg (MD) 2mg (MDD), P
Glykola tonic GSL
Glymese tablets POM
Glymidine POM
Glypressin injection POM
Glytrin spray P
Goddard's Embrocation GSL
Golden eye drops P
Golden eye ointment P
Golden Seal GSL
Gonadorelin POM
Gonal F preparations POM
Gonapeptyl Depot POM
Gopten capsules POM
Goserelin acetate POM
Gramicidin POM but if external maxi-
    mum strength 0.2 per cent, P
Graneodin preparations POM
Granisetron hydrochloride POM
Granocyte injection POM
Gravel Root (Eupatorium purpureum)
    GSL
Grazax POM
Gregoderm ointment POM
Grepafloxacin POM
Grepid tablets POM
Grindelia GSL
Griseofulvin POM
Grisol AF P
Grisovin tablets POM
Ground Ivy GSL
Growth Hormone CD Anab POM
GTN 300mcg tablets P
Guaiacol, external use only GSL
Guaiacum resin, up to 200mg (MD) GSL
Guaifenesin/Guaiphenesin, up to 200mg
    (MD) GSL
Guaiphenesin see Guaifenesin
Guanethidine monosulphate POM
Guanfacine hydrochloride POM
Guanoclor sulphate POM
Guanor preparations P
Guanoxan sulphate POM
Guarem granules P
Guaza see Cannabis
Gum Ammoniacum GSL
Gutta Percha, external use only GSL
Gygel GSL
Gyne T 380 POM
Gynest vaginal cream POM
Gyno-Daktarin preparations POM
Gyno-pevaryl preparations POM
Gynol II GSL
Gynomin P

H

Hactos cough mixture GSL
Haelan preparations POM
Haelan tape POM
Haemaccel infusion solution POM
Haes-steril IV inf POM
Halazepam CD Benz POM
Halciderm Topical POM
Halcinonide POM
Haldol decanoate injection POM
Haldol preparations POM
Half Beta-Prograne POM
Half Sinemet CR POM
Half-Inderal LA capsules POM
Half-Securon SR POM
Halfan tablets POM
Halibut liver oil as for Vitamin A and
    Vitamin D GSL
Halibut-Liver oil capsules BP GSL
Halita GSL
Halls childrens cough pastilles GSL
Halls max strength sore throat relief
    lozenges GSL
Halls Mentho-Lyptus GSL
Halls Soothers GSL
Halofantrine hydrochloride POM
Halogenated phenols, up to maximum

strength 1.0 per cent GSL
Haloperidol POM
Haloperidol decanoate POM
Haloxazolam CD Benz POM
Halquinol, if maximum strength 0.5 per cent (external use only) GSL
Halycitrol vitamin emulsion P
Hamamelis GSL
Happinose GSL
Harmogen tablets POM
Hartmann's solution POM
Hashish see Cannabis
Havrix Junior vaccine POM
Havrix vaccine POM
Haycrom Aqueous eye drops POM
Haycrom Hayfever eye drops P
Hayleve P
Haymine tablets P
HBvaxPRO vaccine POM
HC45 hydrocortisone cream (PL 0327/0039) P
4head GSL
Healonid POM
Healthcheck No1, No 2 P
Healthy feet GSL
Heartsease GSL
Hedex Extra pack sizes 16s GSL; purse pack 12s GSL
Hedex tablets pack sizes 16s GSL; 32s P; purse pack 12s GSL
Hedex ibuprofen GSL
Hedrin P
Heliclear POM
Helicobacter Test HP Plus POM
Helicobacter Test Infai POM
HeliMet triple pack POM
Hemabate I/M solution POM
Heminevrin preparations POM
Hemlock Spruce (Pine Canadian) P but if 400mg (MD), GSL
Hemocane GSL
Hemohes POM
Hep-flush sol POM
Heparin POM but if external use only GSL
Heparin calcium POM but if external GSL
Heparin sodium POM
Heparinoid, if for external use, maximum strength 1% for the relief of bruises, sprains and soft tissue injuries in adults and children aged 6 years and over GSL
Hepatitis A Vaccine POM
Hepatitis B vaccine POM
Hepatyrix vaccine POM
Heplok sol POM
Hepsal sol POM
Hepsera tablets POM
Heptabarbitone CD No Register POM
Herbal Concepts GSL
Herbal Laboratories preps all GSL except comfrey oil
Herbalache P
Herbalhypnos GSL
Herbaloa GSL
Herbulax tabs GSL
Herceptin infusion POM
Heroin see Diamorphine
Herpetad cold sore cream P
Herpid POM
Hespan IV inf POM
Hesperidin Complex GSL
Hewletts cream GSL
Hexachlorophane see Hexachlorophene
Hexachlorophene/Hexachlorophane POM but if external (1) soaps maximum strength 2.0 per cent; (2) aerosols maximum strength 0.1 per cent; (3) preparations other than soaps and aerosols maximum strength 0.75 per cent, P
Hexalen caps POM
Hexamine phenylcinchoninate POM
Hexetidine, if maximum strength 0.1 per cent (external use only) GSL
Hexobarbitone CD No Register POM
Hexobarbitone sodium CD No Register

POM
Hexoestrol POM
Hexoestrol dipropionate POM
Hexopal Forte tablets P
Hexopal suspension P
Hexopal tablets P
Hexyl nicotinate, if maximum strength 2.0 per cent (external use only) GSL
Hexylresorcinol, if external use or internal (pastilles, lozenges, throat tablets maximum strength 2.5mg) GSL
H-F Antidote GSL
Hibicet GSL
Hibiscrub GSL
Hibisol GSL
Hibitane 5% concentrate GSL
Hibitane Obstetric cream GSL
Hill's Balsam Adult expectorant GSL
Hill's Balsam Adult suppressant CD Inv P
Hill's Balsam extra strong 2-in-1 pastilles GSL
Hill's Balsam Junior expectorant GSL
Hill's Balsam pastilles GSL
Hioxyl cream P
Hiprex 1g tabs P
Hirudoid cream P
Hirudoid gel P
Hismanal suspension POM
Histac POM
Histafen POM
Histalix syrup P
Histamine hydrochloride, if maximum strength 0.1 per cent (external use only) GSL
Histergan preps P
L-Histidine hydrochloride POM but if for dietary supplementation, P
Histoacryl tissue adhesive P
Hivid tablets POM
Hollister premium powder POM
Hollister universal remover wipes POM
Hollister skin gel protective dressing wipes POM
Holy Thistle (cnicus benedictus), up to 1.5g (MD) GSL
Homatropine POM but if internal 0.15mg (MD) 0.45mg (MDD); external (except ophthalmic), P
Homatropine hydrobromide POM but if 0.2mg (MD) 0.6mg (MDD), P
Homatropine methylbromide POM but if 2mg (MD) 6mg (MDD), P
Honey, Purified GSL
Honvan preparations POM
Hops (lupulus) GSL
Horehound, white GSL
Hormonin tablets POM
Horse-chestnut (Aesculus), external use only GSL
Horseradish GSL
HRF Ayerst ampoules POM
HRI preparations GSL
Humaject M3 POM
Humaject S POM
Humalog KwikPen POM
Humalog vials and cartridges POM
Human Insulins POM
Humatrope injection CD Anab POM
Humegon injection POM
Humiderm cream P
Humira injection POM
Humulin insulins POM
Hyalase POM
Hyalgan inj POM
Hyaluronidase POM
Hycamtin POM
Hycamtin powder for infusion POM
Hycosan eye drops GSL
Hydergine tablets POM
Hydralazine hydrochloride POM
Hydrangea GSL
Hydrargaphen POM but if for local application to skin, P
Hydrea capsules POM
Hydrex spray GSL
Hydrex surgical scrub GSL
Hydrex peri-operative skin disinfection

GSL
Hydrobromic acid POM
Hydrocare protein remover tabs GSL
Hydrochlorothiazide POM
Hydrocodone; its salts CD POM
Hydrocortisone POM but if external for use either alone or in conjunction with crotamiton in irritant dermatitis, contact allergic dermatitis, insect bite reactions, mild to moderate eczema, and either in combination with clotrimazole or miconazole nitrate for athlete's foot and candidal intertrigo or in combination with lignocaine for anal and perianal itch associated with haemorrhoids in adults and children not less than 10 years, maximum strength 1.0 per cent cream, ointment or spray and container or package contains not more than 15g of medicinal product (cream or ointment) or 30ml (spray), P; if in combination with nystatin for intertrigo, in adults and children not less than 10 years with a maximum strength of 0.5 per cent, P; if for external use in combination with lidocaine hydrochloride for the symptomatic relief of anal and perianal itch, irritation and pain associated with external haemorrhoids in adults and children aged 16 years and over, in a non-pressurised spray with a maximum strength of 0.2 per cent and a maximum pack size 30ml of product, GSL; if for external use for the treatment of insect bite and sting reactions only, in adults and children aged 10 years and over, in a cream with maximum strength of 1 per cent and a maximum pack size of 10g of product, GSL
Hydrocortisone 17-butyrate POM
Hydrocortisone acetate POM but if external for use in irritant dermatitis, contact allergic dermatitis, insect bite reactions, mild to moderate eczema, and in combination with one or more of the following: benzyl benzoate, bismuth oxide, bismuth subgallate, Peru Balsam, pramoxine hydrochloride, zinc oxide, for haemorrhoids or in combination with miconazole nitrate for athletes foot and intertrigo in adults and children not less than 10 years, cream, ointment or suppositories, maximum strength equivalent to 1.0 per cent hydrocortisone and container or package contains not more than 15g of medicinal product; in the case of suppositories, container or package containing no more than 12, P
Hydrocortisone butyrate POM
Hydrocortisone caprylate POM
Hydrocortisone cream (Vantage) P
Hydrocortisone hydrogen succinate POM
Hydrocortisone sodium phosphate POM
Hydrocortisone sodium succinate POM but if external for aphthous ulceration of the mouth for adults and children not less than 12 years in the form of pellets, maximum strength equivalent to 2.5mg hydrocortisone and container or package contains not more than equivalent to 50mg of hydrocortisone, P
Hydrocortistab injection POM
Hydrocortisyl preparations POM
Hydrocortone preparations POM
Hydrocyanic acid POM
Hydroflumethiazide POM
Hydrogen peroxide, external use only GSL
Hydromol Intensive emollient cream GSL

Hydromol preparations GSL
Hydromorphinol; its salts; its esters and ethers; their salts CD POM
Hydromorphone; its salts; its esters and ethers; their salts CD POM
Hydromycin-D ear/eye preparations POM
HydroSaluric tablets POM
Hydrotalcite GSL
Hydrous ointment BP GSL
3-Hydroxy-5a-androstan-17-one CD Anab POM
Hydroxocobalamin POM
4-Hydroxy-n-butyric acid see Gammahydroxy-butyrate (GHB)
Hydroxycarbamide/Hydroxyurea POM
Hydroxychloroquine sulphate POM but if for prophylaxis of malaria, P
2-(3-hydroxycyclohexyl)phenol structurally derived compounds by substitution at the 5-position of the phenolic ring by alkyl, alkenyl, cycloalkylmethyl, cycloalkylethyl or 2-(4-morpholinyl)ethyl, whether or not further substituted in the cyclohexyl ring to any extent CD Lic
9-(Hydroxymethyl)-6, 6-dimethyl-3-(2-methyloctan-2-yl)-6a, 7, 10, 10a-tetrahydrobenzo[c]chromen-1-ol CD Lic
[9-Hydroxy-6-methyl-3-[5-phenylpentan-2-yl] oxy-5, 6, 6a, 7, 8, 9, 10, 10a-octahydrophenanthridin-1-yl] acetate CD Lic
Hydroxypethidine; its salts; its esters and ethers; their salts CD POM
Hydroxyprogesterone POM
Hydroxyprogesterone caproate/ Hydroxyprogesterone hexanoate POM
Hydroxyprogesterone enanthate POM
Hydroxyprogesterone hexanoate see Hydroxyprogesterone caproate
N-Hydroxy-tenamfetamine CD Lic
Hydroxyurea see Hydroxycarbamide
Hydroxyzine embonate POM
Hydroxyzine hydrochloride POM but if (1) For the management of pruritis associated with acute or chronic urticaria or atopic dermatitis or contact dermatitis, in adults and in children not less than 12 years, 25mg (MD) 75mg (MDD) and container or package contains not more than 750mg of hydroxyzine hydrochloride; (2) For the management of pruritis associated with acute or chronic urticaria or atopic dermatitis or contact dermatitis, in children not less than 6 years but less than12 years, 25 mg (MD) 50mg (MDD) and container or package contains not more than 750mg of hydroxyzine hydrochloride, P
Hygroton tablets POM
Hymosa biocream GSL
Hyoscine POM, but if internal maximum strength 0.15 per cent; external (except ophthalmic), for the prevention of travel sickness symptoms, for use in adults and children aged 10 years or over, maximum strength 1.5mg per patch, maximum pack size 2 patches, P, please refer to proprietary names for the classification granted under the marketing authorisation (See Scopoderm preparations)
Hyoscine butylbromide POM but if (1) Internal, (a) by inhaler, (b) otherwise than by inhaler 20mg (MD) 80mg (MDD) and container or package contains not more than 240mg of hyoscine butylbromide; (2) External, P
Hyoscine hydrobromide POM but if (1) internal (a) by inhaler, (b)otherwise than by inhaler 300mcg (MD) 900mcg (MDD); (2) external (except

ophthalmic), P

Hyoscine methobromide POM but if (1) internal (a) by inhaler (b) otherwise than by inhaler 2.5mg (MD) 7.5mg (MDD); (2) external, P

Hyoscine methonitrate POM but if (1) internal (a) by inhaler (b) otherwise than by inhaler, 2.5mg (MD) 7.5mg (MDD); (2) external, P

Hyoscyamine POM but if (1) internal (a) by inhaler (b) otherwise than by inhaler 300mcg (MD) 1mg (MDD); (2) external, P

Hyoscyamine hydrobromide POM but if (1) internal (a) by inhaler (b) otherwise than by inhaler, equivalent of 300mcg of hyoscyamine (MD) equivalent of 1mg of hyoscyamine (MDD); (2) external, P

Hyoscyamine sulphate POM but if (1) internal (a) by inhaler (b) otherwise than by inhaler equivalent of 300mcg of hyoscyamine (MD) equivalent of 1mg of hyoscyamine (MDD); (2) external, P

Hypaque inj/bottle POM

Hypaque sodium powder P

Hypericum (St John's wort), external use only GSL

Hypnomidate POM

Hypnovel injection CD No Register POM

Hypolar Retard POM

Hypolar XL POM

Hypophosphorous acid, external use only GSL

Hypotears P

Hypovase tablets POM

Hypromellose eye drops BPC P

Hypurin insulins POM

Hyssop GSL

Hyteneze tabs POM

Hytrin BPH tablets POM

Hytrin tablets POM

I

Ibandronic acid POM

Ibufac tabs POM

Ibufem tabs GSL

Ibugel P

Ibugel Forte POM

Ibuleve preps P

Ibuleve Speed Relief Gel GSL

Ibumousse P

Ibuprofen POM but if for internal use in rheumatic and muscular pain, backache, neuralgia, migraine, headache, dental pain, dysmenorrhoea, feverishness, symptoms of colds and influenza and either a controlled release preparation with md 600mg and mdd 1,200mg or any other internal preparation with md 400mg and mdd 1,200mg P; or if tablets, capsules, powder or granules for internal use with ms 200mg, md 400mg and mdd 1,200mg in individual containers or packages containing no more than 16 tablets or capsules, or 12 sachets for use in adults and children over 12 years GSL; or if liquid preparations for internal use, maximum strength 2.0%, for the treatment of rheumatic or muscular pain, headache, dental pain, feverishness, or symptoms of colds and influenza for use in children aged under 12 years, 200mg(MD), 800mg(MDD), in the case of liquid preparations of ibuprofen, individual unit doses of not more than 5 millilitres each to a maximum of 20 unit doses GSL; ibuprofen oral suspension with a strength of 2% or less supplied in multidose containers of not more than 100 millilitres GSL; or if for external use with ms 5% P; or if for external use with ms 10%, md 125mg, mdd 500mg in a

container or package containing not more than 50g of medicinal product P; or if for external use with ms 5%, md 125mg, mdd 500mg and in an individual container or package containing not more than 2.5g, for rheumatic pain, muscular aches and pains, swellings such as strains, sprains and sports injuries for use by adults and children over 12 years GSL

Ibuprofen lysine POM but if for rheumatic and muscular pain, pain of non-serious arthritic conditions, backache, neuralgia, migraine, headache, dental pain, dysmenorrhoea, feverishness, symptoms of colds and influenza, (a) in the case of a prolonged release preparation md 600mg and mdd 1,200mg or (b) in any case md 400mg and mdd 1,200mg P; or if maximum strength equivalent to 200mg ibuprofen, in tablet form, for the treatment of rheumatic or muscular pain, backache, neuralgia, migraine, headache, dental pain, dysmenorrhoea, feverishness or symptoms of colds and influenza in adults and in children aged 12 years and over, (MD) equivalent to 400mg ibuprofen, (MDD) equivalent to 1200mg, in an individual container or package containing not more than 16 tablets GSL

Ibuprofen tablets 12s (Galpharm) GSL

Ibuspray P

Ibutop Cuprofen ibuprofen gel P

Icaps GSL

Iceland Moss GSL

Ichthammol, external use only GSL

Icodextrin POM

Icthaband P

Idarubicin hydrochloride POM

Idoxuridine POM

Idrolax sachets P

Ifosfamide POM

Ignatius Bean POM

Ikorel tablets POM

Iloprost POM

Ilosone preparations POM

Ilube POM

Imatinib POM

Imazin XL tabs P

Imbrilon preparations POM

Imdur tablets P

Imidapril POM

Imiglucerase POM

Imigran preparations POM except Imigran Recovery tablets P

Imipenem hydrochloride POM

Imipramine POM

Imipramine hydrochloride POM

Imipramine ion exchange resin bound salt or complex POM

Imiquimod POM

ImmuCyst POM

Immukin POM

Immunoprin tabs POM

Imo LA POM

Imodium POM except for the treatment of acute diarrhoea P; symptomatic treatment of acute diarrhoea in adults and children aged 12 and over, ms 2mg and 4mg (MD) 12mg (MDD), GSL

Imodium Instants tablets 6s GSL; 12s P

Imodium Plus caplets pack sizes 6s GSL; 12s P

Implanon implant POM

Improvera tablets POM

Imuderm oil GSL

Imunovir tablets POM

Imuran preparations POM

Imuvac POM

Inactivated influenza vaccine POM

Inadine GSL

Increlex POM

Indapamide POM

Indapamide hemihydrate POM

Inderal LA capsules POM

Inderal preparations POM

Inderetic capsules POM

Inderex capsules POM

Indian hemp see Cannabis

Indinavir POM

Indivina tablets POM

Indocid PDA POM

Indocid preparations POM

Indocid-R capsules POM

1H-indol-3-yl-(1-naphthyl)methane structurally derived compounds by substitution at the nitrogen atom of the indole ring by alkyl, alkenyl, cycloalkylmethyl, cycloalkylethyl or 2-(4-morpholinyl)ethyl, whether or not further substituted in the indole ring to any extent and whether or not substituted in the naphthyl ring to any extent CD Lic

Indolar SR capsules POM

Indomax capsules POM

Indomax SR capsules POM

Indometacin/Indomethacin POM

Indometacin/Indomethacin sodium POM

Indomethacin see Indometacin

Indomod capsules POM

Indoprofen POM

Indoramin hydrochloride POM

Indotard MR capsules POM

InductOs POM

Inegy tablets POM

Infacol liquid GSL

Infaderm therapeutic body oil GSL

Infadrops P

Infai test POM

Infanrix preparations POM

Infestat susp POM

Inflexal V POM

Infliximab POM

Influenza vaccine POM

Influvac subunit POM

Infukoll POM

Innohep POM

Innovace Melt wafers POM

Innovace tablets POM

Innozide POM

Inosine Pranobex POM

Inositol GSL

Inositol nicotinate P

Inovelon POM

Inoven Caplets P

Inspra tablets POM

Instillagel gel P

Insulatard insulins POM

Insulin POM

Insuman insulins POM

Intal preps POM

Intanza suspension for injection in pre-filled syringe POM

Integrilin solution POM

Intelence POM

Intrafusin preps POM

Intralgin gel P

Intralipid POM

Intraval sodium preparations POM

Intrinsa CD Anab POM

Intron A inj POM

Invanz infusion POM

Invirase capsules POM

Invivac vaccine POM

Iocare balanced salt solution P

Iodamide POM

Iodamide meglumine POM

Iodamide sodium POM

Iodine tincture GSL

Iodine10mg (MDD) GSL

Iodoflex dressing P

Iodoform, if maximum strength 10 per cent in paints, or maximum strength 50 per cent in pastes (external use only) GSL

Iodophenol, if internal (pastilles, lozenges, throat tablets) maximum strength 0.2mg or external maximum strength 0.08 per cent GSL

Iodosorb ointment P

Iodosorb powder P

Iohexol POM

Iomeprol POM

Ionamin capsules CD No Register POM

Ionax scrub P

Ionil T shampoo P

Iopamidol POM

Iopentol POM

Iopidine Ophthalmic POM

Iothalamic acid POM

Ioversol POM

Ioxaglic acid POM

Ipecacuanha GSL

Ipecacuanha and morphine mix (conc) CD Inv P

Ipocol tablets POM

Ipramol POM

Ipratropium bromide POM

Iprindole hydrochloride POM

Iproniazid phosphate POM

Irbesartan POM

Irinotecan HCl POM

Ironorm preps P

Irriclens GSL

Irripod P

Isclofen tabs POM

Isib preps tabs P

Isisfen tabs POM

Ismelin preparations POM

Ismo preparations P

Ismo Retard tablets P

Ismo tabs P

Iso-lysergamide CD Lic

Isoaminile POM

Isoaminile citrate POM

Isocarboxazid POM

Isocard spray P

Isoconazole nitrate POM but if external and in the case of vaginal use only external use for the treatment of vaginal candidiasis, P

Isodur preparations P

Isoetharine POM

Isoetharine hydrochloride POM

Isoetharine mesylate POM

Isoflurane POM

Isogel granules GSL

Isoket ampoules POM

Isoket Retard tablets P

Isomethadone CD POM

Isomide CR POM

Isoniazid POM

Isopentane, external use only GSL

Isoprenaline hydrochloride POM

Isoprenaline sulphate POM

Isopropamide iodide POM but if equivalent of 2.5mg of isopropamide ion (MD) equivalent of 5.0mg of isopropamide ion (MDD), P

Isopropyl alcohol, external use only GSL

Isopropyl myristate, external use only GSL

Isopropyl palmitate, external use only GSL

Isopto Alkaline P

Isopto Atropine POM

Isopto Carbachol POM

Isopto Carpine POM

Isopto Frin P

Isopto Plain P

Isordil tablets P

Isordil Tembids capsules P

Isosorbide dinitrate P

Isosorbide mononitrate P

Isotard preps P

Isotrat tabs P

Isotrate tabs P

Isotretinoin POM

Isotrex gel POM

Isotrexin gel POM

Isovorin injection POM

Ispagel GSL

Ispaghula GSL

Ispaghula Husk GSL

Isradipine POM

Istin tablets POM

Itraconazole POM

Ivabradine POM
Ivemend powder for solution for
  infusion POM

J

Jaap's GSL
Jaborandi POM but if external, P
Jackson's preparations GSL
Jamaica Dogwood GSL
Januvia POM
Jectofer POM
Jeridin tabs P
Jomethid XL capsules POM
Joyrides P
Juniper GSL
Juniper Oil GSL

K

K/L kaolin poultice P
KL preparations P; except magnesium
  sulphate paste GSL
Kabiglobulin POM
Kabikinase injections POM
Kabimix POM
Kaletra preparations POM
Kalms sleep GSL
Kalspare tablets POM
Kalten capsules POM
Kaltostat P
Kamillosan digital thermometer
  dummy/soother GSL
Kamillosan ointment GSL
Kanamycin acid sulphate POM
Kanamycin sulphate POM
Kannasyn preparations POM
Kao-C GSL
Kao-C Child's diarrhoea mixture GSL
Kaodene suspension CD Inv P
Kaolin and morphine mixture BPC CD
  Inv P
Kaolin mixture paediatric BP GSL
Kaolin poultice BPC P
Kaolin, heavy, external use only GSL
Kaolin, light GSL
Kapake preparations CD Inv POM
Kaplon tabs POM
Karvol dropper bottle GSL
Karvol inhalant capsules GSL
Kay-Cee-L syrup P
Kefadim inj POM
Kefadol vials POM
Keflex preparations POM
Keftid capsules POM
Kefzol vials POM
Kelfizine W preparations POM
Keloc SR tablets POM
Kelp GSL
Kemadrin preparations POM
Kemicetine preparations POM
Kenalog injection POM
Kentene caps POM
Kentera POM
Kepivance powder for solution for injec-
  tion POM
Keppra preparations POM
Keral tablets POM
Keri Therapeutic lotion P
Kerlone tablets POM
Ketalar injections CD Benz POM
Ketamine CD Benz POM
Ketanodur tabs POM
Ketazolam CD Benz POM
Ketek tablets POM
Ketil caps POM
Ketobemidone; its salts; its esters and
  ethers; their salts CD POM
Ketocid 200mg caps POM
Ketoconazole POM but if external maxi-
  mum strength 2.0 per cent (a) for the
  prevention and treatment of dandruff
  and seborrhoeic dermatitis of the
  scalp in the form of a shampoo, max-
  imum frequency of application of
  once every 3 days and container or
  package contains not more than
  120ml of medicinal product and con-

taining not more than 2,400mg of
ketoconazole; (b) for the treatment of
the following mycotic infections of
the skin: tinea pedis, tinea cruris and
candidal intertrigo, please refer to
proprietary names for classification
granted under the marketing authorisation (see Dandrazol and Nizoral
products); (c) for the prevention and
treatment of dandruff, in the form of
a shampoo, maximum pack size
100ml GSL; (d) for the treatment of
the following mycotic infection of
the skin: tinea pedis and tinea cruris,
in the form of a cream, maximum
pack size 30g GSL
Ketopine 60ml and 100ml GSL; 120ml
  POM
Ketoprofen POM but if external for rheumatic and muscular pain in adults
  and children not less than 12 for
  maximum period of 7 days, maxi-
  mum strength 2.5 per cent and con-
  tainer or package contains not more
  than 30g of medicinal product, P
Ketorolac trometamol POM
Ketotard 200XL caps POM
Ketotifen fumarate POM
Ketovail caps POM
Ketovite (Supplement) liquid P
Ketovite tablets POM
Ketozip XL 200mg caps POM
Ketpron POM
Ketpron XL caps POM
Kiflone preps POM
Kilkof GSL
Kilkof mix GSL
Kineret injection POM
Kinidin Durules POM
Kivexa POM
KL kaolin preparations P
KL magnesium sulphate paste GSL
Klaricid POM
Klaricid IV POM
Klaricid Paediatric POM
Klaricid XL tablets POM
Klean-Prep sachets P
Kliofem tablets POM
Kliovance tablets POM
Kloref tablets P
Kloref-S sachets P
Kogenate Bayer injection POM
Kogenate vials POM
Kola GSL
Kolanticon gel P
Komil 5/40 tablets POM
Konakion ampoules POM
Konakion MM injection POM
Konakion MM Paediatric POM
Konakion tablets POM
Konsyl powder GSL
Kuvan soluble tablets POM
Kwells tablets P
Kytril preparations POM

L

Labetalol hydrochloride POM
Labiton tonic GSL
Labosept pastilles P
Labrador tea, external use only GSL
Lachesine chloride POM
Lacidipine POM
Lacri-Lube ointment P
Lactic acid, external use only GSL
Lacticare GSL
Lactitol P
Lacto-calamine lotion GSL
Lactugal liquid P
Ladropen preps POM
Lady's Mantle GSL
Lamictal POM
Lamictal chewable and dispersible
  tablets POM
Laminaria GSL
Lamisil AT cream GSL

Lamisil AT gel P
Lamisil AT spray GSL
Lamisil cream POM except OTC 15g GSL
Lamisil Once solution P
Lamisil tablets POM
Lamivudine POM
Lamotrigine POM
Lamprene capsules POM
Lanacane cream GSL
Lanacort cream (PL 3157/0008) P
Lanacort ointment (PL 3157/0011) P
Lanatoside C POM
Lanatoside Complex A, B and C POM
Langdale's tablets GSL
Lanolin BP GSL
Lanoxin preparations POM
Lanoxin-PG preparations POM
Lanreotide POM
Lansoprazole POM
Lantus injection POM
Lanvis tablets POM
Lappa (Burdock) GSL
Laractone tablets POM
Larafen CR caps 200mg POM
Larapam preparations POM
Laratrim preps POM
Largactil Forte suspension POM
Largactil preparations POM
Lariam tablets POM
Laronidase POM
Laryng-O-Jet POM
Lasikal tablets POM
Lasilactone capsules POM
Lasix + K POM
Lasix preparations POM
Lasma tablets P
Lasonil ointment P
Lasoride tablets POM
Latanoprost POM
Latanoprost eye drops POM
Lauromacrogols, external use only GSL
Lauryl alcohol, ethoxylated, external use
  only GSL
Lavender oil GSL
Laxoberal P
Laxose P
Lecithin, internal use GSL
Ledclair injection POM
Lederfen preparations POM
Lederfolin injection POM
Lederfolin solution POM
Ledermycin capsules POM
Lederspan injections POM
Lefetamine; it salts CD POM
Leflunomide POM
Lemlax (lactulose) P
Lemon GSL
Lemon oil GSL
Lemsip preparations GSL except Cold &
  Flu sinus 12hr (ibuprofen and pseu-
  doephedrine) P
Lemsip max preparations GSL except
  Lemsip Max Flu 12hr (ibuprofen and
  pseudoephedrine) P
Lenium P
Lenograstim see Granocyte
Lentard MC insulin POM
Lentaron depot POM
Lentaron injection POM
Lentizol capsules POM
Lepirudin injection POM
Lercanidipine hydrochloride POM
Lercanidipine tablets POM
Lescol POM
Lescol XL tablets POM
Letrozole POM
Letrozole tablets POM
Lettuce (Lactuca sativa) GSL
Leucomax injection POM
Leucovorin POM
Leukeran tablets POM
Leuprorelin acetate preparations POM
Leustat POM
Levallorphan tartrate POM
Levemir preparations POM
Levetiracetam POM
Levitra tablets POM
Levobunolol hydrochloride POM

Levobupivacaine POM
Levocabastine hydrochloride POM but if
  maximum strength equivalent of 0.05
  per cent levocabastine (1) nasal
  sprays for the symptomatic treatment
  of seasonal allergic rhinitis and container or package contains not more
  than 10ml of medicinal product; (2)
  aqueous eye drops for the symptomatic treatment of seasonal allergic
  conjunctivitis and container or package contains not more than 4ml of
  medicinal product, P
Levocetirizine tablets POM
Levodopa POM
Levofloxacin preparations POM
Levomepromazine/Methotrimeprazine
  POM
Levomepromazine/Methotrimeprazine
  maleate POM
Levomethorphan; its salts CD POM
Levomoramide; its salts CD POM
Levonelle 1500 POM
Levonelle One-Step P
Levonorgestrel POM but if maximum
  strength 1.5mg and for use as an
  emergency contraceptive in women
  aged 16 years and over P
Levophed POM
Levophenacylmorphan; its salts, esters
  and ethers CD POM
Levorphanol; its salts, esters and ethers
  CD POM
Levothyroxine sodium/thyroxine sodi-
  um POM
Lexotan tablets CD Benz POM
Lexpec syrup POM
Lexpec syrup with Iron POM
Lexpec syrup with Iron-M POM
LH see Luteinising Hormone
LH-RH see Gonadorelin
Li-liquid POM
Libanil tablets POM
Liberim HB POM
Liberim T POM
Liberim Z POM
Libetist syrup POM
Librium preparations CD Benz POM
Librofem tablets pack sizes 12s GSL; 24s
  P
Lidifen tablets POM
Lidocaine/Lignocaine POM but for non-
  ophthalmic use, P; internal (teething
  gel maximum strength 0.6 per cent)
  or external maximum strength 2.0
  per cent, except local ophthalmic use,
  in adults and in children aged 12
  years and over, GSL
Lidocaine/Lignocaine hydrochloride
  POM but if non-ophthalmic use, P;
  internal (teething gel maximum
  strength 0.7 per cent) or external
  (except local ophthalmic use maximum strength 0.7 per cent), or external (except local ophthalmic use for
  adults and children aged 12 years and
  over, all preparations except sprays,
  maximum strength 2.0 per cent) GSL,
  or external (except local opthalmic
  use for adults and children aged 16
  years and over, in combination with
  hydrocortisone for symptomatic relief
  of anal and perianal itch, irritation
  and pain associated with external
  haemorrhoids, in a non pressurised
  spray with a maximum strength of
  1%) GSL, please refer to proprietary
  names for the classification granted
  under the marketing authorisation
  (See Germoloids HC products)
Lidoflazine POM
Light liquid paraffin, external use only
  GSL
Lignocaine see Lidocaine
Lignospan POM
Lignostab injection POM
Lignostab-A injection POM
Limclair injection POM

Lime Oil GSL
Lincomycin POM
Lincomycin hydrochloride POM
Lingraine tablets POM
Linseed GSL
Linseed oil, external use only GSL
Linus powder GSL
Lioresal intrathecal POM
Lioresal liquid POM
Lioresal tablets POM
Liothyronine sodium POM
Lipantil capsules POM
Lipantil Micro capsules POM
Lipase POM
Lipiodol Ultra fluid P
Lipitor tablets POM
Lipobase P
Lipobay tablets POM
Lipofundin S POM
Liposic P
Liposomal Daunorubicin POM
Liposomal Doxorubicin Citrate POM
Lipostat tablets POM
Lippes Loop intrauterine contraceptive device POM
Liprinal capsules POM
Liqufruta cough medicines GSL
Liqui-Char P
Liquifilm Tears P
Liquivisc gel P
Liquorice GSL
Liquorice extract deglycyrrhizinised GSL
Lisicostad tablets POM
Lisinopril POM
Liskonum tablets POM
Lisuride/Lysuride maleate POM
Litarex tablets POM
Lithium carbonate POM but if equivalent of 5mg of lithium (MD) equivalent of 15mg of lithium (MDD), P
Lithium citrate POM
Lithium succinate POM
Lithium sulphate POM but if equivalent of 5mg of lithium (MD) equivalent of 15mg of lithium (MDD), P
Lithonate POM
Liver extract GSL
Livial tablets POM
Livostin Direct P
Livostin eye drops POM
Livostin nasal spray POM
Lloyd's cream GSL
Lobelia, up to 65mg (MD) GSL
Lobeline POM but if internal 3mg (MD) 9mg (MDD); external, P
Lobeline hydrochloride POM but if internal equivalent of 3mg of lobeline (MD) equivalent of 9mg of lobeline (MDD); external, P
Lobeline sulphate POM but if internal equivalent of 3mg of lobeline (MD) equivalent of 9mg of lobeline (MDD); external, P
Locabiotal aerosol POM
Loceryl cream POM
Loceryl nail lacquer POM
Locoid C preparations POM
Locoid Crelo POM
Locoid Lipocream POM
Locoid preparations POM
Locorten-Vioform ear drops POM
Lodiar POM
Lodine preparations POM
Lodine SR tablets POM
Lodoxamide trometamol POM but if maximum strength equivalent of 0.1% lodoxamide, for the treatment of ocular signs and symptoms of allergic conjunctivitis, in adults and in children aged 4 years and over P
Loestrin 20 tablets POM
Loestrin 30 tablets POM
Lofensaid preparations POM
Lofentanil; its stereoisomers, salts, esters and ethers CD Lic
Lofepramine POM
Lofepramine hydrochloride POM
Lofexidine hydrochloride POM

Logynon ED tablets POM
Logynon tablets POM
Lomefloxacin hydrochloride POM
Lomexin pessaries POM
Lomont POM
Lomotil preparations CD Inv POM
Lomustine POM
Loniten tablets POM
Lopace POM
LoperaGen capsules POM
Loperamide hydrochloride POM; but if for treatment of acute diarrhoea, P; symptomatic treatment of acute diarrhoea, in adults and children aged 12 years and over, maximum strength 2mg and 4mg (MD) 12mg (MDD) maximum pack size 6 tablets or capsules GSL; or for the symptomatic treatment of acute episodes of diarrhoea associated with irritable bowel syndrome in adults aged 18 years and over following initial diagnosis by a doctor, maximum strength 2mg, 4mg (MD),12mg (MDD) maximum pack size 6 tablets or capsules GSL
Lopid preparations POM
Lopinavir POM
Lopranol LA POM
Loprazolam CD Benz POM
Lopresor SR tablets POM
Lopresor tablets POM
Loratadine POM; but if 10mg (MDD) P; or if maximum strength 10mg, in tablet form for the symptomatic relief of perennial rhinitis, seasonal allergic rhinitis and idiopathic chronic urticaria, in adults and children aged 2 years and over and weighing 30kg or more, 10mg (MDD), in an individual container or package containing not more than 14 tablets GSL
Lorazepam CD Benz POM
Lormetazepam CD Benz POM
Lornoxicam POM
Loron preparations POM
Losartan POM
Losartan potassium POM
Losec preparations POM
Lotemax eye drops POM
Lotriderm cream POM
Loxapac capsules POM
Loxapine succinate POM
LSD see Lysergide
Luborant Saliva P
Lubri-Tears ointment P
Lucentis POM
Lucerne (Alfalfa) GSL
Ludiomil tablets POM
Lumigan eye-drops POM
Lung Surfactant Porcine POM
Lungwort GSL
Lustral tablets POM
Lustys preparations GSL
Luteinising hormone POM
Luveris POM
Luvinsta XL tablets
Lyclear preparations P
Lyflex POM
Lymecycline POM
Lynoestrenol POM
Lypressin POM
Lypsyl preparations GSL
Lyrica capsules POM
Lyrinel XL POM
Lysergamide; its salts CD Lic
Lysergide and other N-alkyl derivatives of lysergamide; their salts CD Lic
Lysine hydrochloride GSL
Lysodren POM
Lysovir capsules POM
Lysuride see Lisuride

M

M&M tulle GSL
Maalox Plus tablets and suspension GSL
Maalox suspension GSL
MabCampath preparations POM

Mabron tablets POM
Mabthera vials POM
Mac Throat lozenges GSL
MacKenzies smelling salts GSL
Macrobid capsules POM
Macrodantin capsules POM
Macrogol P
Macugen injection POM
Madopar CR capsules POM
Madopar preparations POM
Mafenide POM
Mafenide acetate POM
Mafenide hydrochloride POM
Mafenide propionate POM but if eye drops maximum strength 5.0 per cent, P
Magaldrate GSL
Magnapen preparations POM
Magnesia, cream of (Magnesium hydroxide) GSL
Magnesium alginate GSL
Magnesium carbonate, heavy GSL
Magnesium carbonate, light GSL
Magnesium citrate P
Magnesium fluoride POM
Magnesium glycerophosphate GSL
Magnesium hydroxide GSL
Magnesium metrizoate POM
Magnesium oxide, heavy GSL
Magnesium oxide, light GSL
Magnesium phosphate GSL
Magnesium stearate GSL
Magnesium sulphate GSL
Magnesium sulphate paste GSL
Magnesium trisilicate GSL
Magnesium trisilicate compound tablets BPC GSL
Magnesium trisilicate mixture BP GSL
Magnesium trisilicate oral powder BP GSL
Maize GSL
Malarivon syrup POM but if for the prevention of malaria P
Malarone Paediatric tablets POM
Malarone tablets POM
Malathion P
Malix tablets POM
Maloprim tablets POM
Malt Extract GSL
Malted Milk GSL
Maltose GSL
Mandafen ibuprofen suspension P
Mandafen ibuprofen 400mg tablets pack sizes 24s, 48s, 84s P; 250s POM
Mandafen ibuprofen 600mg tablets pack sizes 100s POM
Mandalyn preparations P
Mandanol 6+ suspension SF P
Mandanol caplets blister pack 500mg pack sizes 16s GSL; 32s P
Mandanol infant suspension SF P
Mandanol Plus P
Mandanol tablets 500mg pack sizes 32s PO; 100s POM
Mandanol tablets blister pack 500mg pack sizes 16s GSL; 32s PO
Mandragora Autumnalis POM
Manerix tablets POM
Manevac granules P
Manganese glycerophosphate, if MDD equivalent to 1mg elemental manganese GSL
Manganese sulphate, if MDD equivalent to 1mg elemental manganese GSL
Mannitol injection POM
Mannomustine hydrochloride POM
Manorfen P
Manusept antibacterial hand rub GSL
Maprotiline hydrochloride POM
Marcain injection POM
Marcain Polyamp Steripak POM
Marcain with Adrenaline injection POM
Marevan tablets POM
Marshmallow Root GSL
Marvelon tablets POM
Masculine balance GSL
Masnoderm cream P
Mastaflu POM

Mastic, external use only GSL
Mate GSL
Matricaria (German Chamomile) GSL
Matrifen patches CD POM
Maxalt preparations POM
Maxepa capsules and liquid P
Maxidex eye drops POM
Maximet capsules POM
Maxitrol preparations POM
Maxivent POM
Maxolon preparations POM
Maxolon SR capsules POM
Maxtrex tablets POM
Mazindol CD No Register POM
MCR 50 capsules P
Meadow Sweet GSL
Measles vaccine (live attenuated) POM
Mebanazine POM
Mebendazole POM but for oral use in the treatment of enterobiasis in adults and in children not less than 2 years, 100mg (MD) and container or package contains not more than 800mg of Mebendazole, P
Mebeverine hydrochloride POM but if (a) for the symptomatic relief of irritable bowel syndrome 135mg (MD) 405mg (MDD); (b) for uses other than the symptomatic relief of irritable bowel syndrome 100mg (MD) 300mg (MDD), P
Mebeverine pamoate POM
Mebhydrolin POM
Mebhydrolin napadisylate POM
Mebolazine CD Anab POM
Mecamylamine hydrochloride POM
Mecillinam POM
Meclofenoxate hydrochloride POM
Mecloqualone CD POM
Meclozine P
Medazepam CD Benz POM
Medi-Test preparations GSL
Medical Interporous GSL
Medicinal opium CD POM but if in, (a) any preparations from which the opium cannot be readily recovered in amounts which constitute a risk to health and with ms 0.2% (calculated as anhydrous morphine base) CD Inv POM; (b) if in a powder containing 10% opium, 10 % ipecacuanha root and 80% of another powdered ingredient (not a controlled drug) CD Inv POM; (c) if for non-parenteral use in unit preparations diluted to at least one part in a million (6X) in response to a specific request, CD Inv P; or (d) if for non-parenteral use in unit preparations diluted to at least one part in a million million (6C), CD Inv P
Medicoal GSL
Medicoal granules P
Medicross burn gel sachets GSL
Medijel gel GSL
Medijel pastilles P
Medikinet IR CD POM
Medikinet XL CD POM
Medinex P
Medinol Over 6 P
Medinol Paediatric P
Medinol Under 6 P
Medised suspension P
Medocodene 30/500 capsules CD Inv POM
Medomet preparations POM
Medrone preparations POM
Medroxyprogesterone acetate POM
Mefenamic acid POM
Mefenorex; its salts; its stereoisomers; their salts CD Benz POM
Meflam preparations POM
Mefloquine hydrochloride POM
Mefoxin injection POM
Mefruside POM
Megace tablets POM
Megestrol acetate POM
Meggezones lozenges GSL

Meglumine iothalamate POM
Melaleuca oil, external use only GSL
Melleril preparations POM
Meloxicam POM
Melphalan hydrochloride POM
Meltus adult chesty coughs (original and SF/colour free) GSL
Meltus adult dry coughs P
Meltus baby cough linctus GSL
Meltus decongestant P
Meltus junior chesty coughs GSL
Meltus junior dry coughs P
Meltus adult chesty coughs and congestion P
Meltus family honey & lemon GSL
Memantine POM
Mendys capsules POM
Mengivac (A+C) POM
Meningitec POM
Meningococcal Polysaccharide Vaccine POM
Menitorix POM
Menjugate POM
Menogon POM
Menopur POM
Menorest Transdermal patches POM
Menoring 50 POM
Menotrophin POM
Menthodex mixture GSL
Menthodex original lozenges GSL
Menthol GSL
Menthol and eucalyptus inhalation GSL
Menthol BP GSL
Mentholatum Antiseptic lozenge GSL
Mentholatum Deep Heat max strength 35g GSL
Mentholatum Deep Heat spray GSL
Mentholatum ibuprofen gel pack sizes 50g GSL; 100g P
Mentholatum Rub GSL
Mentholatum Vapour rub GSL
Menthyl valerate up to 100mg (MS), 200mg (MD) GSL
Menveo vaccine POM
Menyanthes (bogbean, buckbean) GSL
Mepitiostane CD Anab POM
Mepivacaine hydrochloride POM but any use except ophthalmic use, P
Mepradec POM
Mepranix POM
Meprate tablets CD No Register POM
Meprobamate CD No Register POM
Meptazinol POM
Meptid injection POM
Meptid tablets POM
Mepyramine maleate, if external use for the symptomatic relief of insect stings and bites, and nettle stings and jellyfish stings, in adults and children aged two years and over and maximum strength 2.0% in a pack containing no more than 22g of the product GSL
Mequitazine POM
Merbentyl syrup POM
Merbentyl tablets POM
Mercaptamine bitartrate POM
Mercaptopurine POM
Mercilon tablets POM
Merieux vaccine POM
Merional injection POM
Merocaine lozenges P
Merocet lozenges GSL
Merocets Plus GSL
Meronem preparations POM
Meropenem POM
Mersalyl POM
Mersalyl acid POM
Mesabolone CD Anab POM
Mesalazine POM
Mesna POM
Mesocarb CD Benz POM
Mesren MR POM
Mesterolone CD Anab POM
Mestinon preparations POM
Mestranol POM
Metalyse injection POM
Metanium cradle cap cream GSL

Metanium ointment GSL
Metaraminol tartrate POM
Metastron (radioactive isotope) POM
Metatone tonic GSL
Metazocine; its salts; its esters and ethers; their salts CD POM
Meted shampoo P
Metenix 5 tablets POM
Meterfolic tablets P
Metergoline POM
Metformin hydrochloride POM
Methacycline POM
Methacycline calcium POM
Methacycline hydrochloride POM
Methadole see Dimepheptanol
Methadone; its salts CD POM
Methadose diluent POM
Methadose oral concentrate CD POM
Methadyl acetate; its salts CD POM
Methallenoestril POM
Methamphetamine see Methylamfetamine
Methandienone CD Anab POM
Methandriol CD Anab POM
Methaqualone; its salts CD POM
Metharose CD POM
Methcathinone CD Lic
Methenamine hippurate P
Methenolone CD Anab POM
Methenolone enanthate CD Anab POM
Methex CD POM
Methicillin sodium POM
Methixene POM
Methixene hydrochloride POM
Methocarbamol POM
Methocidin POM but if throat lozenges and throat pastilles, P
Methohexital see Methohexitone
Methohexitone sodium POM
Methoin POM
Methoserpidine POM
Methotrexate POM
Methotrexate sodium POM
Methotrimeprazine see Levomepromazine
Methoxamine hydrochloride POM but if nasal sprays or nasal drops not containing liquid paraffin as a vehicle maximum strength 0.25 per cent, P
Methoxymethane, external use only GSL
Methsuximide POM
Methyclothiazide POM
Methyl cellulose GSL
Methyl nicotinate, external use only GSL
Methyl salicylate, if internal (nasal inhalations except aerosols) or internal (pastilles, lozenges, throat tablets maximum strength 1mg) or external GSL
Methylamfetamine; its salts CD POM
4-Methyl-aminorex CD Lic
4-Methylmethcathinone CD Lic
Methylated spirits industrial, if external use or internal (nasal inhalations to be inhaled from a handkerchief or other soft material) GSL
Methylbenzethonium chloride, external use only GSL
Methylcysteine P
Methyldesorphine; its salts; its esters and ethers; their salts CD POM
Methyldihydromorphine (6-methyldihydromorphine); its salts; its esters and ethers; their salts CD POM
Methyldihydromorphinone see Metopon
Methyldopa POM
Methyldopa hydrochloride POM
Methylephedrine hydrochloride POM but if 30mg (MD) 60mg (MDD), P
2-Methyl-3-morpholino-1,1-diphenyl-propanecarboxylic acid; its salts, ethers and esters CD POM
Methylphenidate; its salts CD POM
Methylphenobarbital/Methylphenobarbitone CD No Register POM
Methylphenobarbitone see Methylphenobarbital
1-Methyl-4-phenylpiperidine-4-car-

boxylic acid CD POM
Methylprednisolone POM
Methylprednisolone acetate POM
Methylprednisolone sodium succinate POM
Methyltestosterone CD Anab POM
Methylthiouracil POM
Methyprylone CD No Register POM
Methysergide maleate POM
Metipranolol POM
Metirosine POM
Metoclopramide hydrochloride POM
Metoject POM
Metolazone POM
Metomidate hydrochloride POM
Metopirone capsules POM
Metopon; its salts; its esters and ethers; their salts CD POM
Metoprolol fumarate POM
Metoprolol succinate POM
Metoprolol tartrate POM
Metosyn FAPG cream POM
Metosyn FAPG ointment POM
Metosyn ointment POM
Metosyn scalp lotion POM
Metribolone CD Anab POM
Metrodin High Purity POM
Metrogel POM
Metrolyl preparations POM
Metronidazole POM
Metronidazole benzoate POM
Metrosa POM
Metrotop gel POM
Metrozol IV inf POM
Metsol POM
Metvix cream POM
Metyrapone POM
Mexenone, external use only GSL
Mexiletine hydrochloride POM
Mexitil POM
Mezlocilin sodium POM
Miacalcic injection POM
Mianserin hydrochloride POM
Mibolerone CD Anab POM
Micanol cream 1 per cent P
Micanol cream 3 per cent POM
Micardis tablets POM
MicardisPlus tablets POM
Micolette Micro-enema P
Miconazole POM but if external and in the case of vaginal use only external use for the treatment of vaginal candidiasis, P; in the case of creams or powders, including spray powders for the treatment of tinea pedis (athlete's foot) only maximum strength 2.0% (for spray powders this shall be weight for weight excluding any propellants) GSL
Miconazole nitrate POM but if external and in the case of vaginal use only external use for the treatment of vaginal candidiasis, P
Micralax Micro-enema P
Microcrystalline wax, external use only GSL
Microgynon 30 tablets POM
Microgynon ED tablets POM
Micronor HRT tablets POM
Micronor tablets POM
Micropirin P
Microval tablets POM
Mictral granules POM
Midazolam CD No Reg POM
Midrid capsules pack sizes 15s P; 30s POM
Mifegyne tablets POM
Mifepristone POM
Migard tablets POM
Miglitol POM
Miglustat POM
Migrafen tablets P
Migraleve pack sizes 12s, 24s CD Inv P; 48s CD Inv POM
Migramax sachets POM
Migranal nasal spray POM
Migravess forte tablets POM
Migravess tablets POM

Migril tablets POM
Mildison Lipocream POM
Milk of Magnesia liquid GSL
Milk of Magnesia tablets GSL
Milpar P
Milrinone POM
Milrinone lactate POM
Mimpara tablets POM
Min-I-Jet preparations POM except Min-I-Jet morphine CD POM
Minalka GSL
Minihep ampoules POM
Minihep-Calcium injection POM
Minims amethocaine hydrochloride POM
Minims artificial tears P
Minims atropine sulphate POM
Minims benoxinate (oxybuprocaine) hydrochloride POM
Minims chloramphenicol POM
Minims cyclopentolate hydrochloride POM
Minims dexamethasone POM
Minims ephedrine hydrochloride P
Minims fluorescein sodium P
Minims gentamicin P
Minims homatropine hydrobromide POM
Minims hyoscine hydrobromide POM
Minims lidocaine and fluorescein POM
Minims metipranolol POM
Minims neomycin sulphate POM
Minims oxybuprocaine POM
Minims phenylephrine hydrochloride P
Minims pilocarpine nitrate POM
Minims prednisolone POM
Minims proxymetacaine POM
Minims proxymetacaine and fluorescein POM
Minims Rose Bengal P
Minims sodium chloride P
Minims tetracaine POM
Minims tetracaine hydrochloride POM
Minims tropicamide POM
Minitran patches P
Minocin MR capsules POM
Minocin tablets POM
Minocycline POM
Minocycline hydrochloride POM
Minodiab tablets POM
Minoxidil POM; but (1) if for external use, maximum strength 5%, for the treatment of alopecia androgenetica in men aged 18 to 65 (but not women) P; (2) if for external use, maximum strength 2% P; (3) if for external use for the treatment of alopecia androgenetica in men and women aged between 18 and 65 years, in a solution or gel with a maximum strength 2% and a maximum pack size of 60ml, GSL, please refer to proprietary names for classification granted under the marketing authorisation (see Regaine products)
Mintec capsules GSL
Mintezol tablets POM
Minulet tablets POM
Miochol E POM
Mirapexin tablets POM
Mirena intrauterine system POM
Mirtazapine POM
Misoprostol POM
Mistamine tablets POM
Mitobronitol POM
Mitomycin POM
Mitomycin C Kyowa POM
Mitomycin injection POM
Mitotane POM
Mitoxana injection POM
Mitoxantrone/Mitozantrone hydrochloride POM
Mitozantrone see Mitoxantrone
Mivacron injection POM
Mivacurium chloride POM
Mixtard insulins POM
Mizolastine POM
Mizollen tablets POM

MMR II vaccine POM
Mobic preparations POM
Mobiflex tablets POM
Mobiflex vials POM
Mobigel spray gel POM
Moclobemide POM
Modafinil POM
Modalim tablets POM
Modaplate POM
Modecate concentrate injection POM
Modecate injection POM
Modern Herbals preparations GSL
Modisal LA preparations P
Modisal XL tablets P
Moditen preparations POM
Modrasone cream, and ointment POM
Modrenal capsules POM
Moducren tablets POM
Moduret 25 POM
Moduretic solution POM
Moduretic tablets POM
Moexipril POM
Mogadon preparations CD Benz POM
Moisture-eyes P
Molcer ear drops P
Molgramostim POM
Molindone hydrochloride POM
Molipaxin preparations POM
Mometasone furoate POM
Monit LS tablets P
Monit SR tablets P
Monit tablets P
Monit XL tablets P
Mono-Cedocard 10 tablets P
Mono-Cedocard 20 tablets P
Mono-Cedocard 40 tablets P
Monoclate-P injection POM
Monocor tablets POM
Monodur tabs POM
Monoethanolamine oleate POM
Monomax SR capsules P
Monomax XL tablets P
Monomil POM
Mononine POM
Monoparin preparations POM
Monosorb XL 60 tablets P
Monotard insulins POM
Monotrim preparations POM
Monovent preparations POM
Monozide 10 tablets POM
Monphytol P
Montelukast POM
Moorland GSL
Moracizine hydrochloride POM
Moraxen suppositories POM
Morazone hydrochloride POM
Morcap SR capsules CD POM
Morhulin ointment GSL
Morpheridine; its salts CD POM
Morphgesic SR CD POM
Morphine; its salts; its esters and ethers; their salts; its pentavalent nitrogen derivatives; their esters and ethers CD POM; but for morphine salts if in, (a) any preparations from which the morphine cannot be readily recovered in amounts which constitute a risk to health and with ms 0.2% (calculated as anhydrous morphine base) CD Inv POM; (b) if for non-parenteral use in unit preparations diluted to at least one part in a million (6X) in response to a specific request, CD Inv P; or (c) if for non-parenteral use in unit preparations diluted to at least one part in a million million (6C), CD Inv P
Morphine acetate see Morphine
Morphine and ipecacuanha mixture BPC CD Inv P
Morphine hydrochloride see Morphine
Morphine methobromide, morphine N-oxide and other pentavalent nitrogen morphine derivatives CD POM
Morphine N-oxide; its esters and ethers CD POM
Morphine sulphate Rapiject CD POM
Morphine sulphate see Morphine

Morphine tartrate see Morphine
Morpholinoethylnorpethidine see Morpheridine
Motens tablets POM
Motherwort GSL
Motherwort compound tabs GSL
Motifene capsules POM
Motilium 10 tablets P
Motilium suppositories POM
Motilium suspension POM
Motilium tablets POM
Motipress tablets POM
Motival tablets POM
Motrin tablets POM
Movelat preparations P
Movicol Paediatric plain sachets POM
Movicol Sachets P
Movicol-Half sachets P
Moviprep P
Moxifloxacin POM
Moxisylyte/Thymoxamine POM
Moxisylyte/Thymoxamine hydrochloride POM
Moxonidine POM
Mozobil solution for injection POM
MST Continus tablets CD POM
MST suspension CD POM
Mucaine POM
Mucodyne preparations POM
Mucogel suspension GSL
Mucron tablets P
Multibionta infusion POM
Multiload IUDs POM
Multiparin injection POM
Mumpsvax vaccine POM
Mupirocin POM
Mupirocin calcium POM
Murine P
Muscinil tablets POM
Muse system POM
Mustard oil, volatile, if maximum strength 0.1 per cent (external use only) GSL
Mustine see Chlormethine
MXL capsules CD POM
Mycamine POM
Mycardol tablets P
Mycifradin preparations POM
Mycil Gold P
Mycil preparations GSL
Mycobutin capsules POM
Mycophenolate mofetil POM
Mycophenolic acid POM
Mycota preparations GSL
Mydriacyl eye drops POM
Mydrilate eye drops POM
Myelobromol tablets POM
Myfortic tablets POM
Myleran tablets POM
Myocet POM
Myocrisin injections POM
Myotonine chloride tablets POM
Myrophine; its salts CD POM
Myrrh GSL
Myrrh tincture BPC GSL
Mysoline preparations POM

N

Nabilone CD POM
Nabumetone POM
Nadolol POM
Nafarelin acetate POM
Naftidrofuryl oxalate POM
Naftifine hydrochloride POM
Nalbuphine hydrochloride POM
Nalcrom capsules POM
Nalidixic acid POM
Nalorex tablets POM
Nalorphine hydrobromide POM
Naloxone hydrochloride POM
Naltrexone hydrochloride POM
Nandrolone CD Anab POM
Nandrolone decanoate CD Anab POM
Nandrolone laurate CD Anab POM
Nandrolone phenylpropionate CD Anab POM
Naphazoline hydrochloride POM but if nasal sprays or nasal drops not containing liquid paraffin as a vehicle, maximum strength 0.05 per cent; eye drops maximum strength 0.015 per cent, P
Naphazoline nitrate POM but if nasal sprays or nasal drops not containing liquid paraffin as a vehicle maximum strength 0.05 per cent, P
3-(1-Naphthoyl)indole structurally derived compounds by substitution at the nitrogen atom of the indole ring by alkyl, alkenyl, cycloalkylmethyl, cycloalkylethyl or 2-(4-morpholinyl)ethyl, whether or not further substituted in the indole ring to any extent and whether or not substituted in the naphthyl ring to any extent CD Lic
3-(1-Naphthoyl)pyrrole structurally derived compounds by substitution at the nitrogen atom of the pyrrole ring by alkyl, alkenyl, cycloalkylmethyl, cycloalkylethyl or 2-(4-morpholinyl)ethyl, whether or not further substituted in the pyrrole ring to any extent and whether or not substituted in the naphthyl ring to any extent CD Lic
1-(1-Naphthylmethyl)indene structurally derived compounds by substitution at the 3-position of the indene ring by alkyl, alkenyl, cycloalkylmethyl, cycloalkylethyl or 2-(4-morpholinyl)ethyl, whether or not further substituted in the indene ring to any extent and whether or not substituted in the naphthyl ring to any extent CD Lic
Napratec tablets POM
Naprosyn preparations POM
Naprosyn SR tablets POM
Naproxen POM but if for the treatment of primary dysmenorrhoea in women aged between 15 and 50 years, maximum strength 250mg, 500mg (MD), 750mg (MDD), for a maximum of 3 days treatment, in a maximum pack size of 9 tablets, P
Naproxen sodium POM
Napsalgesic tablets CD Inv POM
Naramig tablets POM
Naratriptan POM
Narcan ampoules POM
Narcan Neonatal ampoules POM
Nardil tablets POM
Naropin preparations POM
Narphen preparations CD POM
Nasacort spray POM
Naseptin cream POM
Nasivin GSL
Nasobec aqueous spray POM
Nasobec Hayfever P
Nasofan allergy POM
Nasonex aqueous nasal spray POM
Natalizumab POM
Natamycin POM
Natecal D3 tablets P
Nateglinide POM
Natracalm tabs GSL
Natramid POM
Natrasleep GSL
Natravene GSL
Natrilix SR tablets POM
Natrilix tablets POM
Navelbine injection POM
Navidrex tablets POM
Navispare tablets POM
Navoban preparations POM
Nebcin vials POM
Nebido solution for injection CD Anab POM
Nebilet tablets POM
Nebivolol hydrochloride POM
Nedocromil sodium POM but if for the prevention, relief and treatment of seasonal and perennial allergic conjunctivitis maximum strength 2.0 per

cent and container or package contains not more than 3ml of medicinal product, P
Nefazodone hydrochloride POM
Neflinavir POM
Nefopam hydrochloride POM
Negaban powder for solution for injection/infusion POM
Negram preparations POM
NeisVac-C POM
Nelfinavir POM
Nelsons preparations GSL
Neo-Bendromax POM
Neo-Cantil preparations POM
Neo-Cortef preparations POM
Neo-Cytamen injection POM
Neo-Mercazole tablets POM
Neo-NaClex tablets POM
Neo-NaClex-K POM
Neo-planotest 200 P
Neoclarityn oral solution 0.5mg/ml POM
Neoclarityn syrup POM
Neoclarityn tablets POM
Neofel XL POM
Neogest tablets POM
Neomycin POM
Neomycin oleate POM
Neomycin palmitate POM
Neomycin sulphate POM
Neomycin undecanoate POM
Neoral capsules POM
Neoral oral solution POM
NeoRecormon preparations POM
Neosporin eye drops POM
Neostigmine bromide POM
Neostigmine methylsulphate POM
Neotigason capsules POM
Neotren MR POM
Nephril tablets POM
Nerisone Forte preparations POM
Nerisone preparations POM
Nestargel powder P
Netillin injection POM
Netilmicin sulphate POM
Nettle (Urtica dioica) GSL
Neulactil preparations POM
Neulasta injection POM
Neupogen injection POM
Neupogen Singleject POM
Neupro transdermal patch POM
Neurobloc injection POM
Neurontin preparations POM
Neutrogena dermatological cream GSL
Nevanac eye drop suspension POM
Nevirapine POM
New Era preparations GSL
Nexavar POM
Nexium preparations POM
Niaspan tablets POM
Nicam gel P
Nicardipine hydrochloride POM
Nice 'n Clear head lice lotion GSL
Nicef caps POM
Nicergoline POM
Niceritrol POM
Nicobrevin caps GSL
Nicocodine CD POM but if for non parenteral use and: (a) in undivided preparations with ms 2.5% (calculated as base) CD Inv POM; or (b) in single dose preparations with ms per dosage unit 100mg (calculated as base) CD Inv POM
Nicodicodine (6-nicotinoyldihydrocodeine) CD POM but if for non parenteral use and: (a) in undivided preparations with ms 2.5% (calculated as base) CD Inv POM; or (b) in single dose preparations with ms per dosage unit 100mg (calculated as base) CD Inv POM
Nicomorphine; its salts CD POM
Nicorandil POM
Nicorette Combi GSL
Nicorette gum (all flavours and pack sizes) GSL
Nicorette inhalator GSL
Nicorette InvisiPatch GSL

Nicorette microtab P and GSL
Nicorette nasal spray GSL
Nicorette patches GSL
Nicotinamide tablets BP GSL
Nicotinamide, up to 300mg (MDD) GSL; or 4% topical gel for treatment of mild to moderate acne vulgaris GSL
Nicotine GSL if for the relief of nicotine withdrawal symptoms as an aid to smoking cessation only, chewing gum maximum strength 4mg, lozenges maximum strength 4mg, sublingual tablets maximum strength 2mg, transdermal patches for continuous application to the skin for a period of 16 hours maximum strength 25mg in 16hrca, transdermal patches for continuous application to the skin for a period of 24 hours maximum strength 21mg in 24 hrca, inhalation cartridge for oromucosal use maximum strength 10mg per cartridge; if for the relief of nicotine withdrawal symptoms as an aid to smoking reduction with the aim of cessation, chewing gum maximum strength 4mg, inhalation cartridge for oromucosal use maximum strength 10mg per cartridge GSL; if nicotine nasal spray delivering 0.5mg nicotine per spray as an aid to smoking cessation for adults and children over 12 years of age GSL; if in a combination pack comprising transdermal patches releasing a maximum of 15mg in 16 hours of continuous application AND gum with a maximum strength of 2mg as an aid to smoking cessation only GSL
Nicotinell preparations GSL
Nicotinic acid POM but any use, except for the treatment of hyperlipidaemia 600mg (MDD), P 100mg (MDD), GSL
Nicotinyl alcohol P
Nicoumalone see Acenocoumarol
Nicrondil POM
Niddaryl tablets POM
Nifedipine POM
Nifedipress MR POM
Nifedotard 20MR POM
Nifelease tablets POM
Nifenazone POM
Niferex preparations F
Nifopress retard tabs POM
Nifopress MR POM
Night Nurse preparations P
Night time formula P
Nightcalm tablets P
Nikethamide POM
Nilutamide POM
Nimbex Forte injection POM
Nimbex injection POM
Nimetazepam CD Benz POM
Nimodipine POM
Nimodrel XL POM
Nimotop preparations POM
Nindaxa 2.5 POM
Niopam POM
Nipent vials POM
NiQuitin CQ preparations GSL
NiQuitin Minis lozenges GSL
Niridazole POM
Nirolex preparations P
Nisoldipine POM
Nitrados tablets CD Benz POM
Nitrazepam CD Benz POM
Nitrendipine POM
Nitro-dur P
Nitrocine POM
Nitrofurantoin POM
Nitrofurazone POM
Nitrolingual spray P
Nitromin P
Nitronal injection POM
Nitropatch POM
Nitroprusside POM
Nitroxoline POM
Nivaquine injection POM

Nivaquine syrup and tablets POM but when supplied for the prevention of malaria, P
Nivaten Retard POM
Nivemycin tablets POM
Nix pencil GSL
Nizatidine POM but if for the prevention and treatment of the symptoms of food-related heartburn and meal-induced indigestion in adults and children not less than 16 years 75mg (MD) 150mg (MDD) for a maximum period of 14 days, P
Nizoral Anti-dandruff shampoo 50ml P
Nizoral Cream POM
Nizoral shampoo 120ml POM
Nizoral shampoo 100ml P
Nizoral suspension POM
Nizoral tablets POM
Nocutil nasal spray POM
Nolvadex-D POM
Nomifensine maleate POM
Non-human chorionic gonadotrophin CD Anab POM
Nonivamide, if maximum strength 0.1 per cent (external use only) GSL
Nonoxinols, external use only GSL
Nootropil preparations POM
Noracymethadol; its salts CD POM
Noradran syrup P
Noradrenaline POM
Noradrenaline acid tartrate POM
19-Nor-4-androstene-3,17-dione CD Anab POM
19-Nor-5-androstene-3,17-diol CD Anab POM
19-Norandrostenedione CD Anab POM
19-Norandrosterone CD Anab POM
Norboletone CD Anab POM
Norclostebol CD Anab POM
Norcodeine CD POM but if for non-parenteral use and: (a) in undivided preparations with ms 2.5% (calculated as base) CD Inv POM; or (b) in single dose preparations with ms per dosage until 100mg (calculated as base) CD Inv POM
Norcuron injection POM
Nordazepam CD Benz POM
Norditropin injection CD Anab POM
Norditropin SimpleXx CD Anab POM
Norelgestromin POM
Norepinephrine see Noradrenaline
Norethandrolone CD Anab POM
Norethisterone POM
Norethisterone acetate POM
Norethisterone enanthate POM
Norethynodrel POM
19-Noretiocholanolone CDAnab POM
Norfloxacin POM
Norgalax P
Norgestimate POM
Norgeston tablets POM
Norgestrel POM
Noriday tablets POM
Norimin tablets POM
Norimode tabs POM
Norinyl-1 tablets POM
Noristerat injection POM
Norit GSL
Noritate cream POM
Norlevorphanol; its salts; its esters and ethers; their salts CD POM
Normacol Plus preparations GSL
Normacol preparations GSL
Normaloe P
Normasol P
Normax preparations POM
Normegon injection POM
Normethadone; its salts CD POM
Normorphine; its salts; its esters and ethers; their salts CD POM
Normosang infusion POM
Norphyllin preparations POM
Norpipanone; its salts CD POM
Norplant implant POM
Norprolac tablets POM
Nortriptyline hydrochloride POM

Norvir capsules POM
Norvir oral solution POM
Norzol POM
Noscapine POM
Noscapine hydrochloride POM
Novantrone injection POM
Novaprin P
Novobiocin calcium POM
Novobiocin sodium POM
Novofem POM
Novolizer budesonide POM
NovoMix 30 preparations POM
NovoNorm tablets POM
Novorapid injections POM
Novoseven POM
Nowax GSL
Noxafil POM
Noxyflex S vials P
Noxytiolin P
Nozinan POM
Nplate powder for solution for injection POM
Nu-Hope prolapse overbelt P
Nu-Seals Aspirin 300mg pack sizes 100s POM
Nu-Seals Aspirin 75mg pack sizes 56s P
Nubain injection POM
Nucare 300mg aspirin pack sizes 32s P; 100s POM
Nucare co-codamol 8/500 pack size 32s P
Nucare dispersible aspirin 75mg pack size 100s P
Nucare dispersible aspirin 300mg pack size 32s P
Nucare ibuprofen preparations P
Nucare paracetamol caplets pack size 16s GSL
Nucare rehydration sachets GSL
Nucare Sigma Codeine linctus P
Nucare Sigma Paracetamol paediatric P
Nucare Sigma Paracetamol suspension 6 plus P
Nucare Sigma Pholcodine linctus P
Nucare Sigma Simple linctus P
Nucare Sigma Simple linctus paediatric P
Nuelin preparations P
Nulacin tablets GSL
Numark allergy eye drops P
Numark allergy relief and hayfever tablets GSL
Numark allergy relief syrup P
Numark anti-dandruff shampoo GSL
Numark antihistamine oral solution P
Numark baby cream GSL
Numark chloramphenicol 0.5% antibiotic eye-drops P
Numark cold remedy night time P
Numark cold sore cream P
Numark constipation relief GSL
Numark cough mixture adult chesty P/GSL (depending on ingredients)
Numark cough mixture adult dry P
Numark cystitis relief GSL
Numark diarrhoea & dehydration relief GSL
Numark flu relief capsules GSL
Numark flu strength all-in-one P
Numark heartburn relief tablets POM
Numark herbal constipation relief GSL
Numark loratadine liquid P
Numark max strength cold and flu sachets GSL
Numark medicated pastilles GSL
Numark muscle rub GSL
Numark muscle spray GSL
Numark sleep aid 50mg P
Nupercainal P
Nurofen Advance tablets P
Nurofen back pain capsules P
Nurofen Caplets pack sizes 12s, 16s GSL; 24s P
Nurofen Cold and Flu tablets P
Nurofen extra strength P
Nurofen for Children singles sachets GSL
Nurofen for Children oral suspension 3 mths to 9 yrs GSL
Nurofen for Children sugar-free suspension 100ml, 150ml P

Nurofen Gel Maximum Strength P
Nurofen ibuprofen gel 5% 35g GSL
Nurofen liquid capsules pack sizes 10s, 16s GSL; 30s P
Nurofen Long Lasting capsules P
Nurofen Meltlets GSL
Nurofen Micro Granules P
Nurofen migraine pain caplets P
Nurofen migraine pain tablets GSL
Nurofen mobile tablets GSL
Nurofen Muscular pain relief gel GSL
Nurofen Plus tablets CD Inv P
Nurofen recovery GSL
Nurofen tablets 200mg pack sizes 12s, 16s GSL; 24s, 48, 96s P
Nurofen tension headache GSL
Nurse Harvey's gripe mixture GSL
Nurse Sykes bronchial balsam GSL
Nurse Sykes powders pack sizes 4s, 8s GSL
Nutmeg GSL
Nutmeg Oil GSL
Nutracel preparations POM
Nutraplus cream P
NuTRIflex preparations POM
Nutrizym 10 P
Nutrizym 22 P
Nutrizym GR capsules P
NutropinAq CD Anab POM
Nuvaring POM
Nuvelle Continuous tablets POM
Nuvelle tablets POM
Nuvelle TS patches POM
Nux Vomica Seed POM
Nycopren tablets POM
Nylax with senna tablets pack sizes 10s GSL; 30s PO
Nyogel eye gel POM
Nyspes pessaries POM
Nystadermal preparations POM
Nystaform preparations POM
Nystaform-HC preparations POM
Nystamont oral suspension POM
Nystan preparations POM
Nystatin POM
Nytol Caplets P
Nytol herbal tablets GSL
Nytol One-a-Night P
Nytol tablets P

O

Oak Bark GSL
Occlusal P
Octacosactrin POM
Octagam POM
Octaphonium chloride, external use only GSL
Octim injection POM
Octim nasal spray POM
Octreotide POM
Ocufen ophthalmic solution POM
Oculotect eye drops P
Ocusert preparations POM
Ocuvite tablets GSL
Ocuvite lutein GSL
Odrik capsules POM
Oestradiol see Estradiol
Oestrifen tablets POM
Oestriol see Estriol
Oestrogel POM
Oestrogen POM
Oestrogenic Substances Conjugated POM
Oestrone see Estrone
Ofloxacin POM
Oftaquix POM
Oilatum cream GSL
Oilatum emollient GSL
Oilatum gel GSL
Oilatum junior cream 500ml GSL
Oilatum junior emollient bath additive GSL
Oilatum cream pump dispenser GSL
Oilatum Plus GSL
50:50 ointment P
Okacyn eye-drops POM
Olanzapine POM

Olbas inhaler sticks GSL
Olbas oil GSL
Olbas pastilles GSL
Olbetam capsules POM
Old tuberculin POM
Oleic acid, external use only GSL
Oleyl alcohol, external use only GSL
Olive Oil GSL
Olmesartan medoxomil POM
Olmetec tablets POM
Olmetex Plus tablets POM
Olopatadine POM
Olsalazine sodium POM
Omacor capsules P
Omalizumab powder and solvent for
    injection POM
Omeprazole POM but if for the relief of
    reflux-like symptoms (eg heartburn)
    in sufferers aged 18 and over please
    refer to proprietary names for the
    classification granted under the mar-
    keting authorisation (see Omeprazole
    10mg Gastro-resistant Tablets
    [Galpharm])
Omeprazole 10mg gastro-resistant
    tablets (Galpharm) P
Omnic MR POM
Omnikan preparations POM
Omniscan vials POM
Oncovin vials POM
Ondansetron hydrochloride POM
Ondemet preparations POM
One-Alpha capsules POM
One-Alpha injection POM
One-Alpha solution POM
Onglyza tablets POM
Onkotrone injection POM
Opas preparations GSL
Opatanol eye-drops POM
Opazimes CD Inv P
Ophthaine solution POM
Opilon preparations POM
Opium, raw CD Lic
Opizone POM
Oprisine tablets POM
Opticrom Allergy eyedrops P
Opticrom eye drops POM
Optil preparations POM
Optilast eye drops POM
Optimax tablets POM
Optimine syrup P
Optimine tablets P
Optipen Pro 1 Green POM
Optrex allergy eye drops P
Optrex infected eyes eye drops P
Optrex red eyes eye drops P
Optrex sore eyes eye drops P
Opumide tablets POM
Orabet tablets POM
Orajel dental gel GSL
Orajel mouth gel P
Orajel extra strength dental gel P
Oral B sensitive toothpaste GSL
Oral gel 15g P
Oral gel 80g POM
Oraldene GSL
Oramorph Concentrated oral solution
    CD POM
Oramorph oral solution CD Inv POM
Oramorph SR tablets CD POM
Oramorph vials 100mg/5ml CD POM
Oramorph vials 10mg/5ml CD Inv POM
Oramorph vials 30mg/5ml CD POM
Orange GSL
Orap tablets POM
Oraquix periodontal gel POM
Orbifen oral suspension pack sizes
    100ml P; 500ml POM
Orbifen oral suspension sachets GSL
Orciprenaline sulphate POM
Orelox POM
Orelox suspension POM
Orencia injection POM
Orgafol injection POM
Orgalutran POM
Orgaran injection POM
Orimeten tablets POM
Oripavine CD POM

Orlept preparations POM
Orlistat POM; but please refer to propri-
    etary names for the classification
    granted under the marketing authori-
    sation
Orovite 7 sachets GSL
Orovite tablets GSL
Orphenadrine citrate POM
Orphenadrine hydrochloride POM
Ortho Gyne-T intrauterine copper con-
    traceptive device POM
Ortho-Creme GSL
Ortho-Gynest cream POM
Ortho-Gynest pessaries POM
Ortho-Novin preparations POM
Orthoforms pessaries GSL
Orudis capsules POM
Orudis suppositories POM
Oruvail capsules POM
Oruvail gel pack sizes 100g POM
Oruvail gel pack sizes 30g P
Oruvail IM injection POM
Oseltamivir POM
Osmanil transdermal patches CD POM
Ossopan granules P
Ossopan tablets P
Ostex Plus GSL
Ostram sachets P
OTC Concepts preparations GSL
Otex ear drops P
Otodex GSL
Otomize ear spray POM
Otosporin ear drops POM
Otrivine antistin drops P
Otrivine Mu-Cron tablets P
Otrivine preparations GSL
Ovandrotone CD Anab POM
Ovarian Gland Dried POM
Ovestin cream POM
Ovestin tablets POM
Ovex P
Ovitrelle injection CD anab POM
Ovran 30 tablets POM
Ovran tablets POM
Ovranette tablets POM
Ovysmen tablets POM
Oxabolone CD Anab POM
Oxactin POM
Oxamniquine POM
Oxandrolone CD Anab POM
Oxantel embonate POM
Oxaprozin POM
Oxatomide POM
Oxazepam CD Benz POM
Oxazolam CD Benz POM
Oxcarbazepine POM
Oxedrine tartrate POM
Oxerutins P
Oxetacaine/Oxethazaine POM but if
    10mg (MD) 30mg (MDD) container
    or package contains not more than
    400mg of oxethazaine, P
Oxethazaine see Oxetacaine
Oxis turbohaler POM
Oxitropium bromide POM
Oxivent inhaler POM
Oxolinic acid POM
Oxpentifylline see Pentoxifylline
Oxprenolol hydrochloride POM
Oxy Daily cleanser GSL
Oxy daily face wash GSL
Oxy in the shower GSL
Oxy on the spot GSL
Oxy wipeout pads GSL
Oxy 10 P
Oxy-gen products GSL
Oxybuprocaine hydrochloride POM but
    if non-ophthalmic use, P
Oxybutynin hydrochloride POM
Oxycodone; its salts; its esters and
    ethers; their salts CD POM
Oxycontin tablets CD POM
Oxydon tablets POM
Oxygen GSL
Oxymesterone CD Anab POM
Oxymetazoline hydrochloride, if non-
    oily nasal sprays and nasal drops
    maximum strength 0.05 per cent GSL

Oxymetazoline, if non-oily nasal sprays
    and nasal drops maximum strength
    0.05 per cent GSL
Oxymetholone CD Anab POM
Oxymorphone; its salts; its esters and
    ethers; their salts CD POM
Oxymycin tablets POM
Oxynorm preparations CD POM
Oxypertine POM
Oxypertine hydrochloride POM
Oxyphenbutazone POM
Oxyphencyclimine hydrochloride POM
Oxyphenonium bromide POM but if
    5mg (MD) 15mg (MDD), P
Oxysept 1-step neutralising tablets GSL
Oxysept saline 90ml GSL
Oxytetracycline POM
Oxytetracycline calcium POM
Oxytetracycline dihydrate POM
Oxytetracycline hydrochloride POM
Oxytetramix tablets POM
Oxytocin, natural POM
Oxytocin, synthetic POM

P

P2S POM
Pabal injections POM
Pabrinex injections POM
Pacifene Maximum Strength tablets P
Pacifene tablets 200mg pack sizes 12s
    GSL; 24s, 48s, 96s P
Paclitaxel POM
Padimate 0, external use only GSL
Paedo-Sed syrup POM
Palacos LV POM
Palacos R POM
Palfermin POM
Palfium preparations CD POM
Palivizumab POM
Palladone capsules CD POM
Palladone SR capsules CD POM
Palonosetron POM
Paludrine P
Paludrine/avloclor travel packs P
Pamergan P100 injection CD POM
Pamidronate disodium POM
Pamine tablets POM
Panadeine CD Inv P
Panadol Actifast pack sizes 8s, 16s GSL;
    30s P; compack GSL
Panadol capsules pack sizes 16s GSL
Panadol elixir P
Panadol Extra Soluble pack sizes 24s GSL
Panadol Extra tablets pack sizes 12s, 16s
    GSL; 32s P
Panadol Night tablets P
Panadol OA tablets POM
Panadol Soluble tablets pack sizes 12s,
    24s GSL
Panadol tablets pack sizes 12s, 16s GSL;
    32s P
Panadol Ultra tablets 20s CD Inv P
Pancrease capsules P
Pancrease HL POM
Pancreatin POM but if capsules maxi-
    mum strength 21,000 European
    Pharmacopoeia units of lipase per
    capsule; powder maximum strength
    25,000 European Pharmacopoeia
    units of lipase per gram, P
Pancrex granules P
Pancrex V preparations P
Pancuronium bromide POM
Panoxyl preparations P
Pantoloc Control tablets P
Pantoprazole POM
Pantoprazole sodium POM
Pantothenic acid GSL
Papain GSL
Papaveretum see Medicinal opium
Papaverine POM but if (1) by inhaler; (2)
    otherwise than by inhaler 50mg (MD)
    150mg (MDD), P
Papaverine hydrochloride POM but if (1)
    by inhaler; (2) otherwise than by
    inhaler equivalent of 50mg of

papaverine (MD) equivalent of
    150mg of papaverine (MDD), P
Papulex P
Paracetamol tablets, capsules, powders,
    granules, liquid preparations, see
    tables pp69-70
Paracetamol suppositories pack size 10s
    P
Paracets capsules pack size 16s GSL
Paracets Plus capsules GSL
Paracets powders pack size 5s GSL
Paracodol capsules CD Inv P
Paracodol soluble tablets CD Inv P
Paradote pack sizes 24s P; 96s POM
Paraffin white & yellow soft BP, external
    use only GSL
Paraffin, hard, external use only GSL
Paraffin, liquid, all preparations except
    nasal drops, nasal sprays, nasal
    inhalations and oral laxatives GSL
Parake tablets CD Inv POM
Paraldehyde POM
Paramax sachets POM
Paramax tablets POM
Paramed GSL
Paramethadione POM
Paramethasone acetate POM
Paramol tablets CD Inv P
Paranorm P
Paraplatin injection POM
Parathyroid Gland POM
Pardelprin MR capsules POM
Parecoxib POM
Paregoric BP CD Inv POM
Pargyline hydrochloride POM
Pariet tablets POM
Parlodel preparations POM
Parmid preparations POM
Parnate tablets POM
Paromomycin sulphate POM
Paroven capsules P
Paroxetine hydrochloride POM
Parsley GSL
Parsley piert GSL
Parstelin tablets POM
Partobulin POM
Partobulin SDF POM
Parvolex injection POM
Passiflora GSL
Patent Blue VE131 GSL
Pavacol-D pack sizes 150ml P; 300ml CD
    Inv P
Pavulon ampoules POM
Paxene concentrate POM
Paxidorm tablets P
Paxoran POM
Pecilocin POM
Pectin GSL
Pediacel vaccine POM
Peditrace POM
Peg-Intron POM
Pegaptanib POM
Pegasys injection POM
Pegfilgrastim POM
Peginterferon alfa POM
Pegvisomant POM
Pellitory GSL
Pemetrexed POM
Pemoline CD Benz POM
Penamecillin POM
Penbritin preparations POM
Penbutolol sulphate POM
Penciclovir POM; but if for external use
    for the treatment of herpes simplex
    virus infections of the lips and face
    (Herpes labialis) in adults and chil-
    dren aged 12 or more; maximum
    strength 1%; maximum pack size 2g,
    P
Pendramine tablets POM
Penicillamine POM
Penicillamine hydrochloride POM
Penicillin POM
Pennsaid topical solution POM
Pentacarinat POM
Pentamidine injection BP POM
Pentamidine isethionate POM
Pentasa enemas POM

Paracetamol legal status: Tablets, capsules, powders and granules (*see* Note 1)

Product	Container size	Legal status	Where it can be sold	Maximum that can be sold to a person at any one time (*see* Note 2)
Non-effervescent tablets and capsules				
Paracetamol (non-effervescent) tablets and capsules up to 120mg (*see* Note 3)	Up to 16	GSL (for the treatment of children aged less than 6 years)	Pharmacies and non-pharmacy retail outlets	Not more than 100 tablets or capsules (*see* Note 4)
Paracetamol (non-effervescent) tablets and capsules up to 250mg	Up to 16	GSL (for the treatment of children aged 6 years and over)	Pharmacies and non-pharmacy retail outlets	Not more than 100 tablets or capsules (*see* Note 4)
Paracetamol (non-effervescent) tablets and capsules up to 250mg	Between 17 and 32 inclusive	P (if wholly or mainly for children aged less than 12 years)	Pharmacies only	Not more than 100 tablets or capsules (*see* Note 4)
Paracetamol (non-effervescent) tablets and capsules up to 500mg (*see* Note 3)	Up to 16	GSL (for the treatment of adults)	Pharmacies and non-pharmacy retail outlets	Not more than 100 tablets or capsules (*see* Note 4)
Paracetamol (non-effervescent) tablets and capsules up to 500mg	Between 17 and 32 inclusive	If wholly or mainly for adults and children not less than 12 years, *see* Note 6(i)	Pharmacies only	Not more than 100 tablets or capsules (see Note 4)
Paracetamol (non-effervescent) tablets and capsules up to 500mg	Greater than 32	POM	Pharmacies only	To be sold or supplied only in accordance with a prescription
Effervescent tablets (*see* Note 5)				
Paracetamol (effervescent) tablets up to 120mg (*see* Note 3)	Up to 30	GSL (for children aged less than 6 years)	Pharmacies and non-pharmacy retail outlets	No legal limit
Paracetamol (effervescent) tablets up to 120mg (*see* Note 3)	Greater than 30	For children aged less than 6 years, *see* Note 6(ii)	Pharmacies only	No legal limit
Paracetamol (effervescent) tablets up to 250mg	Up to 30	GSL (for children aged 6 and over	Pharmacies and non-pharmacy retail outlets	No legal limit
Paracetamol (effervescent) tablets up to 250mg	Greater than 30	For children aged 6 and over, *see* Note 6(i)	Pharmacies only	No legal limit
Paracetamol (effervescent) tablets up to 500mg (*see* Note 3)	Up to 30	GSL (for the treatment of adults)	Pharmacies and non-pharmacy retail outlets	No legal limit
Paracetamol (effervescent) tablets up to 500mg (*see* Note 3)	Greater than 30	For the treatment of adults, *see* Note 6(i)	Pharmacies only	No legal limit
Powders and granules				
Paracetamol powders and granules up to 240mg (see Note 3)	Up to 10	GSL (for the treatment of children)	Pharmacies and non-pharmacy retail outlets	No legal limit
Paracetamol powders and granules up to 1000mg (see Note 3)	Up to 10	GSL (for the treatment of adults)	Pharmacies and non-pharmacy retail outlets	No legal limit

Note 1: When paracetamol is in combination with a pharmacy medicine (eg, low-strength codeine) or a prescription-only medicine (eg, dextropropoxyphene), the more stringent legal category applies

Note 2: While several products have no legal limit for the amount that may be sold or supplied, pharmacists are expected to exercise professional control to limit the amount of paracetamol which may be stored in a patient's home

Note 3: For product containing paracetamol except when combined with methionine DL

Note 4: The quantity of non-effervescent tablets, capsules or a combination of both, sold or supplied to a person at any one time shall not exceed 100

Note 5: Effervescent preparations in relation to a tablet, means containing not less than 75 per cent, by weight of the tablet, of ingredients included wholly or mainly for the purpose of releasing carbon dioxide when the tablet is dissolved or dispersed in water

Note 6: Strictly speaking, paracetamol is classified as a POM or a GSL product, but is limited to sale through pharmacies under certain conditions and exemptions. Products marked 6(i) would be P medicines and 6(ii) GSL medicines, unless specific products are otherwise licensed

Paracetamol legal status: Liquids (*see* Note 1)

Product	Container size	Legal status	Where it can be sold	Maximum that can be sold to a person at any one time (*see* Note 2)
Liquids				
Paracetamol liquid preparations, up to 2.4 per cent (*see* Note 3)	In unit doses of not more than 5ml and no more than 20 unit doses (100ml)	GSL (for children under 12 years) MD 480mg, MDD 1,920mg	Pharmacies and non-pharmacy retail outlets	No legal limit
Paracetamol liquid preparations, up to 2.4 per cent (*see* Note 3)	In multidose containers of not more than 100ml	GSL (for children under 12 years) MD 480mg, MDD 1,920mg	Pharmacies and non-pharmacy retail outlets	No legal limit
Paracetamol liquid preparations, up to 2.5 per cent (*see* Note 3)	Greater than 160ml	*see* Note 6(i)	Pharmacies only	No legal limit
Paracetamol liquid preparations, up to 5 per cent	In unit doses of not more than 5ml and no more than 12 unit doses	GSL (for persons aged 6 years and over)	Pharmacies and non-pharmacy retail outlets	No legal limit
Paracetamol liquid preparations, up to 5 per cent	In multidose containers of not more than 80ml	GSL (for persons aged 6 years and over)	Pharmacies and non-pharmacy retail outlets	No legal limit
Paracetamol liquid preparations, up to 5 per cent	Up to 160ml	GSL (for the treatment of adults and children aged 12 years and over)	Pharmacies and non-pharmacy retail outlets	No legal limit

Note 1: When paracetamol is in combination with a pharmacy medicine (eg, low-strength codeine) or a prescription-only medicine (eg, dextropropoxyphene), the more stringent legal category applies

Note 2: While several products have no legal limit for the amount that may be sold or supplied, pharmacists are expected to exercise professional control to limit the amount of paracetamol which may be stored in a patient's home

Note 3: For product containing paracetamol except when combined with methionine DL

Note 4: The quantity of non-effervescent tablets, capsules or a combination of both, sold or supplied to a person at any one time shall not exceed 100

Note 5: Effervescent preparations in relation to a tablet, means containing not less than 75 per cent, by weight of the tablet, of ingredients included wholly or mainly for the purpose of releasing carbon dioxide when the tablet is dissolved or dispersed in water

Note 6: Strictly speaking, paracetamol is classified as a POM or a GSL product, but is limited to sale through pharmacies under certain conditions and exemptions. Products marked 6(i) would be P medicines and 6(ii) GSL medicines, unless specific products are otherwise licensed

Pentasa sachets POM
Pentasa suppositories POM
Pentasa Sustained Release tablets POM
Pentaspan IV infusion POM
Pentazocine CD No Register POM
Penthienate bromide POM but if 5mg (MD) 15mg (MDD), P
Pentobarbitone CD No Register POM
Pentobarbitone sodium CD No Register POM
Pentolinium tartrate POM
Pentostam injection POM
Pentostatin POM
Pentoxifylline/Oxpentifylline POM
Pentrax shampoo P
Pep tablets GSL
Pepcid AC indigestion tablets GSL
Pepcid PM tablets POM
Pepcid tablets POM
Pepcidtwo chewable tablets GSL
Peppermint GSL
Peppermint oil GSL
Peptac liquid PO
Peptimax tablets POM
Pepto-bismol P
Peralvex P
Percutaneous Bacillus Calmette-Guerin vaccine POM
Percutol ointment P
Perdix tablets POM
Perflagan POM
Perfan injection POM
Perfluamine POM
Pergolide mesylate POM
Pergonal injection POM
Perhexiline maleate POM

Periactin tablets P
Pericyazine POM
Perinal spray (0173/0049) P
Perindopril POM
Perindopril erbumine POM
Perio.aid GSL
Periostat tablets POM
Permethrin cream (Sandoz) P
Peroxyl GSL
Perphenazine POM
Persantin ampoules POM
Persantin Retard tablets POM
Persantin tablets POM
Pertussis vaccine POM
Peru, balsam of, external use only GSL
Pethidine-scopolamine CD POM
Pethidine; its salts CD POM
Pevaryl P
Pevaryl TC cream POM
Pharmalgen Venom vaccines POM
Pharmaton capsules GSL (100 pack size P and GSL)
Pharmorubicin Rapid Dissolution injection POM
Pharmorubicin Solution for Injection POM
Phasonit LA 50 P
Phenacetin POM but if maximum strength 0.1 per cent, P
Phenadone see Methadone
Phenadoxone; its salts CD POM
Phenampromide; its salts CD POM
Phenazocine; its salts; its esters and ethers; their salts CD POM
Phenazone POM but if external P
Phenazone salicylate POM

Phenbutrazate hydrochloride POM
Phencyclidine; its salts; its esters; their salts CD POM
Phendimetrazine; its salts CD No Register POM
Phenelzine sulphate POM
Phenergan elixir P
Phenergan injection POM
Phenergan Nightime tablets P
Phenergan tablets P
Phenethicillin potassium POM
Phenethylamine derivatives formed by substitution in the ring to any extent with alkyl, alkoxy, alkylenedioxy or halide substituents, whether or not further substituted in the ring by one or more other univalent substituents, also derivatives formed by such substitution of the following (except methoxyphenamine); N-alkylphenethylamines, alpha-methylphenethylamine, N-alkyl-alpha-methylphenethylamine, alpha-ethylphenethylamine, or N-alkyl-alpha-ethylphenethylamine; their salts; their esters and ethers; their salts CD Lic
Phenformin hydrochloride POM
Phenglutarimide hydrochloride POM
Phenindamine tartrate POM
Phenindione POM
Phenmetrazine hydrochloride CD POM
Phenmetrazine theoclate CD POM
Phenmetrazine; its salts CD POM
Phenobarbital/Phenobarbitone CD No Register POM Note: emergency sup-

ply at request of patient not permitted except for use in the treatment of epilepsy
Phenobarbital/Phenobarbitone sodium CD No Register POM Note: emergency supply at request of patient not permitted except for use in the treatment of epilepsy
Phenobarbitone see Phenobarbital
Phenol, if internal (except smelling salts) maximum strength 1.0 per cent, or smelling salts maximum strength 5.0 per cent or external maximum strength 2.5 per cent GSL
Phenolphthalein POM
Phenomorphan; its salts; its esters and ethers; their salts CD POM
Phenoperidine; its salts; its esters and ethers; their salts CD POM
Phenoxybenzamine hydrochloride POM
Phenoxymethylpenicillin POM
Phenoxymethylpenicillin calcium POM
Phenoxymethylpenicillin potassium POM
Phenprocoumon POM
Phensic original tablets pack sizes 12s GSL; 24s P
Phensuximide POM
Phentanyl see Fentanyl
Phentermine CD No Register POM
Phentolamine hydrochloride POM
Phentolamine mesylate POM
3-Phenylacetylindole structurally derived compounds by substitution at the nitrogen atom of the indole ring with alkyl, alkenyl, cycloalkylmethyl,

cycloalkylethyl or 2-(4-morpholinyl)ethyl, whether or not further substituted in the indole ring to any extent and whether or not substituted in the phenyl ring to any extent CD Lic

Phenylbutazone POM

Phenylbutazone sodium POM

Phenylephrine hydrochloride, if internal (all preparations except nasal drops, nasal sprays and nasal inhalations equivalent to 10 mg phenylephrine [MD]) GSL

Phenylephrine injection BP POM

Phenylmethylbarbituric acid CD No Register POM

1-Phenylpiperazine structurally derived compounds by modification in any of the following ways - (i) by substitution at the second nitrogen atom of the piperazine ring with alkyl, benzyl, haloalkyl or phenyl groups; (ii) by substitution in the aromatic ring to any extent with alkyl, alkoxy, alkylenedioxy, halide or haloalkyl groups CD lic

4-Phenylpiperidine-4-carboxylic acid ethyl ester CD POM

Phenylpropanolamine hydrochloride POM but if internal (1) all preparations except prolonged release capsules, nasal sprays and nasal drops, 25mg (MD) 100mg (MDD); (2) prolonged release capsules 50mg (MD) 100mg (MDD); (3) nasal sprays and nasal drops maximum strength 2.0 per cent, P

Phenytoin POM

Phenytoin sodium POM

Phillips preparations GSL

Phillips Milk of Magnesia GSL

Phimetin POM

Pholcodine CD POM but if for non-parenteral use and (a) in undivided preparations with ms 2.5% (calculated as base) CD Inv POM; or (b) in single dose preparations with ms per dosage unit 100mg (calculated as base) CD Inv POM; or (c) in unit preparations diluted to at least one part in a million (6X) in response to a specific request, CD Inv P; or (d) in unit preparations diluted to at least one part in a million million (6C), CD Inv P

Pholcodine citrate see Pholcodine

Pholcodine tartrate see Pholcodine

Phor Pain pack sizes 30g, 50g GSL; 100g P

Phor Pain Forte P

Phortinea paint P

Phosex tablets POM

Phosphate-Sandoz tablets P

Phospholine iodide POM

Photofrin injection POM

Phthalylsulphathiazole POM

Phyldrox tablets CD No Register POM

Phyllocontin Continus tablets P

Phyllocontin Forte Continus tablets P

Phyllocontin Paediatric Continus tablets P

Physeptone preparations CD POM

Physiotens tablets POM

Physostigmine POM

Physostigmine aminoxide salicylate POM

Physostigmine salicylate POM

Physostigmine sulphate POM

Phytex P

Phytomenadione POM but any use except the prevention or treatment of haemorrhagic disorders, P

Pickles foot ointment P

Pickles soothake toothache gel and tincture GSL

Picolax powder P

Picrotoxin POM

Pilewort GSL

Pilocarpine POM

Pilocarpine hydrochloride POM

Pilocarpine nitrate POM

Pilogel POM

Pimecrolimus POM

Pimento Oil GSL

Piminodine; its salts CD POM

Pimozide POM

Pinadone mixture CD POM

Pinazepam CD Benz POM

Pindolol POM

Pinefeld XL POM

Pini silvestris oil, if external use or inhalant capsules [maximum strength 9mg], or pastilles, lozenges, throat tablets [maximum strength 6mg], or cough syrups [maximum strength 0.05mg/5ml] GSL

Pioglitazone POM

Pipenzolate bromide POM but if 5mg (MD) 15mg (MDD), P

Piperacillin sodium POM

Piperacillin/tazobactam powder for solution for injection or infusion POM

Piperazine estrone/Oestrone sulphate POM

Piperidolate hydrochloride POM but if 50mg (MD) 150mg (MDD), P

Piperonal GSL

Piportil Depot injection POM

Pipothiazine see Pipotiazine

Pipotiazine/Pipothiazine palmitate POM

Pipradol; its salts CD No Register POM

Pipril injection POM

Piracetam POM

Pirbuterol acetate POM

Pirbuterol hydrochloride POM

Pirenzepine dihydrochloride monohydrate POM

Pirenzepine hydrochloride POM

Piretanide POM

Piriject injection POM

Piriteze Allergy tablets pack sizes 7s GSL; 30s P

Piriteze allergy syrup GSL

Piriton Allergy tablets P

Piriton Duolets P

Piriton injection POM

Piriton syrup P

Piritramide; its salts CD POM

Piroflam POM

Piroxicam POM but if external for the relief of rheumatic pain, pain of non-serious arthritic conditions and muscular aches, pains and swellings such as strains, sprains and sports injuries for use in adults and children not less than 12 years for maximum period of 7 days maximum strength 0.5 per cent and container or package containing not more than 30g of medicinal product, P

Piroxicam beta-cyclodextrin POM

Pirozip capsules POM

Pitressin injection POM

Pituitary anterior lobe POM

Pituitary Gland (Whole Dried) POM but if by inhaler, P

Pituitary Powdered (Posterior Lobe) POM but if by inhaler, P

Pivampicillin POM

Pivampicillin hydrochloride POM

Pivmecillinam POM

Pivmecillinam hydrochloride POM

Pizotifen POM

Pizotifen malate POM

Placidex liquid P

Plague vaccine POM

Plaquenil tablets POM

Plasmalyte POM

Platinex POM

Plavix tablets POM

Plendil POM

Plesmet syrup P

Pletal tablets POM

Pleurisy root GSL

Plicamycin POM

Pneumococcal vaccine (bacterial antigen) POM

Pneumovax vaccine POM

Pnu-imune vaccine POM

Pnu-Imune vials POM

Podophyllin paint, compound BP POM

Podophyllotoxin POM

Podophyllum POM

Podophyllum Indian POM

Podophyllum resin POM but if external ointment or impregnated plaster maximum strength 20.0 per cent, P

Poke root (Phytolacca), if external use or internal 120mg (MD) GSL

Poldine methylsulphate POM but if 2mg (MD) 6mg (MDD), P

Polidexide POM

Poliomyelitis vaccine (inactivated) POM

Poliomyelitis vaccine (oral) POM

Poliomyelitis vaccine, live (oral) BP POM

Pollenase preparations P

Pollenshield hayfever 7s GSL; 30 P

Pollinex POM

Pollon-eze tablets POM

Poloxamer POM

Polyestradiol phosphate POM

Polyethoxyethanol, external use only GSL

Polyfax ointment POM

Polyfax ophthalmic ointment POM

Polyfax preparations POM

Polygeline P

Polyhexedrine POM

Polymyxin B sulphate POM

Polynoxylin P

Polyoestradiol phosphate POM

Polytar preparations GSL

Polytar AF GSL

Polytar Plus GSL

Polythiazide POM

Polytrim preparations POM

Polyvidone P

Pondocillin preparations POM

Ponstan forte POM

Ponstan preparations POM

Poplar (Aspen) GSL

Poppy capsule POM

Poractant alfa POM

Poregon injection POM

Porfimer sodium POM

Pork insulin POM

Posalfilin ointment P

Posiject POM

PostMI preparations P

Potaba preparations P

Potassium acid tartrate GSL

Potassium aminobenzoate P

Potassium arsenite POM but if 0.0127 per cent, P

Potassium benzoate P

Potassium bicarbonate GSL

Potassium bromide POM

Potassium canrenoate POM

Potassium carbonate GSL

Potassium chloride and sodium chloride injection POM

Potassium chloride, if external use, or internal use for the treatment of acute diarrhoea, maximum strength 0.15 per cent GSL

Potassium citrate GSL

Potassium citrate mixture BP GSL

Potassium clavulanate POM

Potassium clorazepate see Dipotassium clorazepate

Potassium edetate, external use only GSL

Potassium gluconate GSL

Potassium glycerophosphate GSL

Potassium hydroxide, external use only GSL

Potassium hydroxyquinoline sulphate, if maximum strength 0.6 per cent (external use only) GSL

Potassium iodide, if MDD equivalent to 10mg iodine GSL

Potassium molybdate, if MDD equivalent to 200mcg elemental molybdenum GSL

Potassium nitrate, up to 100mg (MD) GSL

Potassium perchlorate POM

Potassium phosphate POM

Potassium sulphate GSL

Potassium thiocyanate, external use only GSL

Potters day and night P

Potters decongestant GSL

Potters Gees linctus CD Inv P

Potter's Herbal supplies all GSL except cleansing herbs, cough remover, malt extracts, skin lotion and ointment and tabritis rubbing oils

Potters pholcodine CD Inv P

Povidone P

Povidone-iodine, all preparations for external use, except those for vaginal use or for use in surgical operations GSL

Powergel POM

PR spray GSL

Practolol POM

Pradaxa capsules POM

Pragmatar ointment P

Pralenal tablets POM

Pralidoxime chloride POM

Pralidoxime iodide POM

Pralidoxime mesylate POM

Pramipexole hydrochloride POM

Prandin POM

Prasterone CD Anab POM

Pravastatin sodium POM

Praxilene preparations POM

Prazepam CD Benz POM

Prazosin hydrochloride POM

Preconceive tablets GSL

Precortisyl tablets POM

Pred Forte eye drops POM

Predenema POM

Predfoam POM

Prednesol tablets POM

Prednisolone POM

Prednisolone 21-steaglate POM

Prednisolone acetate POM

Prednisolone butylacetate POM

Prednisolone hexanoate POM

Prednisolone metasulphobenzoate POM

Prednisolone metasulphobenzoate sodium POM

Prednisolone pivalate POM

Prednisolone sodium phosphate POM

Prednisolone steaglate POM

Prednisone POM

Prednisone acetate POM

Predsol eye/ear drops POM

Predsol preparations POM

Predsol-N eye/ear drops POM

Pregabalin POM

Pregaday tablets P

Pregnyl injections CD Anab POM

Prelude GSL

Premarin preparations POM

Premique Cycle tablets POM

Premique Low Dose tablets POM

Premique tablets POM

Premjact P

Prempak POM

Prempak-C tablets POM

Prenalterol hydrochloride POM

Prenylamine lactate POM

Preotact POM

Prepadine tablets POM

Preparation H preparations GSL

Prepidil gel POM

Prepulsid Quicklet tablets POM

Prepulsid suspension POM

Prepulsid tablets POM

Prescal tablets POM

Preservex tablets POM

Presinex nasal spray POM

Pressimmune injection POM

Prestim tablets POM

Prevenar preparations POM

Prexige tablets POM

Prezista POM

Priadel preparations POM

Prialt POM

Prickly Ash Bark (Zanthoxylum clavaher-culis) GSL
Prilocaine hydrochloride POM but if non-ophthalmic use, P
Primacor injection POM
Primalan tablets POM
Primaquine phosphate tablets (ICI) P
Primaxin infusion POM
Primaxin Monovial POM
Primene POM
Primidone POM
Primolut N tablets POM
Primoteston Depot CD Anab POM
Primperan preparations POM
Primula Rhizome Extract GSL
Prioderm cream shampoo P
Prioderm lotion P
Priorix MMR vaccine POM
Pripsen preparations P
Pro-Banthine preparations POM
Pro-Epanutin POM
Pro-Epanutin concentrate for injection POM
ProPlus GSL
Pro-Viron tablets CD Anab POM
Probenecid POM
Probeta-LA capsules POM
Probucol POM
Procainamide hydrochloride POM
Procaine benzylpenicillin/Procaine penicillin POM
Procaine hydrochloride POM but if non-ophthalmic use, P
Procaine penicillin see Procaine benzylpenicillin
Procarbazine hydrochloride POM
Prochlorperazine POM
Prochlorperazine edisylate POM
Prochlorperazine maleate POM but buccal tablets for the treatment of nausea and vomiting in cases of previously diagnosed migraine only. For use in persons aged 18 years and over, with MDD 12mg, in a container or package containing not more than 8 tablets P
Prochlorperazine mesylate POM
Procorolan tablets POM
Proctocream HC P
Proctofoam HC aerosol POM
Proctosedyl preparations POM
Procyclidine hydrochloride POM
Profasi injection CD Anab POM
Proflavine hemisulphate, external use only GSL
Proflex cream 100g P
Proflex cream 30g GSL
Progesterone POM
Prograf capsules POM
Proguanil P
Progynova preparations POM
Proheptazine; its salts CD POM
Prolactin POM
Proladone preparations CD POM
Proleukin infusion POM
Proligestone POM
Prolintane hydrochloride POM
Proluton Depot injection POM
Promazine embonate POM
Promazine hydrochloride POM
Promethazine injection POM
Prominal tablets CD No Register POM
Promixin powder for nebuliser solution POM
Pronestyl preparations POM
Prontosan GSL
Propaderm preparations POM
Propafenone POM
Propafenone hydrochloride POM
Propain Caplets pack sizes 16s, 32s CD Inv P
Propain Plus CD Inv P
Propamidine P
Propanidid POM
Propanix SR capsules POM
Propantheline bromide POM but if 15mg (MD) 45mg (MDD), P
Propecia tablets POM

Properidine; its salts CD POM
Propess pessaries POM
Propetandrol CD Anab POM
Propicillin potassium POM
Propine eye drops POM
Propiram; its salts CD POM but if in preparations containing, per dosage unit, not more than 100mg of propiram (calculated as base) and compounded with at least the same amount of methylcellulose CD Inv POM
Propiverine hydrochloride POM
Propofol POM
Propranolol hydrochloride POM
Propress RS POM
Propylene glycol, external use only GSL
Propylene phenoxetol, external use only GSL
Propylthiouracil POM
Proquazone POM
Prosaid POM
Proscar tablets POM
Prosparol emulsion P
Prostaglandin F2 alpha tromethamine POM
Prostanozol CD Anab POM
Prostap 3 depot injection POM
Prostap SR injection POM
Prostin preparations POM
Prosulf ampoules POM
Protamine sulphate POM
Protease POM
Protelos granules POM
Prothiaden preparations POM
Prothionamide see Protionamide
Protionamide/Prothionamide POM
Protirelin POM
Protium IV vials POM
Protium tablets POM
Protopic ointment POM
Protriptyline hydrochloride POM
Provera tablets POM
Provigil tablets POM
Proxymetacaine hydrochloride POM but if non-ophthalmic use, P
Prozac preparations POM
Proziere tablets POM
Prozit POM
Pseudoephedrine hydrochloride POM but if internal (a) In the case of a prolonged release preparation 120mg (MD) 240mg (MDD) (b) in any other case 60mg (MD) 240mg (MDD), P
Pseudoephedrine sulphate POM but if 60mg (MD) 180mg (MDD), P
Psilocin; its salts; its esters and ethers; their salts CD Lic
Psoriderm preparations P
Psorigel P
Psorin preparations P
Psyllium GSL
Pulmicort preparations POM
Pulmo Bailly CD Inv P
Pulmozyme POM
Pulsatilla GSL
Pulvinal beclometasone dipropionate dry powder inhaler POM
Pulvinal salbutamol dry powder inhaler POM
Pumilio Pine Oil GSL
Pump-Hep injection POM
Pure Health aspirin dispersible tablets P
Pure Health saline nasal drops GSL
Puregon POM
Puri-Nethol tablets POM
Pylobactell POM
Pylorid tablets POM
Pyralvex solution P
Pyrantel embonate POM but if (a) For the treatment of enterobiosis, in adults and children not less than 12 years 750mg MDD (as a single dose) and container or package contains not more than 750mg of pyrantel embonate; (b) For the treatment of enterobiosis, in children less than 12 years but not less than 6 years 500mg

MDD (as a single dose) and container or package contains not more than 750mg of pyrantel embonate; (c) For the treatment of enterobiosis in children less than 6 years but not less than 2 years 250mg MDD (as a single dose) and container or package contains not more than 750mg of pyrantel embonate, P
Pyrantel tartrate POM
Pyrazinamide POM
Pyrethrum (Chrysanthemum), external use only GSL
Pyridostigmine bromide POM
Pyridoxine hydrochloride GSL
Pyrimethamine POM
Pyrithione zinc, external use only GSL
Pyrogastrone preparations POM
Pyrovalerone; its salts; its stereoisomers; their salts CD Benz POM
Pyroxylin P

Q

Qlaira film-coated tablets POM
Quassia GSL
Queen's Delight, up to 320mg (MD) GSL
Quellada M preparations P
Questran POM
Questran Light POM
Quetiapine fumarate POM
Quiet Life GSL
Quinaband P
Quinagolide POM
Quinalbarbitone see Secobarbital
Quinapril POM
Quinapril hydrochloride POM
Quinbolone CD Anab POM
Quinestradol POM
Quinestrol POM
Quinethazone POM
Quingestanol POM
Quinicardine tablets POM
Quinidine POM
Quinidine bisulphate POM
Quinidine polygalacturonate POM
Quinidine sulphate POM
Quinil POM
Quinine POM but if 100mg (MD) 300mg (MDD), P; quinine base 35mg (MD), GSL
Quinine and urea hydrochloride POM
Quinine bisulphate POM but if equivalent of 100mg of quinine (MD) equivalent of 300mg of quinine (MDD), P
Quinine cinchophen POM but if equivalent of 100mg of quinine (MD) equivalent of 300mg of quinine (MDD), P
Quinine dihydrochloride POM but if equivalent of 100mg of quinine (MD) equivalent of 300mg of quinine (MDD), P
Quinine ethyl carbonate POM but if equivalent of 100mg of quinine (MD) equivalent of 300mg of quinine (MDD), P
Quinine glycerophosphate POM but if equivalent of 100mg of quinine (MD) equivalent of 300mg of quinine (MDD), P
Quinine hydrobromide POM but if equivalent of 100mg of quinine (MD) equivalent of 300mg of quinine (MDD), P
Quinine hydrochloride POM but if equivalent of 100mg of quinine (MD) equivalent of 300mg of quinine (MDD), P
Quinine in combination with urea hydrochloride POM
Quinine iodobismuthate POM but if equivalent of 100mg of quinine (MD) equivalent of 300mg of quinine (MDD), P
Quinine phosphate POM but if equivalent of 100mg of quinine (MD) equivalent of 300mg of quinine (MDD), P

Quinine salicylate POM but if equivalent of 100mg of quinine (MD) equivalent of 300mg of quinine (MDD), P
Quinine sulphate POM but if equivalent of 100mg of quinine (MD) equivalent of 300mg of quinine (MDD), P; equivalent to 35 mg quinine (MD), GSL
Quinine tannate POM but if equivalent of 100mg of quinine (MD) equivalent of 300mg of quinine (MDD), P
Quinocort cream POM
Quinoderm cream P
Quinoderm Lotio-Gel P
Quinoped cream P
Quinupristin POM
Qvar POM

R

Rabeprazole POM
Rabies vaccine POM
Rabipur POM
Racemethorphan; its salts CD POM
Racemoramide; its salts CD POM
Racemorphan; its salts; its esters and ethers; their salts CD POM
Radian-B preparations GSL
Ralgex preparations GSL
Raloxifine hydrochloride POM
Raltitrexed POM
Ramipril POM
Ramysis POM
Ranace POM
Ranclav POM
Ranexa prolonged release tablets POM
Ranflutin POM
Ranitic POM
Ranitidine hydrochloride POM but if for the short term symptomatic relief of heartburn, dyspepsia, indigestion, acid indigestion and hyperacidity or the prevention of these symptoms when associated with consuming food and drink, equivalent to 75mg of ranitidine (MD) equivalent to 300mg of ranitidine (MDD) for a maximum period of 14 days, P; for short term symptomatic relief of heartburn, indigestion, acid indigestion and hyperacidity, max strength 75mg, mdd 150mg, max pack size 12, GSL
Ranitil POM
Rantec POM
Ranvera MR POM
Ranzac 7s GSL
Ranzolont POM
Rap-eze tablets GSL
Rapamune oral solution POM
Rapamune tablets POM
Rapifen injection CD POM
Rapifen Intensive Care injection CD POM
Rapilysin POM
Rapitil eye drops POM
Rapolyte GSL
Rappell pump spray GSL
Rapranol SR POM
Raptiva POM
Rapydan medicated plasters POM
Rasagiline POM
Rasburicase POM
Rasilex POM
Raspberry GSL
Rastinon preparations POM
Ratiograstim POM
Raudixin tablets POM
Rautrax tablets POM
Rauwiloid + Veriloid tablets POM
Rauwiloid tablets POM
Rauwolfia Serpentina POM
Rauwolfia Vomitoria POM
Raxar tablets POM
Razoxane POM
RBC cream GSL
Rebetol capsules POM
Rebetol 40mg/ml oral solution POM

Rebif injection POM
Reboxetine mesilate POM
Recombinate POM
Rectogesic rectal ointment POM
Rectubes CD Benz POM
Redoxon tablets GSL
Reductil capsules POM
Refacto injection POM
ReFacto AF injection POM
Refludan vials POM
Refolinon POM
Refolion preparations POM
Refresh P
Regaine Extra Strength P
Regaine gel for men GSL
Regaine hair supplements for women GSL
Regaine Regular Strength topical solution GSL
Regaine Regular Strength for Women GSL
Regranex gel POM
Regulan sachets GSL
Regulose P
Regurin tablets POM
Rehidrat sachets P
Relaxit P
Relaxyl capsules P
Relcofen tablets P
Relefact LH-RH ampoules POM
Relenza inhalation powder POM
Relestat eye-drops POM
Relifex preparations POM
Relistor POM
Relpax tablets POM
Remedeine preparations CD Inv POM
Remegel chewy squares GSL
Remegel tablets GSL
Remegel Wind Relief tablets GSL
Remicade infusion POM
Remifentanil CD POM
Reminyl preparations POM
Remnos tablets CD Benz POM
Remoxipride hydrochloride POM
Renagel preparations POM
Rennie Deflatine GSL
Rennie Duo preparations PO
Rennie Fruit GSL
Rennie preparations GSL
Rennie soft chews GSL
ReoPro POM
Repaglinide POM
Repevax vaccine POM
Replenate POM
Replenine POM
Replens GSL
Reproterol hydrochloride POM
Requip tablets POM
Rescinnamine POM
Rescue flow infusion POM
Reserpine POM
Resolve Extra sachets GSL
Resolve granules GSL
Resonium A P
Respacal syrup POM
Repaglinide POM
Respontin nebules POM
Resorcinol P
Resprin POM
Restandol capsules CD Anab POM
Retcin tablets POM
Reteplase POM
Retin-A preparations POM
Retinova cream POM
Retrovir preparations POM
Revanil tablets POM
Revasc injection POM
Revatio tablets POM
Revaxis vaccine POM
Reviparin POM
Rexocaine POM
Reyataz capsules POM
Rheomacrodex preparations POM
Rheumacin LA capsules POM
Rheumatac Retard POM
Rheumox preparations POM
Rhinacort Aqua POM
Rhinolast Allergy P

Rhinolast Hayfever P
Rhinolast nasal spray POM
Rhophylac 300 POM
Rhubarb rhizome GSL
Rhumalgan tablets POM
Rhumalgan SR capsules POM
Rhumalgan XL capsules POM
Riamet tablets POM
Ribavirin/Tribavirin POM
Riboflavin/Riboflavine GSL
Riboflavin/Riboflavine sodium phosphate GSL
Riboflavine see Riboflavin
Ricola herb cough lozenges GSL
Ridaura tablets POM
Rideril POM
Rifabutin POM
Rifadin preparations POM
Rifamide POM
Rifampicin POM
Rifampicin sodium POM
Rifamycin POM
Rifater tablets POM
Rifinah tablets POM
Rilutek tablets POM
Riluzole POM
Rimacillin POM
Rimactane preparations POM
Rimactazid tablets POM
Rimafen POM
Rimapam tablets POM
Rimapurinol tablets POM
Rimexolone POM
Rimiterol hydrobromide POM
Rimonabant POM
Rimoxacillin preparations POM
Rimso-50 POM
Rinatec inhaler POM
Rinatec nasal spray POM
Ringer's injection POM
Rinstead gel P
Rinstead pastilles GSL
Risedronate sodium POM
Risperdal preparations POM
Risperidone POM
Ritalin CD POM
Ritodrine hydrochloride POM
Ritonavir POM
Rituximab POM
Rivastigmine POM
Rivotril preparations CD Benz POM
Rizatriptan POM
Roaccutane capsules POM
RoActemra concentrate for solution for infusion POM
Robaxin 750 tablets POM
Robaxin Injectable POM
Robinul injection POM
Robinul-Neostigmine injection POM
Robitussin Chesty Cough 100ml PO
Robitussin Chesty Cough with Congestion P
Robitussin Dry Cough P
Robitussin dry cough pastilles P
Robitussin Junior P
Robitussin Night-Time P
Rocaltrol capsules POM
Rocephin vials POM
Rocuronium POM
Roferon prefilled syringes POM
Roferon-A POM
Rogitine ampoules POM
Rohypnol tablets CD No Register POM
Rolicyclidine CD Lic
Rolitetracycline nitrate POM
Rommix preparations POM
Rondomycin preparations POM
Ronicol tablets P
Ronicol Timespan tablets P
Ropinirole hydrochloride POM
Ropivacaine POM
Rose Fruit GSL
Rosemary GSL
Rosemary Oil GSL
Rosiglitazone POM
Rosuvastatin POM
Rotarix POM
Rotigotine POM

Rovamycin preparations POM
Rowachol POM
Rowatinex POM
Roxibolone CD Anab POM
Rozex gel POM
Rubella vaccine (live attenuated) POM
Rubella, mumps, measles vaccine POM
Rubellin GSL
Rue, if maximum strength 0.1 per cent (external use only) GSL
Rupafin tablets POM
Rusyde POM
Rynacrom preparations P
Rythmodan preparations POM

S

Sabadilla POM
Sabril tablets POM
Saflutan POM
Sage GSL
Sage Oil GSL
Saizen injection CD Anab POM
Salactol P
Salagen tablets POM
Salamol CFC-Free inhaler POM
Salamol Easi-Breathe POM
Salapin syrup POM
Salatac gel P
Salazopyrin preparations POM
Salazosulphadimidine POM
Salbutamol POM
Salbutamol sulphate POM
Salcatonin see Calcitonin (Salmon)
Salicylic acid if (1) internal: maximum strength 0.06 per cent antiseptic liquid, pastilles, lozenges, throat tablets GSL (2) external: corn plasters GSL (3) external: all other preparations for treatment of corns and calluses maximum strength 12.5 per cent GSL (4) external: dusting powder maximum strength 3.0 per cent GSL (5) external: cream, ointment or gel maximum strength 2.0 per cent GSL (6) external: medicated pads maximum strength 0.5 per cent in the impregnating solution GSL (7) external: antiseptic liquid maximum strength 0.06 per cent GSL (8) external liquids neither for the treatment of corns or calluses, nor antiseptic liquids maximum strength 0.05 per cent GSL (9) external: soap maximum strength 3.0 per cent GSL (10) external: wart plasters GSL (11) external: for the treatment of warts, verrucas, corns and calluses in adults and children over 2 years maximum strength 12% (in combination with lactic acid 4%) maximum pack size 8g GSL
Salmefamol POM
Salmeterol xinafoate POM
Salofalk preparations POM
Salonpas medicated plaster GSL
Salsalate POM
Saluric tablets POM
Salzone P
Sambucus GSL
Samsca POM
Sanderson's throat specific GSL
Sandimmun preparations POM
Sando-K effervescent tablets P
Sandocal effervescent tablets P
Sandoglobulin POM
Sandostatin POM
Sandostatin LAR POM
Sandrena gel POM
Sanomigran preparations POM
Saquinavir POM
Saralasin acetate POM
Sarsaparilla GSL
Savene POM
Saventrine tablets POM
Savlon antiseptic cream GSL
Savlon antiseptic wipes GSL
Savlon bites & stings gel GSL
Savlon blister plasters GSL

Savlon concentrated liquid GSL
Savlon disinfectant liquid GSL
Savlon Dry GSL
Savlon First Aid kit GSL
Savlon Liquid antiseptic GSL
Savlon Nappy Rash cream GSL
Savlon wound wash GSL
Saw Palmetto GSL
Scandonest POM
Schering PC4 tablets POM
Scheriproct preparations POM
Schick control POM
Schick test toxin POM
Scholl's athletes foot range GSL
Scholl's callous removal pads GSL
Scholl's corn & callous removal liquid - GSL
Scholl's corn and callous salve P
Scholl's corn removal pads GSL
Scholl's corn removal plasters GSL
Scholl's polymer gel corn removers GSL
Scholl's verruca removal gel seal & heal GSL
Scholl's verruca removal system - GSL
Scoline injection POM
Scopoderm TTS POM
Scopoderm 1.5mg Patch P
Scullcap GSL
Sea-legs tablets P
Seatone 500mg capsules GSL
Sebco GSL
Sebomin capsules POM
Sebren MR POM
Secadrex tablets POM
Secbutobarbitone CD No Register POM
Secbutobarbitone sodium CD No Register POM
Secobarbital/Quinalbarbitone CD POM
Secobarbital/Quinalbarbitone sodium CD POM
Seconal sodium capsules CD POM
Secron suspension P
Sectral preparations POM
Securon preparations POM
Securopen injection POM
Sedonium tablets P
Select-A-Jet Dopamine POM
Selegiline hydrochloride POM
Selenase POM
Selenium sulphide P
Selexid POM
Selsun P
Semi-Daonil tablets POM
Semisodium valproate POM
Semprex capsules POM
Senega GSL
Senna fruit GSL
Senna leaf GSL
Sennosides A and B, up to 15mg (MD) GSL
Senokot direct relief suppositories GSL
Senokot dual relief tablets GSL
Senokot granules PO
Senokot hi-fibre GSL
Senokot max strength tablets GSL
Senokot syrup 150ml GSL
Senokot tablets pack sizes 20s, 40s GSL; 60s, 100s PO
Sensodyne total care toothpaste gel 75ml GSL
Sential cream POM
Sential E cream P
Seominal tablets CD No Register POM
Septex cream No.1 P
Septex cream No.2 POM
Septopal Chains POM
Septrin preparations POM
Sera and antisera: Botulin antitoxin POM Diphtheria antitoxin POM; Gas-gangrene antitoxin (oedematiens) POM; Gas-gangrene antitoxin (perfringens) POM; Gas-gangrene antitoxin (septicum) POM; Mixed gas-gangrene antitoxin POM; Leptospira antiserum POM; Rabies antiserum POM; Scorpion venom antiserum POM; Snake venom antiserum POM; Tetanus antitoxin POM

Seractil tablets POM
Serc POM
Serdolect tablets POM
Serenace preparations POM
Seretide Accuhaler POM
Seretide Evohaler POM
Serevent preparations POM
Sermorelin POM
Serophene tablets POM
Seroquel tablets POM
Serotulle dressing P
Seroxat preparations POM
Sertindole tablets POM
Sertraline POM
Serum gonadotrophin POM
Setlers hearburn and indigestion liquid GSL
Setlers tablets GSL
Setlers Tums GSL
Sevelamer POM
Seven Seas cod liver oil GSL
Seven Seas cod liver oil & orange syrup GSL
Seven Seas cod liver oil capsules GSL
Seven Seas One a Day Pure cod liver oil capsules GSL
Seven Seas vitamin & mineral tonic GSL
Sevoflurane POM
Sevredol concentrated oral solution CD POM
Sevredol oral solution CD Inv POM
Sevredol tablets CD POM
Shark liver oil, if maximum strength 3.0g for suppositories, or all preparations for external use except suppositories (external use only) GSL
Shepherd's Purse GSL
Siberian fir oil, external use only GSL
Sibutramine POM
Silandrone CD Anab POM
Sildenafil POM
Silkis POM
Silver sulfadiazine/sulphadiazine POM
Simeco tablets P
Simple eye ointment P
Simple linctus BP GSL
Simple linctus paed BP GSL
Simplene eye drops POM
Simpson's foot ointment GSL
Simulect infusion POM
Simvador POM
Simvastatin POM, but where maximum strength 10mg, maximum daily dose 10mg and maximum pack size 28 tablets, P, please refer to proprietary names for the classification granted under the marketing authorisation (see Zocor Heart-Pro preparations)
Simzal POM
Sinemet preparations POM
Sinepin POM
Sinequan capsules POM
Singulair Paediatric granules POM
Singulair Paediatric tablets POM
Singulair tablets POM
Sinthrome tablets POM
Sinutab tablets P
Siopel cream GSL
Sirolimus POM
Sissomicin POM
Sissomicin sulphate POM
Sitaxentan POM
Skelid tablets POM
Skin traction kit GSL
Skinoren cream POM
Skintex GSL
Skunk Cabbage (Symplocarpus) GSL
Slippery Elm powdered bark GSL
Slippery Elm tabs GSL
Slocinx XL POM
Slo-Indo POM
Slo-phyllin capsules P
Slofedipine XL tablets POM
Slofenac POM
Sloprolol capsules POM
Slow Sodium tablets GSL
Slow-Fe Folic tablets POM
Slow-Fe tablets P

Slow-K tablets P
Slow-Trasicor tablets POM
Slozem capsules POM
Smallpox vaccine POM
Snake Venoms POM
Sno Phenicol eye drops POM
Sno Tears P
Sno-Pilo preparations POM
Snowfire Healing tablet GSL
Snufflebabe vapour rub GSL
Snug GSL
Sodiofolin POM
Sodium acetrizoate POM
Sodium acid phosphate GSL
Sodium acid pyrophosphate, external use only GSL
Sodium alginate GSL
Sodium alkylsulphoacetate P
Sodium amidiatrizoate preparations POM except powder P
Sodium aminosalicylate POM
Sodium amytal preparations CD No Register POM
Sodium antimonylgluconate POM
Sodium arsanilate POM
Sodium arsenate POM
Sodium arsenite POM but if 0.013 per cent, P
Sodium ascorbate GSL
Sodium aurothiomalate POM
Sodium bicarbonate GSL
Sodium bromide POM
Sodium calcium edetate POM
Sodium carbonate GSL
Sodium chloride GSL
Sodium chloride and dextrose injection POM
Sodium chloride BP tablets GSL
Sodium chloride injection POM
Sodium citrate GSL
Sodium citrate oral solution 0.3M (Viridian Pharma) POM
Sodium clodronate POM
Sodium cromoglicate/Sodium cromoglycate POM but if (a) for nasal administration; (b) for the treatment of acute seasonal allergic conjunctivitis or perennial allergic conjunctivitis in the form of aqueous eye drops maximum strength 2.0 per cent and container or package contains not more than 10ml of medicinal product; (c) for the treatment of acute seasonal allergic conjunctivitis in the form of an eye ointment maximum strength 4.0 per cent and container or package contains not more than 5g of medicinal product, P; or (d) for the relief and treatment of eye symptoms of hayfever, in the form of aqueous eye drops maximum strengh 2.0 per cent and container or package contains not more than 10ml of medicinal product, GSL
Sodium cromoglycate see Sodium cromoglicate
Sodium ethacrynate POM
Sodium feredate P
Sodium fluoride POM but if tablets or drops for prevention of dental caries with mdd 2.2mg P; external use, if maximum strength 0.33 per cent dentifrice or 0.05 per cent daily use mouth rinses for prevention of dental caries, or 0.2 per cent mouth rinses for other than daily use for the prevention of dental caries, GSL
Sodium fusidate POM
Sodium glycerophosphate GSL
Sodium hydroxide, if maximum strength 12.0 per cent (external use only) GSL
Sodium iodide, if MDD equivalent to 10mg iodine GSL
Sodium lactate, external use only GSL
Sodium lauryl ether sulphate, external use only GSL
Sodium lauryl ether sulphosuccinate, external use only GSL

Sodium metrizoate POM
Sodium monofluorophosphate POM but if dentifrice maximum strength 1.14 per cent, GSL (external use only)
Sodium nitrite POM
Sodium oxidronate POM
Sodium para-aminohippurate vials (MSD) POM
Sodium phenylbutyrate POM
Sodium phosphate GSL
Sodium picosulfate/Sodium picosulphate, for adults and children aged 10 years and over maximum stren GSL
Sodium picosulphate see Sodium picosulfate
Sodium potassium tartrate GSL
Sodium pyrophosphate, external use only GSL
Sodium pyrrolidone carboxylate, external use only GSL
Sodium salicylate GSL
Sodium selenite, internal use GSL
Sodium stibocaptate/Stibocaptate POM
Sodium stibogluconate POM
Sodium sulphate GSL
Sodium tetradecyl sulphate POM
Sodium valproate POM
Sofradex preparations POM
Soframycin preparations POM
Soft soap, external use only GSL
Solaquin P
Solarcaine preparations P
Solareze gel POM
Solian tablets POM
Solifenacin POM
Solivito-N vials POM
Soloc tablets POM
Solpadeine Headache preparations GSL
Solpadeine Max CD Inv P
Solpadeine Migraine CD Inv P
Solpadeine Plus CD Inv P
Solpadol preparations CD Inv POM
Solpaflex tablets CD Inv P
Soltamox oral solution POM
Solu-Cortef injection POM
Solu-Medrone vials POM
Solvazinc tablets P
Somatorelin acetate POM
Somatotropin CD Anab POM
Somatrem CD Anab POM
Somatropin CD Anab POM
Somatuline Autogel POM
Somatuline LA POM
Somavert injection POM
Sominex Herbal GSL
Sominex tablets P
Somnite preparations CD Benz POM
Somnwell POM
Sonata capsules POM
Sondate 200EC POM
Soneryl tablets CD No Register POM
Soothake gel GSL
Soothelip cold sore cream P
Sorafenib POM
Soraway P
Sorbichew tablets P
Sorbid SA tablets P
Sorbitol GSL
Sorbitrate tablets P
Sotacor preparations POM
Sotalol hydrochloride POM
Sotol tablets GSL
Southern Wood, external use only GSL
Soya oil GSL
Spasmonal P
Spasmonal Forte capsules P
Spatone GSL
Spectinomycin POM
Spectinomycin hydrochloride POM
SpectraBAN lotion 25 GSL
Spinach GSL
Spiramycin POM
Spiramycin adipate POM
Spiretic tablets POM
Spiriva inhalation capsules POM
Spiro-Co POM
Spiroctan preparations POM

Spiroctan-M injection POM
Spirolone tablets POM
Spironolactone POM
Spirospare tablets POM
Sporanox IV infusion POM
Sporanox preparations POM
Sprilon GSL
Sprycel POM
Squalane, external use only GSL
Squaw Vine GSL
Squill linctus, opiate BPC CD Inv P
Squill Vinegar GSL
Squill, Indian GSL
Squill, White GSL
St. James balm GSL
St Mary's Thistle GSL
Stafoxil capsules POM
Stalevo tablets POM
Stamaril vaccine POM
Stannous fluoride POM but if (a) dentifrice maximum strength 0.62 per cent; (b) dental gels for use in the prevention and treatment of dental caries and decalcification of the teeth maximum strength 0.4 per cent, P
Stanolone CD Anab POM
Stanozolol CD Anab POM
Stantar P
Starch GSL
Staril tablets POM
Starlix tablets POM
Starpax balsam GSL
Stavudine POM
STD injection POM
Stearyl alcohol, ethoxylated, external use only GSL
Stelara solution for injection POM
Stelazine preparations POM
Stemetil preparations POM
Stenbolone CD Anab POM
Ster-Zac preparations GSL
Sterculia GSL
Sterets P
Sterets H P
Steri-Neb Ipratropium POM
Steri-Neb Salamol POM
Stericlens GSL
Steriflex injections POM
Sterillium GSL
Steripaste P
Steripod chlorhexidine/cetrimide P
Steripod topical wound cleanser (sodium chloride 0.9%) P
Steripoules POM
Stesolid rectal tubes CD Benz POM
Stibocaptate see Sodium stibocaptate
Stibophen POM
Stiedex lotion POM
Stiedex LP 0.05% POM
Stiemycin POM
Stilboestrol see Diethylstilbestrol
Stilline POM
Stilnoct tablets CD Benz POM
Stimlor capsules POM
Stingose GSL
Stone root GSL
Stop 'N Grow GSL
Storax GSL
Strattera capsules POM
Strefen lozenges P
Strepsils preparations GSL
Streptase injection POM
Streptodornase POM but if external, P
Streptokinase POM but if external, P
Streptomycin POM
Streptomycin sulphate POM
Stressless GSL
Striant SR tablets CD Anab POM
Stromba preparations CD Anab POM
Stronazon MR capsules POM
Strontium acetate, if dentifrice (external use only) GSL
Strontium chloride hexahydrate, if dentifrice (external use only) GSL
Strontium ranelate POM
Strychnine POM
Strychnine arsenate POM

Strychnine hydrochloride POM
Strychnine nitrate POM
Stud 100 Desensitising spray for men P
Stugeron Forte capsules P
Stugeron tablets P
Stump GSL
Styramate POM
Subcuvia injection POM
Subgam POM
Sublimaze injection CD POM
Suboxone CD No Reg POM
Subutex tablets CD No Register POM
Succinylsulphathiazole POM
Sucralfate POM
Sucrose GSL
Sucrose Octa-acetate GSL
Sudafed Congestion cold & flu tablets P
Sudafed Congestion Relief capsules, non-drowsy GSL
Sudafed decongestant elixir P
Sudafed Dual Relief Max tablets, non-drowsy P
Sudafed Elixir P
Sudafed expectorant P
Sudafed linctus P
Sudafed nasal spray GSL
Sudafed non-drowsy 12-hour tablets P
Sudafed non-drowsy childrens syrup P
Sudafed non-drowsy dual relief capsules 16s GSL
Sudafed Plus preparations P
Sudafed tablets P
Sudafed-Co tablets pack sizes 12s P
Sudocrem preparations GSL
Sufentanil ; its salts; its esters and ethers; their salts CD POM
Sulazine EC tablets POM
Sulbactam Sodium POM
Sulbenicillin POM
Sulbenicillin sodium POM
Sulconazole nitrate POM but if external (except vaginal), P
Suleo-C lotion POM
Suleo-M lotion P
Sulfabenz POM
Sulfabenzamide POM
Sulfacetamide/Sulphacetamide POM
Sulfacetamide/Sulphacetamide sodium POM
Sulfacytine POM
Sulfadiazine/Sulphadiazine POM
Sulfadiazine/Sulphadiazine sodium POM
Sulfadicramide POM
Sulfadimidine/Sulphadimidine POM
Sulfadimidine/Sulphadimidine sodium POM
Sulfadoxine POM
Sulfamerazine POM
Sulfamerazine sodium POM
Sulfamethoxazole/Sulphamethoxazole POM
Sulfametopyrazine POM
Sulfamonomethoxine POM
Sulfapyrazole POM
Sulfapyridine/Sulphapyridine POM
Sulfapyridine/Sulphapyridine sodium POM
Sulfasalazine/Sulphasalazine POM
Sulfathiazole/Sulphathiazole POM
Sulfathiazole/Sulphathiazole sodium POM
Sulfinpyrazone/Sulphinpyrazone POM
Sulindac POM
Sulparex tablets POM
Sulphabromomethazine POM
Sulphacetamide see Sulfacetamide
Sulphachlorpyridazine POM
Sulphadiazine see Sulfadiazine
Sulphadimethoxine POM
Sulphadimidine see Sulfadimidine
Sulphafurazole POM
Sulphafurazole diethanolamine POM
Sulphaguanidine POM
Sulphaloxic acid POM
Sulphamethizole POM
Sulphamethoxazole see Sulfamethoxazole

Sulphamethoxydiazine POM
Sulphamethoxypyridazine POM
Sulphamethoxypyridazine sodium POM
Sulphamoxole POM
Sulphanilamide POM
Sulphaphenazole POM
Sulphapyridine see Sulfapyridine
Sulphasalazine see Sulfasalazine
Sulphathiazole see Sulfathiazole
Sulphatriad preparations POM
Sulphaurea POM
Sulphinpyrazone see Sulfinpyrazone
Sulphur GSL
Sulpiride POM
Sulpitil tablets POM
Sulpor oral solution POM
Sultamicillin POM
Sultamicillin tosylate POM
Sulthiame POM
Sultrin cream POM
Sumatriptan POM; but if tablets for oral use, for the acute relief of migraine attacks, with or without aura, in patients who have a stable well established pattern of symptoms, for adults aged 18 to 65 years, for a maximum period of 1 day, max strength 50mg, max dose 50mg, max daily dose 100mg and with a max pack size of 2 tablets, P
Sumatriptan succinate POM
Sunerven tablets GSL
Sunflower oil GSL
Sunitinib POM
Supralip tablets POM
Suprane POM
Suprax paediatric suspension POM
Suprax suspension POM
Suprax tablets POM
Suprecur injection POM
Suprecur nasal spray POM
Suprefact injection and nasal spray POM
Suprofen POM
Sure-amp ampoules POM
Sure-Lax GSL
Surgam SA capsules POM
Surgam tablets POM
Surmontil preparations POM
Survanta POM
Suscard Buccal tablets P
Sustac tablets P
Sustamycin capsules POM
Sustanon ampoules CD Anab POM
Sustiva preparations POM
Sutent POM
Sutoprofen POM
Suxamethonium bromide POM
Suxamethonium chloride POM
Suxethonium bromide POM
Swarm GSL
Sweet Birch oil GSL
Symbicort Turbohaler POM
Symmetrel preparations POM
Synacthen ampoules POM
Synacthen Depot POM
Synagis injection POM
Synalar C preparations POM
Synalar N preparations POM
Synalar preparations POM
Synandone preparations POM
Synarel nasal spray POM
Synastone injection CD POM
Syndol tablets CD Inv P
Synercid infusion POM
Syner-Kinase POM
Synflex capsules POM
Synflorix vaccine POM
Synphase tablets POM
Syntaris nasal spray POM
Syntex Menophase POM
Synthamin 7S injection POM
Synthamin injections POM
Synthamix POM
Syntocinon preparations POM
Syntometrine ampoules POM
Syntopressin nasal spray POM
Synuretic tablets POM
Syprol oral solution POM

Syscor MR tablets POM
Sytron elixir P

T

T-Zone clear pore body spray GSL
T-Zone clear & restore night gel patches GSL
T-Zone daily skin balancing moisturiser GSL
T/Gel shampoo GSL
Tabphyn MR POM
Tacalcitol monohydrate POM
TachoSil medicated sponge P
Tacrine hydrochloride POM
Tacrolimus POM
Tadalafil POM
Tagamet 100 P
Tagamet Dual Action liquid P
Tagamet preparations POM
Talampicillin POM
Talampicillin hydrochloride POM
Talampicillin napsylate POM
Talc, external use only GSL
Tambocor preparations POM
Tamiflu capsules POM
Tamiflu powder for oral suspension POM
Tamofen tablets POM
Tamoxifen POM
Tamoxifen citrate POM
Tampovagan N pessaries POM
Tampovagan pessaries POM
Tamsulosin POM
Tamsulosin hydrochloride POM; but if for the treatment of functional symptoms of benign prostatic hyperplasia (BPH) in men aged 45 to 75 years for a maximum treatment period of 6 weeks without clinical assessment by a doctor, maximum strength 400 micrograms, maximum daily dose 400 micrograms, maximum pack size 28 capsules P
Tanatril tablets POM
Tannic acid, if internal (pastilles, lozenges, throat tablets maximum strength 5mg) or external GSL
Tar, external use only GSL
Tarceva tablets POM
Tarcortin cream POM
Targinact prolonged release tablets CD POM
Targocid injection POM
Targretin capsules POM
Tarivid preparations POM
Tarka capsules POM
Tarodent GSL
Tartaric acid GSL
Tasigna capsules POM
Tasmar tablets POM
Taumasthman tablets POM
Tavanic IV POM
Tavanic tablets POM
Tavegil elixir P
Tavegil tablets P
Taxol concentrate for solution for infusion POM
Taxotere POM
Taxotere for infusion POM
Tazarotene POM
Tazobactam sodium POM
Tazocin POM
TCP antiseptic cream GSL
TCP cool menthol lozenge GSL
TCP First Aid cream GSL
TCP Liquid Antiseptic GSL
TCP ointment GSL
TCP Sore Throat lozenges GSL
Tea tree & witch hazel cream GSL
Tears Naturale P
Teclothiazide potassium POM
Tegretol preparations POM
Tegretol Retard POM
Teicoplanin POM
Telfast preparations POM
Telithromycin POM
Telmisartan POM
Telzir preparations POM

Temazepam CD No Register POM
Temazepam Gelthix CD No Register POM
Temcapril hydrochloride POM
Temgesic injection CD No Register POM
Temgesic sublingual tablets CD No Register POM
Temocillin sodium POM
Temodal POM
Temoporfin POM
Temozolomide POM
Tenben capsules POM
Tenecteplase POM
Tenif capsules POM
Tenkicin tablets POM
Tenkorex POM
Tenocyclidine CD Lic
Tenofovir POM
Tenoret 50 tablets POM
Tenoretic tablets POM
Tenormin preparations POM
Tenoxicam POM
Tensipine MR tablets POM
Tensium tablets CD Benz POM
Tensopril tablets POM
Teoptic eye drops POM
Terazosin hydrochloride POM
Terbinafine POM but if for external use for the treatment of tinea pedis, tinea cruris and tinea corporis in the form of a gel with maximum strength 1.0%, and in a container or package containing not more than 30g of medicinal product P
Terbinafine hydrochloride POM but (a) preparations, other than spray solutions, for external use of the treatment of tinea pedis and tinea cruris, maximum strength 1.0%, and in a container or package containing not more than 15g of medicinal product, P, but please refer to proprietary names for classification granted under the marketing authorisation (see Lamisil products) ; (b) spray solutions for external use for the treatment of tinea corporis, tinea cruris and tinea pedis, maximum strength 1%, in a container containing not more than 30ml of medicinal product, P, but please refer to proprietary names for classification granted under the marketing authorisation (see Lamisil products); (c) creams, for external use for the treatment of tinea pedis and tinea cruris, maximum strength 1%, in a container containing not more than 15g of medicinal product, GSL, but please refer to proprietary names for classification granted under the marketing authorisation (see Lamisil products) ; (d) sprays for external use for the treatment of tinea pedis and tinea cruris, maximum strength 1%, in a container containing not more than 30ml of medicinal product, GSL, but please refer to proprietary names for classification granted under the marketing authorisation (see Lamisil products) ; (e) cutaneous solution for external use for the treatment of tinea pedis in persons 18 years and over, to be administered as a single application, maximum strength 1%, in a container containing not more than 4g of medicinal product GSL
Terbutaline POM
Terbutaline sulphate POM
Tercolix CD Inv POM
Terebene (Terepene), external use only GSL
Terfenadine POM
Terfinax tablets POM
Teril CR tablets POM
Teriparatide POM
Terlipressin POM
Terodiline hydrochloride POM

Terpineol GSL
Terpoin CD Inv POM
Terra-Cortil Nystatin cream POM
Terra-Cortil preparations POM
Terramycin preparations POM
Tertroxin tablets POM
Testim gel CD Anab POM
Testoderm patches CD Anab POM
Testogel gel CD Anab POM
Testosterone CD Anab POM
Tetabulin POM
Tetanus and pertussis vaccine POM
Tetanus vaccine POM
Tetrabenazine POM
Tetracaine/Amethocaine POM but if
    non-ophthalmic use P
Tetracaine/Amethocaine gentisate POM
    but if non-ophthalmic use P
Tetracaine/Amethocaine hydrochloride
    POM but if non-ophthalmic use P
Tetrachel preparations POM
Tetracosactide/Tetracosactrin POM
Tetracosactide/Tetracosactrin acetate
    POM
Tetracosactrin see Tetracosactide
Tetracycline POM
Tetracycline hydrochloride POM
Tetracycline phosphate complex POM
Tetrahydrocannabinol see Cannabinol
    derivatives
Tetrahydrogestrinone CD Anab POM
Tetralysal preparations POM
Tetrazepam CD Benz POM
Tetroxoprim POM
Teveten tablets POM
Thallium acetate POM
Thallous chloride POM
THC see Cannabinol derivatives
Thebacon; its salts CD POM
Thebaine; its salts CD POM
Thelin POM
Theo-dur tablets P
Thephorin tablets P
Thiabendazole see Tiabendazole
Thiambutosine POM
Thiamine hydrochloride GSL
Thiamine mononitrate GSL
Thiazamide tablets POM
Thiethylperazine malate POM
Thiethylperazine maleate POM
Thiocarlide POM
Thioguanine see Tioguanine
Thiomesterone CD Anab POM
Thiopental/Thiopentone sodium POM
Thiopentone see Thiopental
Thiopropazate hydrochloride POM
Thioproperazine mesylate POM
Thioridazine POM
Thioridazine hydrochloride POM
Thiosinamine POM
Thiosinamine and ethyl iodide POM
Thiostrepton POM
Thiotepa POM
Thiothixene POM
Thiouracil POM
Throaties antibacterial pastilles GSL
Thurfyl salicylate, external use only GSL
Thyme GSL
Thyme Oil GSL
Thymol GSL
Thymoxamine see Moxisylyte
Thyrogen POM
Thyroid POM
Thyrotrophin POM
Thyrotrophin releasing hormone POM
Thyroxine sodium see Levothyroxine
    sodium
Tiabendazole/Thiabendazole POM
Tiagabine POM
Tiamulin fumarate POM
Tiaprofenic acid POM
Tibolone POM
Ticarcillin sodium POM
Ticlid tablets POM
Ticlopidine hydrochloride POM
Tiger Balm GSL
Tigloidine hydrobromide POM
Tilade aerosol POM

Tilarin nasal spray POM
Tildiem LA tablets POM
Tildiem Retard POM
Tildiem tablets POM
Tilia (Lime Flowers) GSL
Tilidate its salts; its esters and ethers;
    their salts CD POM
Tilofyl CD POM
Tiloket POM
Tilolec POM
Tiloryth capsules POM
Tiludronate disodium POM
Tiludronic acid POM
Timecef injection POM
Timentin injection POM
Timodine cream POM
Timolol maleate POM
Timonil Retard tablets POM
Timoptol POM
Timoptol LA ophthalmic solutions POM
Timpron tablets POM
Tinaderm cream GSL
Tinaderm Plus powder GSL
Tinaderm-M cream GSL
Tinazaparin POM
Tinidazole POM
Tinzaparin POM
Tioconazole POM but if external (except
    vaginal) maximum strength 2.0 per
    cent; (2) vaginal for treatment of
    vaginal candidiasis, P
Tioguanine/Thioguanine POM
Tiotropium POM
Tipranavir capsules POM
Tirofiban POM
Tisept solution P
Titanium dioxide GSL
Titanium peroxide, external use only
    GSL
Titanium salicylate, external use only
    GSL
Titralac tablets GSL
Tixycolds cold and allergy nasal drops
    GSL
Tixycolds cold and hayfever inhalant
    capsules GSL
Tixycolds syrup P
Tixylix baby syrup GSL
Tixylix Catarrh syrup P
Tixylix Chesty Cough syrup GSL
Tixylix Cough and Cold linctus CD Inv
    P
Tixylix Daytime linctus CD Inv P
Tixylix dry cough P
Tixylix Night-time linctus CD Inv P
Tixymol suspension P
Tixyplus suspension P
Tizanidine POM
Tobi nebuliser solution POM
Tobradex eye drops POM
Tobramycin POM
Tobramycin sulphate POM
Tocainide hydrochloride POM
Tocopheryl acetate GSL
Toepodo cream P
Tofenacin hydrochloride POM
Tofranil preparations POM
Tofranil with promazine capsules POM
Tolanase tablets POM
Tolazamide POM
Tolazoline hydrochloride POM but if
    external, P
Tolbutamide POM
Tolbutamide sodium POM
Tolcapone POM
Tolfenamic acid POM
Tolmetin sodium POM
Tolnaftate, external use only GSL
Tolperisone POM
Tolterodine tartrate POM
Tolu Balsam GSL
Tolu-flavour solution GSL
Tomudex POM
Tonpular XL capsules POM
Topal tablets GSL
Topamax Sprinkle capsules POM
Topamax tablets POM
Topicycline solution POM

Topiramate POM
Topotecan POM
Toradol injection POM
Toradol tablets POM
Torasemide POM
Torbetol GSL
Torem tablets POM
Toremifene POM
Torisel POM
Totamol tablets POM
Totaretic tablets POM
Toviaz prolonged release tablets POM
Tracleer tablets POM
Tracrium injection POM
Tractocile preparations POM
Tradorec XL POM
Tramacet preparations POM
Tramadol hydrochloride POM
Tramake capsules POM
Tramake Insts sachets POM
Tramazoline POM
Trandate preparations POM
Trandolapril POM
Tranexamic acid POM; but if for oral
    use, for reduction of heavy menstrual
    bleeding over several cycles in
    women aged 18-45 years old with
    regular, 21-35 day cycles with no
    more than 3 days individual variabili-
    ty in cycle duration, maximum
    strength 500mg, 1g (MD), 4g (MDD),
    maximum treatment period 4 days,
    maximum pack size 18 tablets P
Trangina XL POM
Tranquax capsules POM
Tranquilyn tablets CD POM
Transiderm-Nitro P
Transtec transdermal patches CD No
    Register POM
Transvasin cream GSL
Transvasin Heat spray GSL
Tranxene capsules CD Benz POM
Tranylcypromine sulphate POM
Trasicor preparations POM
Trasidrex tablets POM
Trastuzumab POM
Trasylol injection POM
Travasept 100 P
Travatan eye-drops POM
Traveleeze pastilles P
Travogyn vaginal tablets POM
Travoprost POM
Traxam gel POM
Traxam Pain Relief gel P
Traxam Quick Break foam POM
Trazodone hydrochloride POM
Treacle GSL
Tredaptive POM
Trenbolone CD Anab POM
Trental preparations POM
Treosulfan POM
Tretamine POM
Tretinoin POM
TRH-Roche preparations POM
Tri-Adcortyl Otic ointment POM
Tri-Adcortyl preparations POM
Tri-Minulet tablets POM
Triacetyloleandomycin POM
Triadene POM
Triam-Co tablets POM
Triamax-Co tablets POM
Triamcinolone POM
Triamcinolone acetonide POM but if (1)
    for the treatment of common mouth
    ulcers maximum strength 0.1% and
    container or package contains not
    more than 5g of medicinal product,
    or (2) in the form of a pressurised
    nasal spray, for the treatment of
    symptoms of seasonal allergic rhinitis
    in persons aged 18 years and over,
    110mcg per nostril (MD) 110mcg per
    nostril (MDD) for a maximum period
    of 3 months, in a container or pack-
    age containing not more than
    3.575mg of triamcinolone acetonide
    P
Triamcinolone diacetate POM

Triamcinolone hexacetonide POM
Triamterene POM
Triapin Mite tablets POM
Triapin tablets POM
Triazolam CD Benz POM
Tribavirin see Ribavirin
Trichlorofluoromethane (Propellant 11),
    external use only GSL
Triclofos sodium POM
Triclosan, external use only GSL
Tricyclamol chloride POM
Tridene POM
Tridestra tablets POM
Trientine POM
Trientine dihydrochloride POM
Trifluoperazine POM
Trifluoperazine hydrochloride POM
Trifluperidol POM
Trifluperidol hydrochloride POM
Trifyba GSL
Trihexyphenidyl/Benzhexol hydrochlo-
    ride POM
Triiodothyronine injection POM
Trileptal oral suspension POM
Trileptal tablets POM
Trilostane POM
Triludan tablets POM
Trimeperidine; its salts CD POM
Trimeprazine see Alimemazine
Trimetaphan camsylate POM
Trimetazidine POM
Trimetazidine hydrochloride POM
Trimethoprim POM
Trimetrexate glucuronate POM
Trimipramine maleate POM
Trimipramine mesylate POM
Trimogal tablets POM
Trimopan suspension POM
Trimopan tablets POM
Trimovate preparations POM
Trimustine hydrochloride POM
Trinordiol tablets POM
Trinovum ED tablets POM
Trinovum tablets POM
Trintek patches P
Triogesic tablets P
Triominic tablets P
Triprimix tablets POM
Triprolidine P
Triptafen preparations POM
Triptorelin POM
Trisenox POM
Trisequens Forte POM
Trisequens tablets POM
Trisodium edetate POM
Tritace capsules POM
Tritace tablets POM
Trivax vaccine POM
Trivax-AD vaccine POM
Trivax-Hib POM
Trizivir tablets POM
Trobicin vials POM
Tropergen tablets POM
Tropicamide POM
Tropisetron hydrochloride POM
Tropium preparations CD Benz POM
Trosyl nail solution POM
Troxidone POM
Trusopt ophthalmic solution POM
Truvada POM
Tryptizol preparations POM
L-Tryptophan POM but if (1) oral dietary
    supplementation (2) external, P
Trypure POM
Tuberculin purified protein derivative
    POM
Tubocurarine chloride POM
Tuinal capsules CD POM
Tulobuterol POM
Tulobuterol hydrochloride POM
Tums tablets GSL
Tunes GSL
Turpentine oil, if internal (vapour
    inhalations except preparations to be
    applied topically), or external or
    internal (vapour inhalations from
    products to be applied topically maxi-
    mum strength 5%) GSL

Twinrix Adult vaccine POM
Twinrix paediatric POM
Tybamate POM
Tygacil solution for infusion POM
Tylex capsules CD Inv POM
Tylex effervescent CD Inv POM
Tylosin POM
Tylosin phosphate POM
Tylosin tartrate POM
Typherix vaccine POM
Typhim Vi vaccine POM
Typhoid and tetanus vaccine POM
Typhoid vaccine POM
Typhoid-paratyphoid A and B cholera
    vaccine POM
Typhoid-paratyphoid A and B tetanus
    vaccine POM
Typhoid-paratyphoid A and B vaccine
    POM
Typhus vaccine POM
Tyrothricin POM but if throat lozenges
    or throat pastilles, P
Tyrozets lozenges P
Tysabri POM
Tyverb film coated tablets POM

U

Ubretid preparations POM
Ucerax preparations POM
Ucine tablets POM
Uftoral capsules POM
Ukidan injection POM
Ultec tablets POM
Ultiva injection CD POM
Ultra Chloraseptic P
Ultrabase GSL
Ultralanum plain preparations POM
Ultramol soluble tablets CD Inv P
Ultraproct preparations POM
Ultratard insulins POM
Undecenoic acid, external use only GSL
Unguentum M cream GSL
Unichem allergy relief syrup P
Unichem allergy relief tablets P
Unichem bronchial mixture GSL
Unichem childs diarrhoea mixture GSL
Unichem cold relief capsules GSL
Unichem cold relief powders hot lemon
    flu strength GSL
Unichem cystitis relief sachets GSL
Unichem diarrhoea relief capsules 2mg
    GSL
Unichem Hayfever & Allergy non-
    drowsy tablets GSL
Unichem heartburn relief tablets P
Unichem junior paracetamol suspension
    P
Unichem pain relief capsules long last-
    ing P
Unichem Rehydration Treatment GSL
Unichem rehydration treatment sachets
    P
Unichem sleep aid capsule P
Unichem sleep aid extra capsules P
Unichem throat lozenges GSL
Unicorn Root False GSL
Uniflor tablets P
Uniflu with gregovite C CD Inv P
Unigest tablets P
Unihep injection POM
Uniparin injection POM
Uniphyllin Continus tablets P
Unipine XL POM
Uniroid HC preparations POM
Unisept solution P
Univer capsules POM
Uorazepam CD Benz POM
Uprima sublingual tablets POM
Uracil POM
Uramustine POM
Urdox tablets POM
Urea hydrogen peroxide, external use
    only GSL
Urea Stibamine POM
Urea, external use only GSL
Urethane POM
Uriben preparations POM

Uridine 5'-triphosphate POM
Uriflex-G P
Uriflex-R P
Uriflex-S P
Uriflex-SP P
Uriflex-W P
Urispas tablets POM
Urofollitrophin see Urofollitropin
Urofollitropin/Urofollitrophin POM
Urokinase POM
Uromitexan injection POM
Uromitexan tablets POM
Urotainer chlorhexidine 1:5000 P
Ursodeoxychoic Acid POM
Ursofalk capsules POM
Ursofalk suspension POM
Ursogal tablets and capsules POM
Utinor tablets POM
Utovlan tablets POM
Uva Ursi (Bearberry) GSL
Uvacin GSL

V

Vaccine: Bacillus Salmonella Typhi
    POM
Vaccine: Poliomyelitis (Oral) POM
Vadarex rub GSL
Vagifem vaginal tablets POM
Vaginyl tablets POM
Vagisil cream GSL
Valaciclovir POM
Valclair CD Benz POM
Valcyte powder for oral solution
    50mg/ml POM
Valcyte tablets POM
Valdecoxib POM
Valderma GSL
Valdoxan film-coated tablets POM
Valerian GSL
Valerian tabs GSL
Valerina tablets GSL
Valganciclovir POM
Valium preparations CD Benz PCM
Vallergan Forte syrup POM
Vallergan preparations POM
Vallestril tablets POM
Valoid injection POM
Valoid tablets P
Valonorm P
Valpeda GSL
Valpiform POM
Valproic acid POM
Valsartan POM
Valtrex tablets POM
Vamin preparations POM
Vaminolact POM
Vanair cream P
Vancocin preparations POM
Vancomycin hydrochloride POM
Vaniqa cream POM
Vantage Allergy relief preparations P
Vantage Baby cream GSL
Vantage Clearsore cold sore cream P
Vantage clotrimazole cream P
Vantage co-codamol tablets P
Vantage constipation relief tablets P
Vantage cough syrups P
Vantage cystitis relief sachets GSL
Vantage Flu-strength all-in-one P
Vantage haemorrhoid cream GSL
Vantage hayfever relief nasal spray P
Vantage heartburn relief tablets P
Vantage hydrocortisone cream P
Vantage ibuprofen suspension P
Vantage loperamide tablets P
Vantage paracetamol preparations P
Vantage sleep aid tablets P
Vantage thrush treatment capsule P
Vantas implant POM
Vaqta injection POM
Vaqta Paediatric vaccine POM
Vardenafil POM
Varenicline POM
Varicella vaccine POM
Varidase preparations POM
Varilrix vaccine POM
Varivax injection POM

Vascace tablets POM
Vascalpha tablets POM
Vasculit tablets P
Vasodon-A eye drops POM
Vasogen GSL
Vasopressin POM
Vasopressin injection POM
Vasopressin tannate POM
Vasosulf eye drops POM
Vasoxine injection POM
Vectavir cold sore cream POM
Vectibix POM
Vecuronium bromide POM
Veganin tablets pack sizes 10s, 30s CD
    Inv P
Vegetable laxative tablets BPC 1963
    POM
Velbe POM
Velcade injection POM
Velosef preparations POM
Velosulin insulins POM
Venaxx XL modified release capsules
    POM
Venlafaxine POM
Veno's Dry cough mixture GSL
Veno's Expectorant cough mixture GSL
Veno's for Kids GSL
Veno's Honey & Lemon cough mixture
    GSL
Venofer injection POM
Venofundin POM
Ventavis POM
Ventide inhaler POM
Ventmax POM
Ventolin preparations POM
Vepesid preparations POM
Vera-til SR POM
Veracur gel GSL
Verapamil hydrochloride POM
Verapress MR tablets POM
Veratrine POM
Veratrum, Green POM
Veratrum, White PCM
Verbena GSL
Veripaque P
Vermox preparations POM
Verrugon P
Versatis POM
Vertab SR POM
Verteporfin POM
Vesagex cream GSL
Vesanoid capsules POM
Vesicare tablets POM
Vexol ophthalmic suspension POM
Vfend powder for oral suspension POM
Vfend tablets and infusion POM
Viagra tablets POM
Viatim vaccine POM
Viazem XL capsules POM
Vibramycin preparations POM
Vibramycin-D tablets POM
Vicks Action P
Vicks Coldcare P
Vicks First Defence GSL
Vicks inhaler GSL
Vicks Medinite P
Vicks Sinex preparations GSL
Vicks Ultra chloraseptic throat spray P
Vicks VapoRub GSL
Vicks Vaposyrup Chesty Cough GSL
Vicks Vaposyrup Chesty Cough &
    Congestion P
Vicks Vaposyrup Childrens Dry Cough
    P
Vicks Vaposyrup Dry Cough & Nasal
    Congestion P
Victoza solution for injection in prefilled
    pen POM
Vidarabine POM
Vidaza powder for suspension for injec-
    tion POM
Videne preparations P
Videx EC capsules POM
Videx tablets POM
Vidopen preparations POM
Vielle lubricant GSL
Vielle menopause kit GSL
Vigabatrin POM

Vigam liquid POM
Vigam S POM
Vigranon B syrup P
Vikonon GSL
Viloxazine hydrochloride POM
Vinblastine sulphate POM
Vincristine sulphate POM
Vindesine sulphate POM
Vinorelibine tartrate POM
Vioform-hydrocortisone preparations
    POM
Viomycin pantothenate POM
Viomycin sulphate POM
Vioxx preparations POM
VioxxAcute tablets POM
Viracept tablets POM
Viraferon injection POM
Viraferonpeg injection POM
ViraferonPeg prefilled pens POM
Viralief P
Viramune preparations POM
Virasorb cold sore cream GSL
Virazid powder for aerosol POM
Virazole POM
Viread tablets POM
Virgan eye gel POM
Virginiamycin POM
Viridal Duo injection POM
Viridal injection POM
Viroflu vaccine POM
Virormone injections CD Anab POM
Virovir tablets POM
Visclair tablets P
Viscotears liquid gel P
Viscotears single dose units P
Viskaldix tablets POM
Visken tablets POM
Vista-Methasone drops POM
Vista-Methasone-N drops POM
Vistabel POM
Visthesia Intercameral P
Visthesia Light Intercameral P
Vistide solution POM
Visudyne infusion POM
Vitacoll Extra GSL
Vitacoll Gold GSL
Vitalux Plus capsules P
Vitamin A POM but if (1) external, P; (2)
    internal 7,500iu (2,250mcg retinol
    equivalent) (MDD), GSL
Vitamin A acetate POM but if (1) exter-
    nal, P; (2) internal equivalent to
    7,500iu Vitamin A (2,250mcg retinol
    equivalent) (MDD), GSL
Vitamin A palmitate POM but if (1)
    external, P; (2) internal equivalent to
    7,500iu Vitamin A (2,250mcg retinol
    equivalent) (MDD), GSL
Vitamin D (calciferol), up to 400iu
    (10mcg cholecalciferol) (MDD) GSL
Vitlipid Adult POM
Vitlipid Infant POM
Vitlipid N POM
Vitravene injection POM
Vitrimix KV POM
Vivabec P
Vivacor POM
Vivadone POM
Vivaglobin POM
Vivalan tablets POM
Vivazide POM
Vivicrom eye-drops P
Vividrin eye drops POM
Vividrin nasal spray P
Vivioptal capsules P
Vivotif vaccine POM
Vivpryl tablets POM
Viz-on eyedrops POM
Vocalzone throat pastilles GSL
Volmax tablets POM
Volplex POM
Volraman tablets POM
Volsaid Retard tablets POM
Voltarol Emulgel P 30g and 50g P
Voltarol Optha POM
Voltarol Paineze Emulgel GSL
Voltarol preparations POM
Voltarol Rapid tablets POM

Voluven POM
Voriconazole POM

W

Wahoo (Euonymus atropurpureus) GSL
Wala pillules all PO except
    Apis/Levisticum,
    Belladonna/Chamomilla,
    Chamomilla/Nicotiana, Silicea Comp
    and Valeriana Comp GSL
Warfarin POM
Warfarin sodium POM
Wartex ointment (Pickles) P
Warticon preparations POM
Warticon Fem POM
Waspeze aerosol for stings P
Waspeze bites & stings spray GSL
Wate-On P
Water GSL
Water Balance tablets GSL
Water for injection ampoules POM
Watercress GSL
Wax-Aid P
Waxsol GSL
Weleda Aconite/Bryonia drops PO
Weleda Antimony ointment PO
Weleda Apatite 6X Comp tablets PO
Weleda Arnica ointment GSL
Weleda Arnica 6X tablets GSL
Weleda Avena Sativa compound GSL
Weleda Balsamicum ointment PO
Weleda Bidor tablets GSL
Weleda Bolus Eucalypti compound PO
Weleda Calendolon ointment GSL
Weleda Catarrh cream PO
Weleda Chamomilla 3X drops GSL
Weleda Choleodoron drops PO
Weleda Cinnabar 20X/Pyrites 3X tablets
    PO
Weleda Combudoron ointment GSL
Weleda Combudoron spray GSL
Weleda Conchae 5% compound tablets
    PO
Weleda Copper ointment GSL
Weleda Cough drops PO
Weleda Cough drops compound PO
Weleda Crataegus Comp drops PO
Weleda Dermatodoron ointment PO
Weleda Digestodoron drops PO
Weleda Digestodoron tablets PO
Weleda Dulcarmara/Lysamachia drops
    PO
Weleda Erysidoron drops PO
Weleda Ferrum phosphate Co. pillules
    POM
Weleda Ferrum Siderum 6X tablets PO
Weleda Feverfew 6X drops GSL
Weleda Feverfew 6X tablets GSL
Weleda Fragador tablets GSL
Weleda Fragaria/Urtica drops PO
Weleda Fragaria/Vitis tablets PO
Weleda Frost cream PO
Weleda Gencydo ointment PO
Weleda granules GSL
Weleda homoeopathic medicines tablets
    GSL
Weleda Hypericum/Calendula ointment
    GSL
Weleda Infludo drops POM
Weleda juices & elixirs GSL
Weleda Larch resin ointment GSL
Weleda Laxadoron tablets GSL
Weleda lotions GSL
Weleda Mandragora Comp drops PO
Weleda massage balms GSL
Weleda medicinal gargle GSL
Weleda Melissa compound GSL
Weleda Menodoron drops PO
Weleda Mercurius Cyanat 4X POM
Weleda mini medicines massage balm
    GSL
Weleda mini medicines ointments GSL
Weleda nasal spray GSL

Weleda Nausyn tablets POM
Weleda Oleum Rhinale drops PO
Weleda Onopordon Comp A drops PO
Weleda Onopordon Comp B drops PO
Weleda Pertudoron 1 drops POM
Weleda Pertudoron 2 drops PO
Weleda Phosphorus/Tart POM
Weleda Pyrites 3X tablets PO
Weleda Rheumadoron 1 drops PO
Weleda Rheumadoron 102A drops PO
Weleda Rheumadoron 2 drops PO
Weleda Rheumadoron ointment PO
Weleda Rhus Tox ointment GSL
Weleda Ruta ointment GSL
Weleda Scleron tablets PO
Weleda Vitis Comp tablets PO
Weleda W.C.S. dusting powder PO
Welldorm preparations POM
Wellferon POM
Wellvone suspension POM
Wellvone tablets POM
Wheat GSL
Whita preparations GSL
Wild Cherry GSL
Wild Indigo GSL
Wild Lettuce GSL
Willow White GSL
Wilzin POM
Wind-Eze products GSL
Windcheaters capsules GSL
Windsetlers GSL
WinRho SDF POM
Witch Doctor skin treatment gel GSL
Witch Doctor hydrating gel GSL
Witch Doctor radiance serum GSL
Wood Betony GSL
Woodward's gripe water GSL
Woodwards teething gel GSL
Wool alcohols, acetylated, external use
    only GSL
Wool alcohols, external use only GSL
Wool fat, external use only GSL
Wright's vaporiser blocks P
Wright's vaporising fluid P

X

Xagrid tablets POM
Xalacom eye-drops POM
Xalantan eye drops POM
Xamiol gel POM
Xamoterol fumarate POM
Xanax tablets CD Benz POM
Xanthan gum GSL
Xanthomax POM
Xarelto POM
Xatral SR tablets POM
Xatral tablets POM
Xatral XL tablets POM
Xefo tablets and injection POM
Xeloda tablets POM
Xenazine 25 tablets POM
Xenical capsules POM
Xepin cream POM
Xigris infusion POM
Xipamide POM
Xismox XL POM
Xolair POM
Xylocaine 4% topical P
Xylocaine antiseptic gel P
Xylocaine eye drops POM
Xylocaine gel P
Xylocaine injections POM
Xylocaine ointment P
Xylocaine spray P
Xylocaine with adrenaline injections POM
Xylocard injections POM
Xylometazoline hydrochloride, if non-
    oily nasal sprays and nasal drops
    maximum strength 0.1 per cent GSL
Xyloproct preparations POM
Xylotox injections POM
Xyrem oral solution CD Benz POM
Xyzal tablets POM

Y

Yariba GSL
Yarrow GSL
Yasmin tablets POM
Yeast GSL
Yeast-Vite GSL
Yellow Dock GSL
Yellow fever vaccine POM
Yentreve capsules POM
Yohimbine hydrochloride POM
Yomesan tablets P
Yondelis POM
Yutopar preparations POM

Z

Z Span Spansules P
Z-Span P
Zacin cream POM
Zaditen capsules POM
Zaditen elixir POM
Zaditen eye-drops POM
Zaditen tablets POM
Zadstat preparations POM
Zaedoc tablets POM
Zafirlucast POM
Zalcitabine POM
Zaleplon POM
Zamadol 24hr tablets POM
Zamadol Melt tablets POM
Zamadol preparations POM
Zamadol SR capsules POM
Zanaflex tablets POM
Zanamivir POM
Zanidip tablets POM
Zanprol tablets P
Zantac 75 P
Zantac 75 Dissolve P
Zantac 75 Relief GSL
Zantac 75 Relief Dissolve GSL
Zantac preparations POM
Zanza GSL
Zapain capsules CD Inv POM
Zaponex tablets POM
Zarontin preparations POM
Zarzio POM
Zavedos capsules POM
Zavedos injection POM
Zavesca capsules POM
Zeasorb powder P
Zebinix tablets POM
Zeffix preparations POM
Zelapar tablets POM
Zemon XL tablets POM
Zemplar injection POM
Zemtard XL capsules POM
Zenalb solution POM
Zenapax infusion POM
Zenoxone cream (PL 0181/0033) P
Zeranol CD Anab POM
Zerit capsules POM
Zerobase GSL
Zestoretic tablets POM
Zestril tablets POM
Zevalin POM
Ziagen preparations POM
Zibor preparations POM
Zida-Co tablets POM
Zidoval vaginal gel POM
Zidovudine POM
Zileze tablets POM
Zilpaterol CD Anab POM
Zimbacol XL tablets POM
Zimeldine hydrochloride POM
Zimovane POM
Zimovane LS POM
Zinacef preparations POM
Zinamide tablets POM
Zinc carbonate, external use only GSL
Zinc citrate trihydrate, if dentifrice,
    external use only GSL
Zinc gluconate, if MDD equivalent to
    5mg elemental zinc GSL

Zinc oleate, external use only GSL
Zinc oxide, if MDD equivalent to 5mg
    elemental zinc GSL
Zinc stearate, external use only GSL
Zinc sulphate, if internal equivalent to
    5mg elemental zinc (MDD) or exter-
    nal maximum strength 1.0 per cent
    GSL
Zinc undecenoate, external use only GSL
Zincaband P
Zindaclin gel POM
Zineryt application POM
Zinga capsules POM
Zinnat preparations POM
Zipeprol CD POM
Zipzoc P
Zirtek Allergy relief tablets pack sizes 7s
    GSL
Zirtek Allergy solution pack sizes 70ml
    GSL; 150ml P; 200ml P
Zirtek allergy tablets pack sizes 21s P; 30s
    P
Zispin SolTabs POM
Zispin tablets POM
Zita tablets POM
Zithromax preparations POM
Ziz Forte P
Ziz tablets P
Zocor Heart-Pro tablets P
Zocor tablets POM
Zofran Flexi-Amps POM
Zofran preparations POM
Zoladex injection POM
Zoledronic acid POM
Zoleptil tablets POM
Zolmitriptan POM
Zolpidem CD Benz POM
Zolpidem tartrate CD Benz POM
Zolvadex LA Depot injection POM
Zolvera oral solution POM
Zomacton CD Anab POM
Zomepirac sodium POM
Zometa infusion POM
Zomig nasal spray POM
Zomig nasal spray POM
Zomig Rapimelt tablets POM
Zomig tablets POM
Zomorph capsules CD POM
Zonegran capsules POM
Zonisamide POM
Zonivent Aquanasal spray POM
Zopiclone POM
Zorac gel POM
Zotepine POM
Zoton preparations POM
Zovirax 5% pump GSL
Zovirax cold sore cream GSL
Zovirax cream POM
Zovirax dispersible tablets POM
Zovirax Double Strength suspension
    POM
Zovirax IV POM
Zovirax ophthalmic ointment POM
Zovirax suspension POM
Zoxin capsules POM
Zoxycil capsules POM
Zubes lozenges GSL
Zuclopenthixol acetate POM
Zuclopenthixol decanoate POM
Zuclopenthixol dihydrochloride
    POM
Zumenon tablets POM
Zuvogen POM
Zyban tablets POM
Zydol preparations POM
Zydol SR tablets POM
Zydol XL tablets POM
Zyloric 300 tablets POM
Zyloric tablets POM
Zyomet gel POM
Zyprexa IntraMuscular POM
Zyprexa tablets POM
Zyprexa Velotab tablets POM
Zyvox preparations POM

1.4 Non-medicinal poisons

A "non-medicinal poison," or simply a "poison," is a substance that is included in the poisons list made under the Poisons Act 1972, as amended. A reference to a poison includes substances containing that poison. Other substances, no matter how toxic, are not poisons under this Act.

A comprehensive fact sheet on poisons is now available from the Legal and Ethical Advisory Service.

Some substances in the poisons list (eg, arsenic, mercuric oxide) also have medicinal uses. When sold as medicines such substances are controlled by the Medicines Act 1968, as amended, but when sold for non-medicinal purposes they are subject to the Poisons Act 1972, as amended.

The poisons list is divided into two parts. In general, substances included in **Part I** of the list (ie, Part I poisons) may be sold only by persons lawfully conducting retail pharmacy businesses. Such sales must be conducted at a registered pharmacy under the supervision of a pharmacist.

Part II of the list (ie, Part II poisons) may be sold both by persons lawfully conducting a retail pharmacy business and by listed sellers of Part II poisons, that is, by persons whose names appear in a list of sellers maintained by a local authority. A listed seller may nominate one or two deputies who also may effect the sale of Schedule 1 poisons.

Listed sellers may only sell Part II poisons in prepacked containers and sales must be made on the listed premises.

Certain Part II poisons may be sold only by listed sellers if the poison is in a specified form, and some of these poisons may only be sold to persons engaged in the trade or business of horticulture, agriculture or forestry and for the purposes of that trade or business.

Apart from these matters, the requirements for the sale of Part II poisons are substantially the same for listed sellers as for persons lawfully conducting retail pharmacy businesses.

NB: Since 1 September 2006, strychnine no longer has approval for purchase or use for mole control, from the Pesticides Safety Directorate (PSD).

1.4.1 Poisons schedules

The Poisons Rules 1982, as amended, apply or relax the restrictions imposed by the Act in particular circumstances. There are eight schedules to the Rules and they are described, briefly, below (more detailed reference is made to some of them later):

Schedule 1 A list of poisons to which special restrictions apply relating to storage, conditions of sale and keeping of records of sales. The restrictions do not apply to articles which contain barium carbonate or to alpha-chloralose and zinc phosphide when they are prepared for the destruction of rats and mice as described in the individual entries in the alphabetical list (see *Medicines, Ethics and Practice*, Section 1.5).

Schedule 4 A list of articles exempted from control as poisons. There are two groups. Group I comprises classes of articles which contain poisons which are totally exempt from the requirements of the Poisons Act 1972, as amended, and the Poisons Rules 1982, as amended, eg, builders'

materials. Group II lists exemptions for certain poisons when in specified articles or substances, eg, sulphuric acid in accumulators.

Schedule 5 Some Part II poisons may be sold by listed sellers only in certain forms. The details are given in this schedule which also specifies certain poisons which may be sold by listed sellers only to persons engaged in the trade or business of agriculture, horticulture or forestry and for the purpose of that trade or business. In any other circumstances the sale of Schedule 5 poisons is restricted to pharmacies.

Schedule 8 Form of application for inclusion in local authority's list of sellers of Part II poisons.

Schedule 9 Form of the list of listed sellers of Part II poisons kept by a local authority.

Schedule 10 Certificate for the purchase of a non-medicinal poison.

Schedule 11 Form of entry to be made in poisons book on sale of Schedule 1 poison.

Schedule 12 Restriction of sale and supply of strychnine and other substances. Forms of authority required for certain of these poisons.

Schedules 2, 3, 6 and 7 were deleted by a Poisons Rules Amendment Order in 1985.

1.4.2 Sales of poisons

Sales of Schedule 1 poisons

There are certain requirements that must be fulfilled for the lawful sale of Schedule 1 poisons (and no other poisons). These requirements are concerned with record keeping and having knowledge, or confirmation of the identity by way of certification, of the purchaser.

Knowledge of the purchaser

The purchaser of a Schedule 1 poison must be either:

(a) certified in writing in the prescribed manner by a householder to be a person to whom the poison may properly be sold (*see Figure 1.1*). If the householder is not known to the seller to be a responsible person of good character, the certificate must be endorsed by a police officer in charge of a police station. It must be retained by the seller; or,

(b) known by the seller, or by a pharmacist employed by the seller at the premises where the sale is effected, to be a person to whom the poison may properly be sold.

If the purchaser is known by the person in charge of the premises on which the poison is sold, or of the department of the business in which the sale is effected, then the requirement as to knowledge of the purchaser by the seller is deemed to be

```
SCHEDULE 10                    Rule 25

CERTIFICATE FOR THE PURCHASE OF A NON-MEDICINAL POISON

    For the purposes of section 3(2)(a)(i) of the Poisons Act 1972 I, the undersigned,
a householder occupying (a) .................................................................
hereby certify from my knowledge of (b) .................................................
of (a) ..............................................................................................
that he is a person to whom (c) .............................may properly be supplied.
    I further certify that (d) ..................................is the signature of the said
(b) ........................................

                            .................................................
                            Signature of householder giving
                                    certificate.
                        Date ...........................................
                        (a) Insert full postal address.
                        (b) Insert full name of intending purchaser.
                        (c) Insert name of poison.
                        (d) Intending purchaser to sign his name here.

Endorsement required by Rule 25 of the Poisons Rules 1982 to be made by a police
officer in charge of a police station when, but only when, the householder giving the
certificate is not known to the seller of the poison to be a responsible person of good
character.

    I hereby certify that in so far as is known to the police of the district in which
*  .............................................................resides he is a responsible
person of good character.
                        Signature of Police Officer .................................
                        Rank ..........................................................
                        In charge of police station at ..............................
                        Date ...........................................
Office Stamp of
    Police Station.
            * Insert full name of householder giving this certificate.
```

Figure 1.1: Certificate for the purchase of a non-medicinal poison

satisfied in the case of (a) sales made by listed sellers of Part II poisons, and (b) sales exempted by Section 4 of the Act (*see* p81).

The requirements as to knowledge of the purchaser, entry in the poisons book and signature (or signed order) by the purchaser do not apply to:

(a) the sale of poisons to be exported to purchasers outside the United Kingdom;
(b) the sale of any article by its manufacturer or by a person carrying on a business in the course of which poisons are regularly sold by way of wholesale dealing, if
(i) the article is sold to a person carrying on a business in the course of which poisons are sold or regularly used in the manufacture of other articles; and
(ii) the seller is reasonably satisfied that the purchaser requires the article for the purpose of that business.

The requirements which apply to the sale of Schedule 1 poisons apply also to the supply of such poisons in the form of commercial samples. The requirement that the person supplied must be known to the seller is satisfied, for the supply of commercial samples, if the person to be supplied is known by the person in charge of the department of the business through which the sale is made.

Records

The seller must not deliver a Schedule 1 poison until he has made the required entry in the poisons book and the purchaser has signed it. The particulars to be recorded are:

(a) the date of the sale;
(b) the name and quantity of poison supplied;
(c) the name and address of the purchaser;

(d) the business, trade or occupation of the purchaser;
(e) the purpose for which it is stated by the purchaser to be required;
(f) the name and address of the householder, if any, by whom a certificate was given and the date of the certificate.

Entries in the poisons book must be made in the manner prescribed in the Poisons Rules 1982, as amended. The book must be retained for two years from the date on which the last entry was made.

A signed order may be accepted in lieu of the purchaser's signature in the circumstances described below.

The Poisons Rules 1982, as amended, require any authority or certificate to be retained by the seller of the poison to which the authority or certificate relates. As the poisons register must be retained for two years after the date of the last entry, the authority or certificate must also be retained for at least two years.

There is no requirement under the legislation to make an entry of receipts of poisons. Only records of supplies are legally required.

Signed orders

A signed order in writing may be accepted from a person who requires a Schedule 1 poison for the purpose of his trade, business or profession. The seller must be reasonably satisfied that the purchaser carries on the trade, business or profession stated, and that the signature is genuine. In addition to the signature of the purchaser the order must state:

(a) his name and address;
(b) his trade, business or profession;
(c) total quantity to be purchased;
(d) the purpose for which the poison is required.

A signed order is required to be dated. The entry made in the poisons book before delivery of the poison must be dated. The date of the signed order and the words "signed order" must be recorded in place of the signature and be identified by a reference number. In an emergency the seller may deliver the poison on receiving an undertaking that a signed order will be furnished within the next 72 hours. Failure to comply with an undertaking, or the making of false statements to obtain a Schedule 1 poison without a signed order, are contraventions of the Poisons Rules.

Labelling of poisons

Substances in the Poisons List are subject to the legislation concerned with Chemicals and must be labelled accordingly (*see* p87).

Containers for poisons

Substances in the Poisons List are subject to the legislation concerned with Chemicals and must be supplied in an appropriate container (*see* p88).

Storage of Schedule 1 poisons

Schedule 1 poisons in any retail shop, or premises used in connection with such a shop, must be stored in one of the following ways:

(a) in a cupboard or drawer reserved solely for the storage of poisons; or

(b) in a part of the premises which is partitioned off or otherwise separated from the remainder of the premises and to which customers are not permitted to have access; or

(c) on a shelf reserved solely for the storage of poisons, and no food is kept directly under the shelf.

If the poison is to be used in agriculture, horticulture or forestry then:

(a) it must not be stored on any shelf or any part of the premises where food is kept; and

(b) it may only be stored in a cupboard or drawer which is reserved for poisons used in agriculture, horticulture or forestry.

The Control of Substances Hazardous to Health Regulations 2002, made under the Health and Safety at Work etc Act 1974 imposes duties on employers to protect employees and other persons who may be exposed to substances hazardous to health. For this reason a COSSH risk assessment would have to be carried out by a pharmacist before storing and selling poisons.

Schedule 1 poisons subject to special restrictions

Some Schedule 1 poisons are subject to special restrictions on sale or supply as detailed in Schedule 12 of the Poisons Rules 1982, as amended. They may only be sold:

(a) by way of wholesale dealing,

(b) for export to purchasers outside the United Kingdom, or

(c) to persons or institutions concerned with scientific education or research or chemical analysis for the purpose of that education, research or analysis.

Sale or supply of these poisons is also permitted in the circumstances indicated below:

(1) Fluoroacetic acid its salts or fluoroacetamide may be sold:
To a person producing a certificate, in form "A" or form "B" as provided in Schedule 12, which has been issued within the preceding three months. The certificate must specify the quantity of the poison to be used as a rodenticide and identify the places where it is to be used, which may be:

(a) ships or sewers as indicated in the certificate; or

(b) drains identified in the certificate, being drains situated in restricted areas and wholly enclosed and inaccessible when not in use; or

(c) warehouses identified in the certificate which are in restricted dock areas and kept securely locked and barred when not in use

The proper officer of health of a local authority or port health authority may issue forms "A" to employees of the authority for the purpose of purchasing rodenticide for use as in (a), (b) or (c) above.

The proper officer of health of a local authority or port health authority may issue forms "B" to persons carrying on the business of pest control, or to their employees for the purpose of purchasing rodenticide for use as in (a) or (b) above.

For the purchase of rodenticide for use as in (a) or (b) above form "B" may also be issued, in England, by a person duly authorised by the Department for Environment, Food and Rural Affairs (DEFRA), or in Scotland a person authorised by the Scottish Ministers, or in Wales a person authorised by the National Assembly for Wales (NAW), certifying that the substance is required for use by their officers.

(2) Strychnine
Strychnine is no longer approved for purchase or use for the killing of moles, but there is provision for the supply of strychnine for the purpose of killing foxes in an infected area within the meaning of the Rabies (Control) Order 1974, as amended. A request under these circumstances is very unlikely, as there have been no requests for this use in recent years, but would have to be in accordance with a written authority, as detailed in the Poisons Rules.

The sale and supply of thallium salts, potassium and sodium arsenites, and zinc phosphide are also restricted to certain circumstances but no longer have Pesticides Safety Directorate (PSD) approval.

The sale and supply of calcium, potassium and sodium cyanide are also restricted and also no longer have PSD approval.

Sales exempted by Section 4

Section 4 of the Poisons Act 1972, as amended, exempts certain categories of sales of poisons from the provisions of Section 3(1) and 3(2) of the Act, except as provided by the Poisons Rules 1982, as amended. The principal effect is that exempted transactions of any Part 1 poison may be made without the supervision of a pharmacist, provided the sales are not made by a shopkeeper on premises connected with his retail business. The requirements as to signed orders and poisons book records in respect of Schedule 1 poisons also apply.

The exempted categories are:

(1) Sales of poisons by way of wholesale dealing, that is, sales made to a person who buys for the purpose of selling again.

(2) The sale of an article to a doctor, dentist, veterinary surgeon or veterinary practitioner for the purpose of his profession.

(3) The sale of an article for use in or in connection with any hospital infirmary or dispensary or similar institution approved by an order, whether general or special of the Secretary of State.

(4) The sale of an article by a person carrying on a business in the course of which poisons are regularly sold either by way of wholesale dealing or for use by the purchasers in their trade or business to:

(a) a government department or an officer of the Crown requiring the article for the purposes of the public service, or any local authority, requiring the article in connection with the exercise by the authority, of any statutory powers; or

(b) a person or institution concerned with scientific education or research, if the article is required for the purposes of that education or research; or

(c) a person who requires the article for the purpose of enabling him to comply with any requirements with respect to the medical treatment of persons employed by that person in any trade or business carried on by him; or

(d) a person who requires the article for the purpose of his trade or business. A person can be said to be carrying on a business if he engages in full-time or part-time commercial activity with a view to profit.

Sales of poisons to be exported to purchasers outside the United Kingdom are also listed as exempted categories. However, these types of transaction are exempted from the provisions of Section 3(1) and 3(2) of the Act and the Rules requiring signed orders and poisons book records etc.

Wholesale dealing to a shopkeeper

"Sale by way of wholesale dealing" means sale to a person who buys for the purpose of selling again.

It is not lawful to sell by way of wholesale dealing any poison included in Part I of the Poisons List to a person carrying on a business of shopkeeping unless the seller:

(a) has reasonable grounds for believing that the purchaser is a person lawfully conducting a retail pharmacy business; or
(b) has received a statement signed by the purchaser or by a person authorised by him on his behalf to the effect that the purchaser does not intend to sell the poison on any premises used for or in connection with his retail business.

1.5 Alphabetical list of non-medicinal poisons

A

Acetarsol P1; S1 except substances containing less than the equivalent of 0.0075% arsenic (P1 only)

Acetarsone P1; S1 except substances containing less than the equivalent of 0.0075% arsenic (P1 only)

Aldicarb P2; S1; S5 listed sellers of poisons permitted to sell only if in preparations for use in agriculture, horticulture or forestry and such sales are restricted to these trade or business users

Alpha-chloralose see Chloralose

Aluminium phosphide P1; S1

Ammonia P2; S4 in substances, not being solutions of ammonia or preparations containing solutions of ammonia, in substances containing less than 10% w/w ammonia, in refrigerators

Ammonium bifluoride P2

Ammonium fluoride P2

Antimony barium tartrate P1; S1

Arecoline-acetarsol P1; S1 except substances containing less than the equivalent of 0.0075% arsenic (P1 only)

Arsanilic acid P1; S1 except substances containing less than the equivalent of 0.0075% arsenic (P1 only); S4 in reagent kits or reagent devices, supplied for medical or veterinary purposes, substances containing less than 0.1% w/w arsanilic acid

Arsenates, except copper arsenates and lead arsenates P1; S1 except substances containing less than the equivalent of 0.0075% arsenic (P1 only)

Arsenic P1; S1 except substances containing less than the equivalent of 0.0075% arsenic (P1 only)

Arsenic, halides of P1; S1 except substances containing less than the equivalent of 0.0075% arsenic (P1 only)

Arsenic, organic compounds of P1; S1 except substances containing less than the equivalent of 0.0075% arsenic (P1 only)

Arsenic, oxides of P1; S1

Arsenic, oxides of P1; S1 except substances containing less than the equivalent of 0.0075% arsenic (P1 only)

Arsenic sulphides P1; S1 except substances containing less than the equivalent of 0.0075% arsenic (P1 only)

Arsenic tribromide P1; S1 except substances containing less than the equivalent of 0.0075% arsenic (P1 only)

Arsenic trichloride P1; S1 except substances containing less than the equivalent of 0.0075% arsenic (P1 only)

Arsenic triiodide P1; S1 except substances containing less than the equivalent of 0.0075% arsenic (P1 only)

Arsenic trioxide P1; S1 except substances containing less than the equivalent of 0.0075% arsenic (P1 only)

Arsenious acid P1; S1 except substances containing less than the equivalent of 0.0075% arsenic (P1 only)

Arsenious anhydride P1; S1 except substances containing less than the equivalent of 0.0075% arsenic (P1 only)

Arsenious iodide P1; S1 except substances containing less than the equivalent of 0.0075% arsenic (P1 only)

Arsenious oxide P1; S1 except substances containing less than the equivalent of 0.0075% arsenic (P1 only)

Arsenites, except calcium arsenites and copper arsenites P1; S1 except substances containing less than the equivalent of 0.0075% arsenic (P1 only)

Arsenobenzene P1; S1 except substances containing less than the equivalent of 0.0075% arsenic (P1 only)

Arsenobenzol P1; S1 except substances containing less than the equivalent of 0.0075% arsenic (P1 only)

Arsenophenolamine P1; S1 except substances containing less than the equivalent of 0.0075% arsenic (P1 only)

Arsphenamine, silver P1; S1 except substances containing less than the equivalent of 0.0075% arsenic (P1 only)

Azinphos-methyl see Phosphorus compounds

B

Barium antimonyltartrate P1; S1

Barium carbonate P2; S1; S4 in witherite, other than finely ground witherite, when bonded to charcoal for case hardening, in sealed smoke generators containing not more than 25% barium carbonate; S5 listed sellers of poisons permitted to sell only for use in preparations for the destruction of rats or mice, but such sales are not restricted to trade or business users

Barium chloride P1; S1; S4 in fire extinguishers containing barium chloride

Barium, salts of, other than barium sulphate P1; S1

Barium silicofluoride P2; S1

Barium sulphide P1; S1

Bismuth glycollylarsanilate P1; S1 except substances containing less than the equivalent of 0.0075% arsenic (P1 only)

Bromomethane P1; S1; S4 in fire extinguishers

C

Calcium arsenate P1; S1 except substances containing less than the equivalent of 0.0075% arsenic (P1 only)

Calcium arsenites P2; S1 except substances containing less than the equivalent of 0.0075% arsenic (P2 only); S5 listed sellers of poisons permitted to sell only for use as agricultural, horticultural and forestal insecticides or fungicides and such sales are restricted to these trade or business users

Calcium cyanide* P1; S1 except substances containing less than the equivalent of 0.1% w/w hydrogen cyanide (P1 only), and except in the case of a sale exempted by Section 4 of the Poisons Act 1972 it is not lawful to sell or supply calcium cyanide

Carbarsone P1; S1 except substances containing less than the equivalent of 0.0075% arsenic (P1 only)

Carbofuran P2; S1; S4 in granular preparations; S5 listed sellers of poisons permitted to sell only if in preparations for use in agriculture, horticulture or forestry and such sales are restricted to these trade or business users

Chloralose P2; S5 listed sellers of poisons permitted to sell only if in preparations intended for indoor use in the destruction of rats or mice and containing not more than 4% w/w chloralose, preparations intended for indoor use in the destruction of rats or mice and containing not more than 8.5% w/w chloralose, where the preparation is contained in a bag or sachet which is itself attached to the inside of a device in which the preparation is intended to be so used and the device contains not more than 3 grams of the preparation, but such sales are not restricted to trade or business users

Chlorfenvinphos see Phosphorus compounds

Chloropicrin P1; S1

Copper acetoarsenite P2; S1 except substances containing less than the equivalent of 0.0075% arsenic (P2 only); S5 listed sellers of poisons permitted to sell only for use as agricultural, horticultural and forestal insecticides or fungicides, and such sales are restricted to these trade or business users

Copper arsenates P2; S1 except substances containing less than the equivalent of 0.0075% arsenic (P2 only); S5 listed sellers of poisons permitted to sell only for use as agricultural horticultural and forestal insecticides or fungicides and such sales are restricted to these trade or business users

Copper arsenites P2; S1 except substances containing less than the equivalent of 0.0075% arsenic (P2 only); S5 listed sellers of poisons permitted to sell only for use as agricultural, horticultural and forestal insecticides or fungicides and such sales are restricted to these trade or business users

Cyanides (metal) other than ferrocyanides and ferricyanides P1; S1 except substances containing less than the equivalent of 0.1% w/w hydrogen cyanide (P1 only), and except in the case of a sale exempted by Section 4 of the Poisons Act 1972, it is not lawful to sell or supply calcium cyanide, potassium cyanide or sodium cyanide

Cycloheximide P2; S1; S5 listed sellers of poisons permitted to sell only if in preparations for use in forestry, and such sales are restricted to trade or business users

D

Demephion see Phosphorus compounds

Demeton-S-methyl see Phosphorus compounds

Demeton-S-methyl sulphone see Phosphorus compounds

Dialifos see Phosphorus compounds

Dichlorophenarsine hydrochloride P1; S1 except substances containing less than the equivalent of 0.0075% arsenic (P1 only)

Dichlorvos see Phosphorus compounds

Diethylamine acetarsol P1; S1 except substances containing less than the equivalent of 0.0075% arsenic (P1 only)

Diethylamine acetarsone P1; S1 except substances containing less than the equivalent of 0.0075% arsenic (P1 only)

Dinitrocresols (DNOC); their compounds with a metal or a base P2; S1 except winter washes containing not more than the equivalent of 5% dinitrocresols (P2 only); S5 listed sellers of poisons permitted to sell only if in preparations for use in agriculture, horticulture or forestry and except for the above mentioned winter washes, such sales are restricted to these trade or business users

Dinoseb, its compounds with a metal or a base P2; S1; S5 listed sellers of poisons permitted to sell only if in preparations for use in agriculture, horticulture or forestry and such sales are restricted to these trade or business users

Dinoterb, P2; S1; S5 listed sellers of poisons permitted to sell only if in preparations for use in agriculture, horticulture or forestry and such sales are restricted to these trade or business users

Dioxathion see Phosphorus compounds

Diphetarsone P1; S1 except substances containing less than the equivalent of 0.0075% arsenic (P1 only)

Drazoxolon; its salts P2; S1; S4 in treatments on seeds; S5 listed sellers of poisons permitted to sell only if in preparations for use in agriculture, horticulture or forestry and such sales are restricted to these trade or business users

Disulfoton see Phosphorus compounds

E

Endosulfan P2; S1; S5 listed sellers of poisons permitted to sell only if in preparations for use in agriculture, horticulture or forestry, and such sales are restricted to these trade or business users

Endothal, its salts P2; S1; S5 listed sellers of poisons permitted to sell only if in preparations for use in agriculture, horticulture or forestry, and such sales are restricted to these trade or business users

Endrin P2; S1; S5 listed sellers of poisons permitted to sell only if in preparations for use in agriculture, horticulture or forestry, and such sales are restricted to these trade or business users

F

Fentin, compounds of P2; S1; S5 listed sellers of poisons permitted to sell only if in preparations for use in agriculture, horticulture or forestry and such sales are restricted to these trade or business users

Ferric cacodylate P1; S1 except substances containing less than the equivalent of 0.0075% arsenic (P1 only)

Ferrous arsenate P1; S1 except substances containing less than the equivalent of 0.0075% arsenic (P1 only)

Fluoroacetic acid, its salts; fluoroacetamide P1; S1. Rule 12 prohibits sale or supply except in the cases mentioned in Section 1.4.2

Fonofos see Phosphorus compounds

Formaldehyde P2; S4 in substances containing less than 5%w/w formaldehyde, in photographic glazing or hardening solutions

Formic acid P2; S4 in substances containing less than 25% w/w formic acid

H

Hydrochloric acid P2; S4 in substances containing less than 10%w/w hydrochloric acid

Hydrofluoric acid P2

Hydrogen cyanide P1; S1 except substances containing less than 0.15%. w/w hydrogen cyanide (P1 only); S4 in preparations of wild cherry, in reagent kits supplied for medical or veterinary purposes composed of substances which contain less than the equivalent of 0.1% w/w hydrogen cyanide

4-Hydroxy-3-nitrophenyl-arsonic acid P1; S1 except substances containing less than the equivalent of 0.0075% arsenic (P1 only)

L

Lead acetates P1; S4 in substances containing less than the equivalent of 2.5% w/w of elemental lead (Pb)

Lead arsenates P2; S1 except substances containing less than the equivalent of 0.0075% arsenic (P2 only); S5 listed sellers of poisons permitted to sell only for use in agricultural, horticultural or forestal insecticides or fungicides, and such sales are restricted to these trade or business users

Lead arsenite P1; S1 except substances containing less than the equivalent of 0.0075% arsenic (P1 only)

Lead, compounds of, with acids from fixed oils P1; S1

M

Magnesium Phosphide P1; S1

Mecarbam see Phosphorus compounds

Melarsonyl potassium P1; S1 except substances containing less than the equivalent of 0.0075% arsenic (P1 only)

Melarsoprol P1; S1 except substances containing less than the equivalent of 0.0075% arsenic (P1 only)

Mephosfolan see Phosphorus compounds

Mercuric ammonium chloride P1

Mercuric chloride P2; S1 except substances containing less than 1% mercuric chloride (P2 only); S4 in batteries, in treatments on seeds or bulbs; S5 listed sellers of poisons permitted to sell only for use as agricultural, horticultural and forestal fungicides, seed and bulb treatments, insecticides, and such sales are restricted to these trade or business users

Mercuric cyanide P1; S1 except substances containing less than the

equivalent of 0.1% w/w hydrogen cyanide (P1 only)

Mercuric cyanide oxides P1

Mercuric iodide P2; S1 except substances containing less than 2% mercuric iodide (P2 only); S4 in treatments on seeds or bulbs; S5 listed sellers of poisons permitted to sell only for use as agricultural, horticultural and forestal fungicides, seed and bulb treatments, and such sales are restricted to these trade or business users

Mercuric nitrates P1; S1 except substances containing less than the equivalent of 3% w/w mercury (P1 only)

Mercuric oxide, red P1

Mercuric oxide, yellow P1; S4 in canker and wound paints (for trees) containing not more than 3% w/w yellow mercuric oxide

Mercuric oxycyanide see Mercuric cyanide oxides

Mercuric sulphocyanide P1

Mercuric thiocyanate P1

Mercury (metal) not in the Poisons List

Mercury, ammoniated P1

Mercury biniodide see Mercuric iodide

Mercury, nitrates of P1; S1 except substances containing less than the equivalent of 3% w/w mercury (P1 only)

Mercury, oleated P1; S1 in aerosols and in substances containing the equivalent of 0.2% w/w mercury or more (otherwise P1 only)

Mercury, organic compounds of, which contain a methyl group directly linked to the mercury atom P1 (for all other organic compounds of mercury see next entry); S1 in aerosols and in substances containing the equivalent of 0.2% w/w mercury or more (otherwise P1 only); S4 in treatments on seeds or bulbs; S5 listed sellers of poisons permitted to sell only for use as agricultural, horticultural and forestal fungicides, seed and bulb treatments, and such sales are restricted to these trade or business users

Mercury, organic compounds of (except those which contain a methyl group directly linked to the mercury atom for these see previous entry) P2; S1 in aerosols and in substances containing the equivalent of 0.2% w/w mercury or more (otherwise P2 only); S4 in treatments on seeds or bulbs; S5 listed sellers of poisons permitted to sell only for use as agricultural, horticultural and forestal fungicides, seeds and bulb treatments and solutions containing not more than 5% w/v phenylmercuric acetate for use in swimming baths, and except for this last mentioned substance, such sales are restricted to trade or business users

Mercury, organic compounds in aerosols (whether P1 or P2) S1; S4 in treatments on seeds or bulbs; S5 (in the case of P2 aerosols only) listed sellers of poisons permitted to sell only for use as agricultural, horticultural and forestal fungicides, seed and bulb treatments, and such sales are restricted to these trade or business users

Metallic oxalates see Oxalates, metallic

Methidathion see Phosphorus compounds

Methomyl P2; S1; S4 in solid substances containing not more than 1% w/w of methomyl; S5 listed sellers of

poisons permitted to sell only if in preparations for use in agriculture, horticulture or forestry and such sales are restricted to these trade or business users

Mevinphos see phosphorus compounds

N

Neoarsphenamine P1; S1 except substances containing less than the equivalent of 0.0075% arsenic (P1 only)

Nicotine, its salts, its quaternary compounds P2; S1; S4 in tobacco, in cigarettes, the paper of a cigarette (excluding any part of that paper forming part of or surrounding a filter), where that paper in each cigarette does not have more than the equivalent of 10 milligrams of nicotine; in aerosol dispensers containing not more than 0.2% w/w nicotine; in other liquid preparations, and solid preparations with a soap base containing not more than 7.5% w/w nicotine (for Nicotine dusts see next entry)

Nicotine dusts P2; S1 except if present in agricultural and horticultural insecticides containing not more than 4% w/w nicotine; label "Poison" in red but no register entry needed

Nitric acid P2; S4 in substances containing less than 20% w/w nitric acid

Nitrobenzene P2; S4 in substances containing less than 0.1% nitrobenzene, in polishes; S5 listed sellers permitted to sell only for use as agricultural, horticultural and forestal insecticides, but such sales are not restricted to these trade or business users

O

Omethoate see Phosphorus compounds

Oxalates, metallic P2; S4 in laundry blue, polishes, cleaning powders or scouring products, containing the equivalent of not more than 10% oxalic acid dihydrate; S5 (except for potassium quadroxalate), listed sellers of poisons permitted to sell for use only as photographic solutions or materials, but such sales are not restricted to trade or business users

Oxalic acid P1; S4 in laundry blue, in polishes, in cleaning powders or scouring products, containing the equivalent of not more than 10% oxalic acid dihydrate

Oxamyl P2; S1; S4 in granular preparations; S5 listed sellers of poisons permitted to sell only if in preparations for use in agriculture, horticulture or forestry and such sales are restricted to these trade or business users

Oxophenarsine hydrochloride P1; S1 except substances containing less than the equivalent of 0.0075% arsenic (P1 only)

Oxophenarsine tartrate P1; S1 except substances containing less than the equivalent of 0.0075% arsenic (P1 only)

Oxydemeton-methyl see Phosphorus compounds

P

Paraquat, salts of P2; S1; S4 preparations in pellet form containing not more than 5% of salts of paraquat (calculated as paraquat ion); S5 listed sellers of poisons permitted to sell

only if in preparations for use in agriculture, horticulture or forestry and such sales are restricted to these trade or business users

Parathion see Phosphorus compounds

Phenkapton see Phosphorus compounds

Phenols, substances containing 60% w/w phenols (or more) and compounds of phenol with a metal containing the equivalent of 60% w/w phenol (or more) P1 (for all other phenols see next entry)

Phenols, substances containing less than 60% w/w phenols and compounds of phenol with a metal containing the equivalent of less than 60% w/w phenols P2; S4 creosote obtained from coal tar, in liquid disinfectants and antiseptics containing less than 0.5% phenol and containing less than 5% of other phenols, motor fuel treatments not containing phenol and containing less than 2.5% of other phenols, in reagent kits supplied for medical or veterinary purposes, solid substances containing less than 60% of phenols, tar (coal or wood), crude or refined, in tar oil distillation fractions containing not more than 5% of phenols

Phenylmercuric acetate as for Phenylmercuric salts

Phenylmercuric borate P2; S1 in aerosols and in substances containing the equivalent of 0.2% w/w mercury or more (otherwise P2 only); S4 as for Phenylmercuric salts; S5 listed sellers of poisons permitted to sell only for use as agricultural, horticultural and forestal fungicides, seed and bulb treatments, and such sales are restricted to these trade or business users

Phenylmercuric nitrate P2; S1 in aerosols and in substances containing the equivalent of 0.2% w/w mercury or more (otherwise P2 only); S4 as for Phenylmercuric salts; S5 listed sellers of poisons permitted to sell only for use as agricultural, horticultural and forestal fungicides, seed and bulb treatments, and such sales are restricted to these trade or business users

Phenylmercuric salts P2; S1 in aerosols and in substances containing the equivalent of 0.2% w/w mercury or more (otherwise P2 only) S4 in antiseptic dressings on toothbrushes, in textiles containing not more than 0.01% phenylmercuric salts as a bacteriostat and fungicide; S5 listed sellers of poisons permitted to sell only for use as agricultural, horticultural and forestal fungicides, seed and bulb treatments and solutions containing not more than 5% w/v phenylmercuric acetate for use in swimming baths (when S1 restrictions apply), and except for this last mentioned substance, such sales are restricted to these trade or business users

Phorate see Phosphorus compounds

Phosphamidon see Phosphorus compounds

Phosphoric acid P2; S4 in substances containing phosphoric acid, not being descaling preparations containing more than 50% w/w orthophosphoric acid

Phosphorus compounds:
Azinphos-methyl
Demephion
Demeton-S-methyl
Demeton-S-methyl sulphone
Dialifos

Dioxathion
Mecarbam
Mephosfolan
Methidathion
Mevinphos
Omethoate
Phenkapton
Phosphamidon
Quinalphos
Thiometon
Vamidothion
P2; S1; S5 listed sellers of poisons permitted to sell only if in preparations for use in agriculture, horticulture or forestry such sales are restricted to these trade or business users
Disulfoton
Fonofos
Parathion
Phorate
Thionazin
Triazophos
P2; S1; S4 in granular preparations; S5 listed sellers of poisons permitted to sell only if in preparations for use in agriculture, horticulture or forestry, and such sales are restricted to these trade or business users
Chlorfenvinphos
P2; S1; S4 in treatments on seeds, in granular preparations; S5 listed sellers of poisons permitted to sell only if in preparations for use in agriculture, horticulture or forestry, and such sales are restricted to these trade or business users
Dichlorvos
P2; S1; S4 in aerosol dispensers containing not more than 1% w/w dichlorvos, in materials impregnated with dichlorvos for slow release, in granular preparations, in ready for use liquid preparations containing not more than 1% w/v of dichlorvos; S5 listed sellers of poisons permitted to sell only if in preparations for use in agriculture, horticulture or forestry, and such sales are restricted to these trade or business users
Oxydemeton-methyl
P2; S1; S4 in aerosol dispensers containing not more than 0.25% w/w oxydemeton-methyl; S5 listed sellers of poisons permitted to sell only if in preparations for use in agriculture, horticulture or forestry, and such sales are restricted to these trade or business users
Pirimiphos-ethyl

P2; S1; S4 in treatments on seeds; S5 listed sellers of poisons permitted to sell only if in preparations for use in agriculture, horticulture or forestry, and such sales are restricted to these trade or business users
Phosphorus, yellow P1
Pirimiphos-ethyl *see* Phosphorus compounds
Potassium arsenite* P1; S1 except substances containing less than the equivalent of 0.0075% arsenic (P1 only). Rule 12 prohibits sale or supply except in certain circumstances
Potassium cyanide* P1; S1 except substances containing less than the equivalent of 0.1% w/w hydrogen cyanide (P1 only), and except in the case of a sale exempted by Section 4 of the Poisons Act 1972 it is not lawful to sell or supply potassium cyanide
Potassium fluoride P2
Potassium hydroxide P2; S4 in substances containing the equivalent of less than 17% of total caustic alkalinity expressed as potassium hydroxide, in accumulators, in batteries
Potassium oxalate P2; S4 in laundry blue, polishes, cleaning powders or scouring products, containing the equivalent of not more than 10% oxalic acid dihydrate; S5 (except for potassium quadroxalate), listed sellers of poisons permitted to sell for use only as photographic solutions or materials, but such sales are not restricted to trade or business users
Potassium quadroxalate P2; S4 in laundry blue, polishes, cleaning powders or scouring products, containing the equivalent of not more than 10% oxalic acid dihydrate
Potassium tetroxalate *see* Oxalates, metallic

Q

Quinalphos *see* Phosphorus compounds

S

Sodium arsanilate P1; S1 except substances containing less than the equivalent of 0.0075% arsenic (P1 only)
Sodium arsenate P1; S1 except substances containing less than the equivalent of 0.0075% arsenic (P1 only)
Sodium arsenite* P1; S1 except substances containing less than the

equivalent of 0.0075% arsenic (P1 only). Rule 12 prohibits sale or supply except in certain circumstances
Sodium cacodylate P1; S1 except substances containing less than the equivalent of 0.0075% arsenic (P1 only)
Sodium cyanide* P1; S1 except substances containing less than the equivalent of 0.1% w/w hydrogen cyanide (P1 only), and except in the case of a sale exempted by Section 4 of the Poisons Act 1972 it is not lawful to sell or supply sodium cyanide
Sodium dimethylarsonate P1; S1 except substances containing less than the equivalent of 0.0075% arsenic (P1 only)
Sodium fluoride P2; S4 in substances containing less than 3% sodium fluoride as a preservative
Sodium glycarsamate P1; S1 except substances containing less than the equivalent of 0.0075% arsenic (P1 only)
Sodium glycollylarsanilate P1; S1 except substances containing less than the equivalent of 0.0075% arsenic (P1 only)
Sodium hydroxide P2; S4 in substances containing the equivalent of less than 12% of total caustic alkalinity expressed as sodium hydroxide
Sodium methylarsinate P1; S1 except substances containing less than the equivalent of 0.0075% arsenic (P1 only)
Sodium metharsinite P1; S1 except substances containing less than the equivalent of 0.0075% arsenic (P1 only)
Sodium nitrite P2; S4 in substances other than preparations containing more than 0.1% sodium nitrite for the destruction of rats or mice
Sodium oxalate P2; S4 in laundry blue, polishes, cleaning powders or scouring products, containing the equivalent of not more than 10% oxalic acid dihydrate; S5 (except for potassium quadroxalate), listed sellers of poisons permitted to sell for use only as photographic solutions of materials, but such sales are not restricted to trade or business users
Sodium silicofluoride P2; S4 in substances containing less than 3%

sodium silicofluoride as a preservative
Sodium thioarsenate P1; S1 except substances containing less than the equivalent of 0.0075% arsenic (P1 only)
Strychnine; its salts and quaternary compounds P1; S1 except substances containing less than 0.2% strychnine (P1 only). Rule 12 prohibits sale or supply except in the cases mentioned in Section 1.4.2
Sulpharsobenzene P1; S1 except substances containing less than the equivalent of 0.0075% arsenic (P1 only)
Sulpharsphenamine P1; S1 except substances containing less than the equivalent of 0.0075% arsenic (P1 only)
Sulphuric acid P2; S4 in substances containing less than 15% w/w sulphuric acid, in accumulators, in batteries and sealed containers in which sulphuric acid is packed together with car batteries for use in those batteries; in fire extinguishers

T

Thallium*, salts of P1; S1. Rule 12 prohibits sale or supply except in certain circumstances
Thiofanox P2; S1; S4 in granular preparations; S5 listed sellers of poisons permitted to sell only if in preparations for use in agriculture, horticulture or forestry and such sales are restricted to these trade or business users
Thiometon *see* Phosphorus compounds
Thionazin *see* Phosphorus compounds
Triazophos *see* Phosphorus compounds

V

Vamidothion *see* Phosphorus compounds

Z

Zinc phosphide* P2; S1 except preparations used for the destruction of rats or mice; S5 listed sellers of poisons permitted to sell only if in preparations for the destruction of rats or mice, but such sales are not restricted to trade or business users. Rule 12 prohibits sale or supply except in certain circumstances

1.6 Chemicals

Chemicals in Great Britain are classified and labelled and packaged under the Chemicals (Hazard Information and Packaging for Supply) Regulations 2009 (also referred to here as CHIP or CHIP 4). CHIP 4 represents the fourth consolidated version of CHIP and came into force in Great Britain on 6 April 2010. CHIP 4 does not introduce any new overarching duties and consolidates all the amendments to CHIP 3 since 2002.

CHIP 4:
- Implements the Dangerous Substances Directive (No 67/548/EEC) and Dangerous Mixtures Directive (No 1999/45/EC). CHIP 4 reflects the changes to these two directives brought in by both the European REACH and CLP Regulations.
- Reflects the transitional arrangements in the CLP Regulation, as suppliers can choose to apply the CLP criteria and terminology ahead of the mandatory compliance dates (*see* below), as an alternative to CHIP. Therefore, CHIP 4 allows for the enforcement of both CHIP 4 and the CLP Regulation.

Limited future

The duties in CHIP 4 will be replaced by the European Regulation (EC) No 1272/2008 on Classification, Labelling and Packaging of Substances and Mixtures (CLP Regulation) over a transitional period running until 1 June 2015. The CLP Regulation adopts the UN Globally Harmonised System of classification and labelling of chemicals (GHS) throughout the European Union.

Harmonised classifications and the withdrawal of the Approved Supply List (ASL)

The Approved Supply List (ASL) has now been withdrawn. CHIP 4 refers instead to Table 3.2 in Part 3 of Annex VI of the CLP Regulation which lists all the 'harmonised' substance classifications agreed at European level, that used to appear in Annex I of the Dangerous Substances Directive, and were published in Great Britain as the ASL..

Table 3.2 reflects the list of harmonised classifications expressed using the criteria and terminology in the Dangerous Substances Directive and the Dangerous Mixtures Directive. Table 3.1 in Part 3 of Annex VI reflects the same classifications only expressed using the criteria and terminology in the CLP Regulation. When complying with the duties to use harmonised classifications, suppliers should refer to Table 3.2 (when applying CHIP) and Table 3.1 (when applying CLP) in Annex VI when seeking harmonised classifications as the legal source for this information.

Harmonised classifications are legally binding and must be applied by suppliers.

Safety data sheets

CHIP 4 no longer requires safety data sheets (SDS). However, SDSs are still legally required under Article 31 and Annex II of the European REACH Regulation (EC) No 1907/2006.

UN Globally Harmonised System of Classification and Labelling of Chemicals (GHS)

The United Nations (UN) developed the Globally Harmonised System of Classification and Labelling of Chemicals (GHS) which aims to have the same criteria for classifying chemicals worldwide according to their health, environmental, physical hazards, and hazard communication requirements for labelling and safety data sheets. The GHS is not legally binding, and each EU country has to introduce separate legislation to adopt it.

European Regulation (EC) No 1272/2008 on Classification, Labelling and Packaging of Substances and Mixtures (CLP)

The EU has introduced the Regulation (EC) No 1272/2008 on Classification, Labelling and Packaging of Substances and Mixtures (CLP), which adopts the GHS in the EU. The CLP Regulation came into effect on 20 January 2009, subject to a transitional period running until 1 June 2015, and is directly-acting in all Member States. This will replace the Dangerous Substances Directive and the Dangerous Mixtures Directive over a transitional period running until 1 June 2015, when the Regulation will then have wholesale application. As a consequence, the duties in the CHIP regulations will cease to have effect from 1 December 2010 for substances and from 1 June 2015 for mixtures, leaving those provisions which allow the CLP Regulation to be enforced.

The transitional arrangements are:

Substances

20 January 2009 to 1 December 2010 Suppliers have a duty to classify, label and package according to CHIP. However, they may also classify according to CLP, and if they decide to do so, the labelling and packaging requirements of CHIP no longer apply and the labelling and packaging requirements of CLP apply instead.

1 December 2010 to 1 June 2015 Suppliers must classify substances according to both CHIP and CLP. They must label and package according to CLP.

1 June 2015 onwards Suppliers must classify, label and package according to CLP.

Mixtures

20 January 2009 to 1 June 2015 Suppliers have a duty to classify, label and package according to CHIP. However, they may also classify according to CLP, and if they decide to do so, the labelling and packaging requirements of CHIP no longer apply and the labelling and packaging requirements of CLP apply instead. In this case, they must, in addition, continue to classify under Regulation 4 of CHIP, but the requirements on labelling and packaging in regulations 6 to 11 of CHIP no longer apply.

1 June 2015 onwards Suppliers must classify, label and package according to CLP.

Chemicals (Hazard Information and Packaging for Supply) Regulations 2009 (CHIP 4)

CHIP does not apply to certain chemicals such as those that are intended for use as medicinal products, veterinary products, investigational medicinal products, controlled drugs, cosmetic products, substances or mixtures which are in the form of waste to which the Waste Management Licensing Regulations 1994, the Special Waste Regulations 1996, the Hazardous Waste (Wales) Regulations 2005 or the Hazardous Waste (England and Wales) Regulations 2005 apply, food, animal feeding-stuffs, radioactive substances or mixtures, or medical devices. CHIP also does not apply to a substance or mixture which is a sample taken by an enforcement authority. It also does not apply when the substance is under customs control or intended for export as specified in CHIP 4.

Because of the complex nature of CHIP, the information provided below is not comprehensive. Pharmacists involved in the supply, labelling or packaging of chemicals are advised to first consult the Health and Safety Executive (HSE) published guidance (*www.hse.gov.uk/chip/index.htm*). For additional guidance, the HSE can be contacted on 0845 345 0055 (e-mail: *hse.infoline@connaught.plc.uk*).

The main objectives of CHIP are to help protect people and the environment from the ill effects of chemicals by requiring suppliers to:
(a) identify the hazards (dangers) of the chemicals they supply;
(b) give information about the chemicals' hazards to their customers (through hazard labels and, for workers, through a safety data sheet); and
(c) package the chemicals safely.

CHIP requires suppliers of dangerous substances and dangerous mixtures to:
(a) identify the hazards (or dangers) of dangerous substances and dangerous mixtures they supply (this process is called classification);
(b) give information about those hazards to the persons they supply - both on the label and methods of marking, with particular labelling requirements for certain mixtures, and for workers, through a safety data sheet;
(c) package the chemicals safely, including child resistant fastenings, tactile warning devices and other consumer protection measures; and
(d) retain data for dangerous mixtures (this will not apply on or after 1 June 2018).

These requirements are known as the supply requirements. The carriage or transportation of chemicals is not the same as supply. However, similar duties are placed on persons who transport chemicals by road or by rail.

1.6.1 Supply requirements

Classification of dangerous substances and dangerous mixtures

The fundamental requirement of CHIP is to assess whether a particular chemical is hazardous (dangerous) or not. If it is, then it must be classified by precise identification of the hazard by assigning a category of danger (e.g. "Toxic"), and a description of the hazard by allocation of a risk phrase (e.g. "Harmful in contact with skin").

The main categories of danger can be subdivided into substances and mixtures dangerous because of their:
- Physicochemical properties - explosive, oxidising, extremely flammable, highly flammable and flammable.
- Health effects - very toxic, toxic, harmful, corrosive, irritant, sensitising, carcinogenic, mutagenic, toxic for reproduction.
- Environmental effects.

CHIP makes it an offence to supply a dangerous chemical before it is classified. It is important that this process is carried out correctly as failure to do so could lead to errors being made in other requirements of CHIP (i.e. labelling, SDS mixture and packaging). When chemicals are supplied to a pharmacy they should already have been properly classified by that supplier. If this is the case, the pharmacist could use this classification provided he is satisfied that it is correct and the competence of the supplier is known to him.

CHIP requires a supplier to exercise "all due diligence" in complying with its legal requirements. This means that if a pharmacist uses the classification assigned by a manufacturer or supplier higher up the supply chain, then he should consider making appropriate enquiries about the classification to ensure accuracy. If suppliers are known to the pharmacist and there is confidence in their ability, only simple checks may be judged necessary. For example, using a common sense check: if an acid commonly known to cause burns has not been classified as being corrosive, enquiries should be made with the supplier or another person the pharmacist knows to be competent in this area.

CHIP makes suppliers of chemicals responsible for the classification of a chemical right down the supply chain and it must be remembered that pharmacists will be the final supplier.

Labelling

CHIP sets down requirements for the information which has to appear on hazard labels when a dangerous chemical is supplied.

Note: Safety Data Sheet (SDS) requirements are no longer part of CHIP. Regulation 5 of CHIP 4 acts as a 'signpost' to refer suppliers to Article 31 and Annex II of REACH, which now incorporates the duties and obligations to provide an SDS.

For supplies to domestic users, the CHIP label will contain all the information required to be given under CHIP. There may be further specific labelling requirements determined by other regulations relating to other aspects of chemical supply such as transport and general product safety or consumer safety, etc. However, with regard to CHIP, chemicals obtained by a pharmacist in their original packs should already be labelled to comply with CHIP. Where the chemicals are to be decanted from bulk into smaller packages appropriate for the contents, these packages must be correctly labelled in accordance with CHIP. In any case, as the supplier of the product the pharmacist will be responsible for the labelling, and it is advisable to make checks with all "due diligence". As a guide to the labelling requirements in relation to CHIP, *see* below. A common sense check would also be beneficial.

Labels, including the accompanying hazard symbols, must be clearly and indelibly marked, and securely fixed to the package with its entire surface in contact with it. The label itself must be placed so that it may be read horizontally when the package is set down. The colour and nature of the marking must be such that any symbol and the wording stand out clearly from the background and the wording must be of such size and spacing as to be easily read. The regulations also specify the minimum sizes of label depending on the quantity supplied and where the label should be placed (on outer packaging as well as on the container).

CHIP specifies exactly what must appear on the hazard label. This is partially dependent on whether it is a substance (usually a single chemical) or a mixture (in general terms, a mixture of substances) being labelled. It is also dependent on how it has been classified under CHIP.

The particulars required for labelling in relation to a dangerous substance supplied in a package are (Regulation 7(2)):
(a) the name, full address and telephone number of a person in an EEA State who is responsible for supplying the substance, including the pharmacist, whether he be its manufacturer, importer or distributor;
(b) the name of the substance, being:
(i) where the substance appears in Table 3.2 of part 3 of Annex VI of the CLP Regulation, the name or one of the names listed therein for that substance; or
(ii) where the substance does not appear in Table 3.2 of part 3 of Annex VI of the CLP Regulation, an internationally recognised name; and
(c) the following particulars ascertained in accordance with Part I of Schedule 4, namely
(i) any indications of danger together with corresponding symbols;
(ii) the risk phrases, set out in full;
(iii) the safety phrases, set out in full; and
(iv) any EC number and, in the case of a substance which is listed in Table 3.2 of part 3 of Annex VI of the CLP Regulation, the words "EC label".

The particulars required for labelling in relation to a dangerous mixture supplied in a package are (Regulation 7(3)):
(a) the name, full address and telephone number of a person in an EEA State who is responsible for supplying the mixture, including the pharmacist, whether that person be its manufacturer, importer or distributor;
(b) the trade name or other designation of the mixture; and
(c) the following particulars ascertained in accordance with Part I of Schedule 4, namely
(i) identification of the constituents of the mixture which result in it being classified as a dangerous mixture;
(ii) any indications of danger together with corresponding symbols;
(iii) the risk phrases, set out in full;
(iv) the safety phrases, set out in full; and
(v) in the case of a mixture intended for sale to the general public, the nominal quantity (nominal mass or nominal volume).

Indications such as "non-toxic", "non-harmful", "non-polluting", "ecological" or any other statement indicating that the dangerous substance or dangerous mixture is not dangerous or that is likely to lead to underestimation of the dangers of the dangerous substance or dangerous mixture must not appear on the package (Regulation 7(4)).

Where the package contains such small quantities of that substance or mixture that there is no foreseeable risk, under conditions of supply, use and disposal, arising from that hazardous property to persons handling that substance or mixture or to other persons, the packaging of a dangerous substance or dangerous mixture classified in one or more of the categories of danger harmful, extremely flammable, highly flammable, flammable, irritant or oxidising are not required to be labelled in respect of that hazardous property (Regulation 7(5) and 7(6)).

Where the package in which a dangerous substance is supplied does not contain more than 125 millilitres of that substance the risk phrases and safety phrases do not have to be shown if the dangerous substance is classified only in one or more of these categories of danger:
(a) highly flammable, flammable, oxidising or irritant; or
(b) harmful, provided the dangerous substance is not sold to the general public (Regulation 7(8)).

Where the package in which a dangerous mixture is supplied does not contain more than 125 millilitres of that mixture:
(a) the risk phrases and safety phrases do not have to be shown if the dangerous mixture is classified only in one or more of these categories of danger:
(i) irritant (except those assigned the risk phrase R41);
(ii) dangerous for the environment and assigned the N symbol;
(iii) oxidising; or
(iv) highly flammable; and
(b) the safety phrases need not be shown if the dangerous mixture is classified only in one or more of these categories of danger:
(i) flammable; or
(ii) dangerous for the environment and not assigned the N symbol. (Regulation 7(9))

The supply of dangerous mixtures

Dangerous substances must be labelled with the appropriate safety phrases as detailed in the Approved Classification and Labelling Guide (ACLG). In addition, the label on the packaging of dangerous mixtures and substances intended to be supplied to the general public must also contain the relevant safety advice, and bear the relevant safety phrase S1 (Keep locked up), S2 (Keep out of reach of children), S45 (In case of accident or if you feel unwell seek medical advice immediately [show the label where possible]) or S46 (If swallowed, seek medical advice immediately and show the container or label), in accordance with the ACLG. When the dangerous mixtures are classified as very toxic, toxic or corrosive and where it is physically impossible to give the information on the package itself, packages containing such mixtures must be accompanied by precise and easily understandable instructions for use including, where appropriate, instructions for the destruction of the empty package.

Pharmacists involved in preparing labels for dangerous substances and dangerous mixtures should refer to CHIP and HSE guidance and also to Table 3.2 in Annex VI of the CLP Regulation for information on legally binding harmonised classifications that may need to be considered.

Packaging

It is an offence to supply a dangerous chemical, unless it is in a suitable package. The packaging and fastenings should be strong and solid throughout to ensure that they will not loosen when subjected to the stresses and strains of normal handling. The container must not be adversely affected by the chemical or react with the chemical to form other dangerous chemicals. Where the package is fitted with a replaceable closure its integrity must remain with repeated use. Except where a special safety device has been fitted to make the receptacle closable, the package should be designed and constructed so that its contents cannot escape.

There is also a requirement for certain chemicals to be packaged with a child-resistant fastening (CRF) (Regulation 11), although they are not required if it can be shown that a child cannot gain access to the chemical without the help of a tool. CRFs must be used for chemicals which are sold to the public containing any of the following:

(i)   dangerous substances and dangerous mixtures which are required to be labelled with the indications of danger "very toxic", "toxic" or "corrosive" (Regulation 11(3)(a));
(ii) methanol (3% or more by weight) (Regulation 11(3)(b));
(iii) dichloromethane (1% or more by weight) (Regulation 11(3)(c));
(iv) substances which have been assigned the risk phrase (R65) in Table 3.2 of part 3 of Annex VI of the CLP Regulation, which states, "Harmful: may cause lung damage if swallowed", except where the chemical is supplied in an aerosol dispenser or a container fitted with a sealed spray attachment (Regulation 11(3)(d));
(v)   substances and mixtures which are assigned the risk phrase R65 and are classified and labelled according to the approved classification and labelling guide, except where such a substance or mixture is supplied in an aerosol dispenser or a container fitted with a sealed spray attachment (Regulation 11(3)(e)).

A further requirement prohibits supply of a dangerous mixture or a mixture specified in Regulation 11(3) to the general public if the packaging in which that mixture is supplied has:

(a) either a shape or a designation or both likely to attract or arouse the active curiosity of children or to mislead consumers; or
(b) either a presentation or a designation or both used for:
(i)   human or animal foodstuffs;
(ii) medicinal products; or
(iii) cosmetic products.

Chemicals sold to the public which are labelled "toxic", "very toxic", "corrosive", "harmful", "extremely flammable" or "highly flammable" must also have a tactile warning device (TWD - normally a small raised triangle) to alert the blind and partially sighted that they are handling a dangerous product. This does not apply to an aerosol dispenser which is classified and labelled only with the indication of danger "extremely flammable" or "highly flammable" (Regulations 11(7) and (8)).

Pharmacists must check that packaging complies with the above before supplying chemicals to the public. It is important to remember the need for "due diligence" to be exercised and when there is a legal obligation to supply an SDS.

CLP Regulation – guidance

Official guidance on the CLP Regulation has been produced by the European Chemicals Agency (ECHA). The guidance is published at two levels. The first provides an introduction to the Regulation; the second provides much more detailed guidance on how the CLP classification criteria should be applied. The guidance is available on the ECHA web site: *http://echa.europa.eu/clp/clp_help_en.asp*

More information about the CLP Regulation, including the text of the Regulation itself and the technical annexes, its duties, new provisions, harmonised classifications, the classification and labeling inventory etc, can also be found at ECHA: *http://echa.europa.eu/clp_en.asp*

Registration, Evaluation, Authorisation and restriction of Chemicals (REACH)

REACH is the European Regulation on the Registration, Evaluation, Authorisation and Restriction of Chemicals (REACH) Regulation ([EC] No 1907/2006), which came into effect on 1 June 2007. The Regulation runs in parallel to the European CLP Regulation. They have direct application within the EU, however, the enforcement is up to the individual Member State. The REACH Enforcement Regulations 2008 apply to the United Kingdom and provide for the enforcement of REACH.

REACH covers the registration, pre-registration, evaluation, authorisation, restrictions, classification and labelling and information provision of chemicals.

For further guidance pharmacists are advised to contact *www.hse.gov.uk/reach or ukreachca@hse.gsi.gov.uk*.

Substances of Very High Concern (SVHC)

REACH contains a list of substances of very high concern, the registration and use of which is subject to further controls, principally authorisation and the provision of information to downstream users and consumers. SVHCs are substances which are included on the REACH 'Candidate List' – potentially any substance which is:

• classified as carcinogenic, mutagenic or toxic for reproduction (CMR) category 1 or 2;
• persistent, bio-accumulative and toxic (PBT);
• very persistent and very bio-accumulative (vPvB)
• substances not classified as above but where there is scientific evidence of probable serious effects to human health or the environment.

Substances meeting the above criteria may be placed on the Candidate List (published by ECHA). It is possible that a substance that meets the criteria will not appear on either list. Where a substance does appear on the Candidate List, this means that they meet the criteria for authorization and they may eventually be included in the authorization procedure under REACH and added to Annex XIV.

Pharmacists supplying any substance should check with the HSE whether it is a SVHC and for further guidance refer to *www.hse.gov.uk/reach/svhc.pdf*.

Safety data sheets for substances and mixtures (SDS)

The rules relating to Safety Data Sheets (SDS) are now to be found in the REACH regulations. They were previously covered in the CHIP regulations. The supplier of a substance or a mixture must provide the recipient with an SDS compiled in accordance with Annex II where the substance or mixture is:

• classified as dangerous;
• a PBT or vPvB;
• a SVHC or on the Candidate list; or
• hazardous as it contains at least one substance in an individual concentration greater than or equal to: 1% by weight for non-

gaseous mixtures; 0.2% by volume for gaseous mixtures; or greater than or equal to: 0.1% by weight for non-gaseous mixtures which are PBT or vPvB in accordance with specified criteria; or
- there are 'workplace exposure limits'.

Unless one is requested, an SDS does not need to be provided where dangerous substances or mixtures are sold to the general public where sufficient information is given to enable the user to take measures which are necessary for the protection of health and safety and the environment.

The headings under which information must be provided are listed below together with a general description of the information which may be found under the heading. These descriptions are not all encompassing. For further information contact the HSE.

(1) *Identification of the substance/mixture and company/undertaking* The name of the substance/mixture should be identical to the name used on the label. It should indicate the intended or recommended uses of the substance/mixture. The name, full address, telephone number and email address of the competent person responsible for the SDS. Where this person is not in the Member State where the substance or mixture is placed on the market, the full address and telephone number for the person responsible in that member state. An emergency telephone number of the company and/or relevant advisory body should be added if access to advice in the event of an emergency is not available on the number already given and specify if the phone number is available only during office hours.

(2) *Hazards identification* The classification of the substance or mixture under the classification rules should be stated here. The most important hazards of the substance or mixture to man and the environment should be stated.

(3) *Composition/information on ingredients* Sufficient information must be given to enable the recipient to readily identify the hazards of the components of the mixture. The hazards of the mixture itself are listed in (2).

(4) *First aid measures* The information should state whether immediate medical attention or professional assistance by a doctor is needed or advisable. The information should be brief and easy to understand by the victim, bystanders and first aiders. Subheadings should be given for different routes of exposure, eg, skin and eye contact, inhalation or ingestion. If immediate medical attention or if a specific form of treatment is required, that should be stated.

(5) *Fire fighting measures* Suitable extinguishing media should be stated, together with details of extinguishing media which are not safe to be used, and details of special protective equipment for fire fighters. Exposure hazards arising from the substance or mixture, combustion products and resulting gases should be stated.

(6) *Accidental release measures* Information should be provided on personal precautions, eg,"removal of ignition sources", "provision for sufficient ventilation/respiratory protection", environmental precautions, eg, "keep away from drains, surface and ground water and soil", and methods of cleaning up, eg,"use of absorbent material" "sand". Consideration should also be given to using statements such as "Never use with..." or "Neutralise with...."

(7) *Handling and storage* This information relates to the protection of human health, safety and the environment and assist the employer in implementing suitable working procedures and organisational measures. Precautions necessary for safe handling, such as measures to prevent dust generation, fire, etc, and conditions for storage, eg, ventilation, temperature, light and humidity should also be stated. For end products designed for specific use(s), recommendations must refer to the identified use, with reference to industry/sector specific approved guidance.

(8) *Exposure controls and personal protection* This should include the full range of precautionary measures to be taken during use to minimise worker and environmental exposure. It should specify where necessary the type of equipment to afford suitable protection, eg respiratory, eye, skin and hand protection.

(9) *Physical and chemical properties* The following information should be provided: Appearance, eg, white solid; odour, if perceptible a brief description; pH; boiling point/melting range; flash point; flammability (solid, gas); explosive properties; oxidising properties; vapour pressure; relative density; solubility (water or fat); partition coefficient; viscosity; vapour density; evaporation rate; other important safety parameters of the product.

(10) *Stability and reactivity* State the stability of the substance or mixture and the possibility of hazardous reactions occurring under certain conditions of use and also if released into the environment, ie, conditions to avoid (temperature, pressure, shock, etc); materials to avoid (water, air, etc); hazardous materials produced in dangerous amounts on decomposition, addressing specifically the need for and the presence of stabilizers; the possibility of a hazardous exothermic reaction; safety significance, if any, of a change in physical appearance of the substance or mixture, hazardous decomposition products, if any, formed upon contact with water;and the possibility of degradation to unstable products.

(11) *Toxicological information* Provide a concise but complete and comprehensive description of the toxicological effects resulting from contact with the substance or mixture. Known delayed and immediate and chronic effects from short and long term exposure should be stated. Information on different routes of exposure and a description of the symptoms related to the physical, chemical and toxicological characteristics should be given.

(12) *Ecological information* An assessment should be given of the possible effects on the environment in relation to such factors as ecotoxicity, mobility, persistence and degradability, bioaccumulative potential, results of a persistent, bioaccumulative and toxic assessment (PBT) and any other adverse effects.

(13) *Disposal considerations* Information should be provided on the dangers associated with disposal. Safety and appropriate methods of disposal should be given together with references to appropriate legislation.

(14) *Transport information* Details of special precautions relating to transport or conveyance, either within or outside premises.

(15) *Regulatory information* The health, safety and environmental information on the label required by CHIP should be given. Reference to the Control of Substances Hazardous to Health Regulations 2009, as amended (COSHH), may also be made.

(16) *Other information* Advice on other information which may be of importance for health and safety of the user and for the protection of the environment, eg, training advice, recommended restrictions on use, further information, ie, written references and /or technical contact point, sources of key data used to compile the safety data sheet. A list of the relevant R-phrases referred to under headings (2) and (3) above, the full text of which must be written out in full, must appear under this heading on the SDS. A revised SDS should clearly indicate the information which has been added, deleted or revised (unless this has been indicated elsewhere).

Pharmacists may be able to use the SDSs provided by their supplier, who is responsible for the accuracy of the SDS. The pharmacist may wish to make the following "due diligence" checks: that

(i) all the safety headings (as detailed above) are present;

(ii) the SDS is comparable with those for similar products;

(iii) the sections dealing with safe use/storage, etc, are adequate for the intended applications of the pharmacy's customers; and

(iv) the SDS covers foreseeable eventualities.

Substances restricted to professional users

Certain substances specified in Annex XVII of REACH, in addition to the classification, packaging and labelling requirements of dangerous substances and mixtures, must contain the safety labelling phrase, legible and indelibly marked, 'Restricted to professional users'. The substances to which this restriction applies are those classified as "carcinogenic", "mutagenic", or "toxic to reproduction" and are listed as categories 1 or 2. (These products are not normally sold through pharmacies to the general public.)

An SDS and any updated version should be provided free of charge on paper or electronically, and be dated, in an official language of the Member State where the substance or mixture is placed on the market. The suppliers must update the SDS as soon as new information on risks and hazards becomes available or there are changes to the authorisation or restrictions imposed. The new, dated version of the information, identified as "Revision: (date)", including the registration number, must be supplied to all persons who have received the substance or mixture within the preceding 12 months. For this reason it would be wise to keep a record of sales of such products.

Pharmacists are advised to check the HSE website for further details on Safety Data Sheets: *www.hse.gov.uk/reach/resources/reachsds.pdf*.

Detailed guidance on REACH has been produced by the European Chemicals Agency (ECHA) at: *http://echa.europa.eu/home_en.asp*.

Chloroform and certain other halogenated hydrocarbons

Chloroform and certain other halogenated hydrocarbons (including carbon tetrachloride) are listed in Annex XVII of REACH, with specific restrictions on their use (and also in Schedule 2 COSHH). Chloroform and carbon tetrachloride must not be used in concentrations equal to or greater than 0.1% by weight, in substances and mixtures placed on the market, for sale to the general public, and/or in diffusive applications such as in surface cleaning and cleaning of fabrics. In addition to the classification, packaging and labelling requirements of dangerous substances and mixtures the packaging of such substances and mixtures containing them in concentrations equal to or greater than 0.1% must be legible and indelibly marked with: "For use in industrial installations only". This does not however apply to medicinal, veterinary products or cosmetic products as defined in the Directives.

1.7 Denatured alcohol

Denatured alcohol is alcohol that has been made unsuitable for drinking by the addition of denaturants.

Law affecting denatured alcohol

The Denatured Alcohol Regulations 2005 cover the whole of the United Kingdom.

Section 77 of the Alcoholic Liquor Duties Act 1979 gives HM Revenue and Customs the power to make regulations laying down requirements for the manufacture, supply and use of denatured alcohol. Section 78 of the Act prescribes penalties for offences in connection with denatured alcohol. The requirements are set out in the Denatured Alcohol Regulations 2005 (SI 2005/1524) and further implements Articles 27 (1)(a) and (b) of Council Directive 92/83/EEC.

1.7.1 Type of denatured alcohol

There are three approved classes of denatured alcohol in the UK: completely denatured alcohol; industrial denatured alcohol; and trade specific denatured alcohol, although most pharmacists will deal only with the first two.

(a) Completely denatured alcohol (CDA) (formerly known as Mineralised Methylated Spirits - MMS)

Completely denatured alcohol is the most heavily denatured alcohol. CDA is suitable for heating, lighting, cleaning and general domestic use. Pharmacists can obtain CDA from wholesalers in any quantity.

CDA is a mixture of 90 parts by volume of alcohol, 9.5 parts by volume of wood naphtha or a substitute for wood naphtha and 0.5 parts by volume of crude pyridine, to each 1000 litres of the mixture of which is added 3.75 litres mineral naphtha (petroleum oil) and 1.5g of synthetic organic dyestuff (methyl violet). A full list of formulations of CDA used in EU Member States can be found in HM Customs and Excise Notice 473 (April 2010), available from HM Revenue and Customs National Advice Service (0845 010 9000).

(b) Industrial denatured alcohol (IDA) (formerly known as Industrial Methylated Spirits - IMS)

Industrial denatured alcohol is the grade of denatured alcohol designed for industrial use. IDA is usually approved for use in industrial, scientific and external medical applications. A full list of authorised uses can be found in HM Customs and Excise Notice 473 (April 2010). To use IDA in a way not on the approved list, the National Registration Unit should be contacted with the details of the proposed use. They may approve its use as an alternative.

IDA consists of 95 parts by volume of alcohol and 5 parts by volume of wood naphtha, or a substitute for wood naphtha. Where a substitute for wood naphtha is used, the volume mixed with every 95 parts of alcohol may be less than 5 parts depending on: (i) the proportion of the marker in the resulting mixture, and (ii) the resulting mixture contains the other substances that the Commissioners approved when they

approved the substitute for wood naphtha in the proportions that they specify.

Denatured alcohol that is not CDA, which has been made in another Member State, in accordance with a CDA formulation of that Member State and has been incorporated into a product that is not for human consumption, must be accepted in the UK free of duty.

(c) Trade specific denatured alcohol (TSDA) (includes Denatured Ethanol B - DEB)

Trade specific denatured alcohol formulations are types of denatured alcohol approved to meet specific trade needs. TSDA can only be obtained by persons specifically authorised by HM Revenue and Customs to receive them. TSDA can only be used in certain formulations for specific authorised uses. For example, the TDSA formulation for the former Denatured Ethanol B (DEB) - Tertiary Butyl Alcohol 0.1% vol and Denatonium benzoate added to the resulting mixture in the proportion of 10 micrograms per millilitre; is approved for use in the manufacture of skin preparations (perfumes, toiletries, cosmetics and external medical applications such as medicated creams and ointments), printing ink and as a biocide reagent.

There is a list of formulations of, and uses for, TSDA, which have been approved by the Commissioners of HM Revenue and Customs. This list can be found in Section 18 of HM Customs and Excise Notice 473 (April 2010), or contact the National Advice Service Helpline to ensure it is up to date. To use a TSDA in a way that is not on the approved list or to use a new formulation of TSDA, the National Registration Unit should be contacted in writing with the following details:
(i) the proposed TSDA formulation;
(ii) the use; and
(iii) the reason why CDA, IDA and the approved TSDA formulations would be unsuitable for the intended use,
who may then approve this use or formulation as an alternative

1.7.2 Application for authority to receive IDA or TSDA

Pharmacists must be authorised by HM Revenue and Customs to receive IDA or TDSA (except where this is contained in a ready prepared medicinal product containing the denatured alcohol). To obtain authority to receive IDA or TSDA, an application has to be made to HM Revenue and Customs National Registration Unit (NRU). The application form can be found in Section 19 of HM Customs and Excise Notice 473 (April 2010) (see Figure 1, p94). If approved, the Commissioners may authorise a person in writing to receive IDA or TSDA, stating what they are entitled to receive, what it can be used for, and the conditions that must be observed (see 1.7.4 below). The authority and conditions can be changed or revoked by HM Revenue and Customs at any time, but authorised users must comply with any conditions or restrictions imposed by the Commissioners.

The authorisation is valid indefinitely.

The user must notify the National Registration Unit of any changes and may not receive any further supplies of

Application for authorisation to receive and use IDA or TSDA

Application for Authority to receive Industrial Denatured Alcohol/Trade Specific Denatured Alcohol*

Part A *I/We (name of company, partnership, proprietor, as appropriate) apply for authority to receive IDA/TSDA* formulation(s)

....

....

....

for use at (address of premises):

....

....

....

Type of business/activity..

VAT Registration Number...

Part B The *IDA/TSDA is to be used for the following purpose(s):

....

....

Part C (only for requests to use TSDA for a use not previously approved) CDA/IDA is unsuitable because

....

Part D *My/Our estimated annual requirement is:

*Industrial Denatured Alcohol....................................litres

*Trade Specific Denatured Alcohol..............................litres

Signature...

Full name...

Status...

(proprietor, partner, director, company secretary etc.)

Date...

Telephone Number...

Fax Number..

E-mail address..

*Delete as necessary

Figure 1. Application for authorisation to receive and use IDA or TSDA

IDA or TSDA until the National Registration Unit has been notified.

1.7.3 Supply of denatured alcohol by authorised users

Authorised users may supply denatured alcohol or articles containing denatured alcohol as follows:

CDA

CDA can be supplied to anyone including the general public. There are no restrictions on the quantity of CDA that can be supplied nor conditions on its use.

CDA may be received free of duty if the denatured alcohol made in a Member State is in accordance with a formulation of that Member State, or it is made as near as possible in accordance with the UK CDA formulation or a CDA formulation of another Member State. The acceptability of the formulation should be checked with the National Advice Service (See C& E Notice 473 April 2010). CDA may be imported directly to your premises from a Member State if the CDA is denatured in accordance with a CDA formulation of a Member State, otherwise it has to be consigned to an excise warehouse with the relevant approval to hold such goods.From 1 January 2011 there will be changes to the import procedure. (See HMRC Notice 197).

IDA and TSDA

An authorised IDA/TDSA user is a person authorised by Customs and Excise to receive and use IDA/TDSA under the Denatured Alcohol Regulations 2005. IDA and TSDA can only be supplied to producers or distributors who are authorised by HM Revenue and Customs as users. Supply of IDA or TSDA must not be made without holding a copy of the user's authorisation or for a use that is not included in the user's authorisation. Suppliers can only distribute the formulations of denatured alcohol that are on their licence.

An authorised user may supply IDA/TSDA in quantities of less than 20 litres at any one time to another authorised user provided the supplier's authority does not specifically restrict this.

Only licensed, or authorised producers or distributors are permitted to supply denatured alcohol in quantities of greater than 20 litres (wholesale quantities).

Supply of IDA by a pharmacist

Authorised users must furnish the pharmacist (supplier) with a copy of the authorisation before they may receive IDA. Where the IDA is not intended for medical use, it can only be supplied in the quantity and for the purpose stated in the authorisation from HM Revenue and Customs.

When a pharmacist (as a user) supplies IDA for "medical use" on a prescription or order of a medical or veterinary practitioner,(an authorised use), a copy of the person's authorisation to receive and use denatured alcohol is not needed. An authorisation is not required to be held by the patient when receiving denatured alcohol on a prescription but the pharmacist is required to keep records under the alcohol legislation for this supply.

Where a pharmacist makes a supply against an order from a doctor for use in their professional practice, the signed order should be kept to show that it has been dispensed correctly. Users (the pharmacist) have to be able to account for how much denatured alcohol has been received and what has been used.

An "order" is a request to be supplied with a specific quantity of denatured alcohol. There is no set format for an order, but should include the quantity and class of denatured alcohol required.

The definitions for the above section are:

"Pharmacist" has the meaning given in section 132(1) of the Medicines Act 1968;

"Medical or veterinary practitioner" means a person entitled by law to provide medical or veterinary services in the United Kingdom (HM Revenue and Customs have confirmed that this does include a dentist, nurse and chiropodist);

"Medical use" means any medical, veterinary, surgical or dental purpose other than administration internally.

Isle of Man

IDA/TSDA can be supplied to users in the Isle of Man who are authorised to receive that IDA/TSDA in accordance with the laws of the Isle of Man. The user in the Isle of Man must supply the pharmacist with a written statement showing:

(i) the date the user was authorised to receive the denatured alcohol of the formulation requested;

(ii) the intended use(s) for that denatured alcohol;

(iii) any conditions or restrictions imposed on him by his authorisation to receive denatured alcohol; and

(iv) the uses to which he is entitled to put the received denatured alcohol.

Do I need to "make entry" of premises?

If stocks of denatured alcohol are held by the pharmacist, an entry of the premises will need to be made before beginning to hold denatured alcohol (unless the premises are approved as an excise warehouse). To do this, Form EX 103 for a sole trader or partnership, or Form EX 103A for an incorporated company, should be completed.

Each continuation sheet to the EX 103(A) must be signed and dated. To obtain copies of these forms or help in completing them, the HM Revenue and Customs National Advice Service should be contacted.

1.7.4 Use of IDA and TSDA

(a) Storage: All stocks of IDA and TSDA must be kept securely and the security is the pharmacist's responsibility.

(b) Disposal of stock: If the business is discontinued while holding stocks of denatured alcohol, or the authority or licence to hold stocks of denatured alcohol is revoked, the National Advice Service should be contacted to arrange how the stocks must be disposed of and within what time period. Once all stocks are disposed of, the National Registration Unit must be contacted to cancel the licence or the authority. If the discontinuation of the business is caused by the death of a producer or distributor or other person, their personal representative must contact the National Advice Service.

Records and documents to be kept

Authorised persons must keep and preserve records relating to their use of denatured alcohol as specified by the Commissioners, and must also comply with any conditions or restrictions imposed by them.

On receipt of IDA or TSDA the following must be kept:
(i) a record of the amount of denatured alcohol received;
(ii) the receipt details noted on the suppliers dispatch documents and
(iii) one copy of the supplier's dispatch document signed as a receipt and returned to the supplier, and the other copy retained on the premises for records.

When supplies of IDA/TDSA are made the following must be kept:
(i) written statements from authorised users;
(ii) written signed orders from medical practitioners.

These records are required for a supply made against a prescription.

These records and documents will need to be shown to the HM Revenue and Customs officer when the premises are visited.

Distribution

For a pharmacist to be considered a distributor, the following criteria would need to be met:
(a) holds an excise licence for the purpose of Section 75 of the Act;

(b) does not denature alcohol at any premises on which denatured alcohol is kept;
(c) deals or intends to deal wholesale in denatured alcohol.

Only the denatured alcohols which are detailed on the licence may be distributed. To apply for a licence the application form L5 should be sent to the National Registration Unit with a letter stating which denatured alcohol will be distributed. In the "specified trade" section on the licence application, "distributor" must be entered. The licence may cover more than one set of premises and any proposed changes must be notified to the NRU. If stocks of denatured alcohol are held, you will also need an authorisation from HM Revenue and Customs, as a user in order to receive denatured alcohol from producers and other distributors.

An entry of premises must be made where stocks of denatured alcohol are held, and this must be done before holding the stock. An entry of premises is not required if stocks of denatured alcohol are not held. Denatured alcohol can be sold without holding stock, but the distributor would have to be licensed in the same way as a distributor holding stock. A pharmacist may hold stocks of denatured alcohol up to the level for which they are authorised.

Users with multi-premises businesses (eg, retail chains, etc) may apply to be authorised to distribute IDA/TSDA to premises, eg, branches, under their control. A multisite application form must be used for authorisation to receive and use IDA or TSDA (see Section 20 of Customs and Excise Notice 473 April 2010).

Specific record keeping requirements for producers/distributors

Under the Denatured Alcohol Regulations 2005, there is a requirement to keep records which show the following information:
(i) purchases of materials used in the production of denatured alcohol;
(ii) imports of denatured alcohol, including details of the country of origin;
(iii) the class of denatured alcohol held in containers, that is whether it is CDA, IDA or TSDA;
(iv) quantities of alcohols, denaturants, markers, dyes and denatured alcohol held and used on your premises;
(v) the results of stocktakes and action taken to investigate deficiencies and surpluses identified by those stocktakes;
(vi) exports and sales of denatured alcohol;
(vii) copy authorisations received in support of orders for denatured alcohols.

Specific record keeping requirements for users

Under the Denatured Alcohol Regulations 2005, there is a requirement to keep records which show the following information:
(i) purchases of IDA or TSDA;
(ii) imports of IDA or TSDA, including details of the country of origin;
(iii) the class of denatured alcohol held in containers, where IDA or TSDA;
(iv) quantities of IDA or TSDA held and used on the premises;

(v) the results of stocktakes and action taken to investigate deficiencies and surpluses identified by those stocktakes;

(vi) sales of IDA or TSDA to other authorised users;

(vii) copy authorisations received in support of orders for IDA or TSDA.

HM Revenue and Customs will visit from time to time to inspect the premises and examine any denatured alcohol on the premises.

Pharmacists may be liable to penalties, required to repay the duty on the alcohol lost in any unauthorised processes and supplies and could have their authorisation withdrawn, if there are unexplained losses of denatured alcohol where:

(a) as a distributor supplies have been made to users without receiving a copy of the authorisations, or

(b) supplies have been made to persons who are not authorised users, or

(c) as a user the denatured alcohol has not been used in accordance with its authorised use.

For further guidance on assessments and civil penalties see HMRC Notice 208 and 209. There are also review and appeals procedures where you disagree with a decision of the HM Revenue and Customs inspector.

Some EU countries may require a certificate of denaturing for cosmetics or toiletries which are exported to them. The National Advice Service should be contacted for more details.

Surplus/deficiency in stocks of denatured alcohol as a distributor

Any surplus or deficiency would have to be investigated and the reasons recorded for the deficiency/surplus in the business records and the National Advice Service notified in writing. The records would have to be amended to reflect the quantities of alcohols actually in stock.

Surplus/deficiency in stocks of denatured alcohol as a user

Any surplus or deficiency would have to be investigated and the reasons recorded for the deficiency/surplus in the business records and the National Advice Service notified in writing. For any surplus the records must be amended to reflect the quantities if alcohols actually in stock. If the denatured alcohol cannot be accounted for and has been supplied to an unauthorised user, or for an unauthorised purpose, a demand may be issued to pay the duty on the alcohol in the missing amount.

Contacts

For further information on the Denatured Alcohol Regulations 2005 please contact HM Revenue and Customs National Advice Service Helpline (tel 0845 010 9000; for information in Welsh 0845 010 0300; *www.hmrc.gov.uk*).

HM Revenue and Customs, National Advice Service - Written Enquiries Section, Alexander House, 21 Victoria Avenue, Southend, Essex SS99 1BD
National Advice Service - email service: *enquiries.estn@hmrc.gsi.gov.uk*

HM Revenue and Customs, National Registration Unit, Portcullis House, 21 India Street, Glasgow G2 4PZ
e-mail: enquiries.sco@hmrc.gsi.gov.uk

Isopropyl alcohol

Isopropyl alcohol 70% (which is isopropyl alcohol diluted down with water) is not a denatured alcohol and is not covered by the Denatured Alcohol Regulations 2005. Therefore, there is no requirement to be authorised by HM Revenue and Customs to receive or supply isopropyl alcohol 70%.

Ether (Ethyl ether)

Ether does not come under the Denatured Alcohol Regulations 2005; it is classed as a Chemical (see Section 1.6) except when it is licensed as a medicinal product.

Duty Free Spirits (DFS)

Duty free spirits cannot be used for general cleaning and other purposes. Duty free spirits are not permitted to be used for making for sale: any product which contains spirits (other than, subject to special conditions, ethyl esters and ethyl ethers); or use any beverage, foodstuff, flavouring essence, perfumery or cosmetic preparation.

There is no definitive list of allowable medicinal uses of DFS. The HMRC would consider each case on its merits, however the general medical applications and uses for which DFS will be allowed include:

- for the production of recognised medical products, drugs and pharmaceuticals (whether or not the final product contains spirits) including veterinary products, including DFS to be used in the manufacture of any product (including herbal or homoeopathic) which has a Medicines and Healthcare products Regulatory Agency (MHRA) product licence;

- herbal or homoeopathic remedies which do not have an MHRA licence. They must be recognised, by Customs and Excise as having medicinal properties;

- the manufacture of intermediate products used exclusively for the production of medical products (as above);

- for use in hospitals, and, where applicable, dental and veterinary surgeries for specific uses:

DFS can be used in the manufacture of any product prescribed by a doctor to be made up by a pharmacist. This includes "specials" which may be made up on behalf of a pharmacist and which may not have an MHRA product licence.

A pharmacist would have to apply for authorisation to obtain or use duty free spirits. Further details can be obtained from HMRC Notice 47 (April 2010) "Duty free spirits: use in manufacture or for medical or scientific purposes."

The application for authority to receive duty free spirits (Form EX 240) is available from HMRC National Advice Service and should also be returned there.

Surgical Spirit

Surgical Spirit which is a mix of ethyl alcohol and methyl alcohol is not an IDA. It is not covered by the Denatured Alcohol Regulations 2005. There is no restriction on the quantity of surgical spirit that can be sold from a pharmacy.

1.8 Medicines for veterinary use

Section 1.8 covers the following:

A veterinary medicinal product (VMP) is defined in the Veterinary Medicines Regulations 2009 as any substance or combination of substances presented as having properties for treating or preventing disease in animals, or any substance or combination of substances that may be used in, or administered to, animals with a view either to restoring, correcting or modifying physiological functions by exerting a pharmacological, immunological or metabolic action, or to making a medical diagnosis.

The Veterinary Medicines Regulations 2009 which came into force on 1 October 2009 revoked the Veterinary Medicines Regulations 2008. The Veterinary Medicines Regulations replaced the Medicines Act as far as veterinary legislation is concerned. The classes of VMPs include:

1. Prescription-only medicine - veterinarian (POM-V)
2. Prescription-only medicine - veterinarian, pharmacist, suitably qualified person (POM-VPS)
3. Non-food animal - veterinarian, pharmacist, suitably qualified person (NFA-VPS)
4. Authorised veterinary medicine - general sales list (AVM-GSL).

See table, p98, for further information on the different classes of VMPs.

Pharmacists may only supply VMPs classified as a POM-V, POM-VPS or NFA-VPS from registered pharmacy premises and from premises registered as being premises from which a veterinary surgeon supplies VMPs, or, in the case of VMPs classified as POM-VPS or NFA-VPS from premises which are registered under Schedule 3, paragraph 14 of the Regulations

The Veterinary Medicines Regulations 2010 are expected to come into force on 1 October 2010. After this date, pharmacists are advised to consult the Royal Pharmaceutical Society's website, *www.rpsgb.org*, for any additional up-to-date guidance on the sale and supply of veterinary medicinal products.

1.8.1 Prescriptions

A POM-V or POM-VPS may only be supplied by retail in accordance with a prescription (*see* **table, p92**, for guidance on who may prescribe VMPs authorised as either POM-V or POM-VPS). The prescription may be oral (eg, if the pharma-cist prescribing a POM-VPS medicine also supplies it) or written (eg, where a veterinary surgeon issues a prescription to be separately dispensed by a pharmacist). Only veterinary surgeons registered with the Royal College of Veterinary Surgeons (RCVS) can carry out acts of veterinary surgery and are eligible to practise in the UK. Where a VMP is not supplied by the person who has prescribed it, the prescription must be written.

A written prescription must include the following particulars:

(a) the name, address and telephone number of the person prescribing the product;
(b) the qualifications enabling the person to prescribe the product;
(c) the name and address of the owner or keeper;
(d) the identification (including the species) of the animal or group of animals to be treated;
(e) the premises at which the animals are kept if different from that of the owner or keeper;
(f) the date of the prescription;
(g) the signature or other authentication of the prescriber (NB: "other authentication" is not acceptable for a CD);
(h) the name and amount of the product prescribed;
(i) the dosage and administration instructions (NB: the VMD have advised that a dosage of "as directed" is not acceptable);
(j) any necessary warnings;
(k) the withdrawal period if relevant;
(l) if it is prescribed under the cascade, a statement to that effect (*see* Section 1.8.2 for further information.

It is not lawful to alter a written veterinary prescription unless authorised to do so by the person who signed the prescription.

In the case of a repeatable prescription it must specify the number of times the VMP may be supplied.

A prescription for any medicine (which is not a Schedule 1-4 Controlled Drug, is valid for six months or shorter if specified by the prescriber on the prescription.

Controlled Drug prescriptions

Where the VMP prescribed is also a Schedule 2 or 3 Controlled Drug (CD) (except temazepam), the prescription must also include the following:

(a) the address of the prescriber, which must be in the UK (NB: This is a requirement for temazepam prescriptions);
(b) the form of the preparation;
(c) the strength of the preparation (when more than one strength of the preparation is available);
(d) the total quantity (in both words and figures) of the preparation to be supplied. This must be in dosage units;
(e) a declaration written on it that the CD is prescribed for an animal or herd under the veterinary surgeon's or veterinary practitioner's care;
(f) the name and address of the person to whom the CD is to be delivered;
(g) a CD to be dispensed in instalments must contain a direction specifying the amount of the instalment which

Classification of veterinary medicinal products

Legal category	Retail supply and record keeping	Restrictions on supply

POM-V
(POM-veterinarian)
	May be supplied by a veterinary surgeon or pharmacist in accordance with a prescription from a veterinary surgeon. Records must be kept of all supplies for a period of at least five years (see Section 1.8.3)	A pharmacist supplying a POM-V under a written prescription:
		- may only supply the product specified in that prescription
		- must take all reasonable steps to be satisfied that the prescription has been written and signed by a person entitled to prescribe the product; and
		- must take all reasonable steps to ensure that it is supplied to the person named in the prescription.
		- must be present when it is handed over, unless the pharmacist:
		  • authorises each transaction individually before the product is supplied; and
		  • is satisfied that the person handing it over is competent to do so.
		- may only supply the product from registered pharmacy premises, or from premises registered under the Regulations as being premises from which a veterinary surgeon supplies VMPs.

POM-VPS
(POM-veterinarian, pharmacist and suitably qualified person[1])
	May be supplied by a veterinary surgeon, pharmacist or suitably qualified person[2] in accordance with a prescription from one of those persons. Records must be kept of all supplies for a period of at least five years (see Section 1.8.3)	99pharmacist supplying a POM-VPS under a written prescription:
		- may only supply the product specified in that prescription
		- must take all reasonable steps to be satisfied that the prescription has been written and signed by a person entitled to prescribe the product; and
		- must take all reasonable steps to ensure that it is supplied to the person named in the prescription.
		
		A pharmacist supplying a POM-VPS:
		- must be present when it is handed over, unless the pharmacist:
		  • authorises each transaction individually before the product is supplied; and
		  • is satisfied that the person handing it over is competent to do so.
		- may only supply the product from registered pharmacy premises, or from premises registered under the Regulations as being premises from which a veterinary surgeon supplies VMPs, or from premises which are registered under Schedule 3, Paragraph 14 of the Veterinary Medicines Regulations 2009.
		
		A pharmacist prescribing a POM-VPS must:
		- always advise on the safe administration of the product
		- advise as necessary on any warnings or contraindications on the label/package leaflet
		- be satisfied that the person using it is competent, and intends to use it for an authorised use
		- not prescribe more than the minimum amount required for the treatment; unless the product supplied is in a container specified in the marketing authorisation; the manufacturer does not supply that VMP in a smaller container; and he is not a person authorised to break open the package before supply (NB: A pharmacist may break open any package other than the immediate packaging of injectable products).

NFA-VPS
(Non-food animal-veterinarian, pharmacist and suitably qualified person[1])
	May be supplied by veterinary surgeon, pharmacist or suitably qualified person[2]. It is a good practice requirement to keep records of NFA-VPS medicines received or supplied	A pharmacist supplying a NFA-VPS must:
		- always advise on the safe administration of the product
		- advise as necessary on any warnings or contraindications on the label/package leaflet
		- be satisfied that the person using it is competent, and intends to use it for an authorised use
		- not supply more than the minimum amount required for the treatment; unless the product supplied is in a container; and he is not a person authorised to break open the package before supply (NB: A pharmacist may break open any package other than the immediate packaging of injectable products)
		- be present when it is handed over, unless the pharmacist:
		  • authorises each transaction individually before the product is supplied; and
		  • is satisfied that the person handing it over is competent to do so.
		- may only supply the product from registered pharmacy premises, or from premises registered under the Regulations as being premises from which a veterinary surgeon supplies VMPs, or from premises which are registered under Schedule 3, Paragraph 14 of the Veterinary Medicines Regulations 2009.

AVM-GSL (Authorised veterinary medicine-GSL)	There are no restrictions on supply	No additional restrictions

[1] Suitably qualified person who must be registered with Animal Medicines Training Regulatory Agency (AMTRA)
[2] In accordance with paragraph 14 of the Regulations

may be supplied and the intervals to be observed when supplying.

The requirement to use standardised private prescription forms when prescribing Schedule 2 and 3 CDs does not apply to veterinary prescriptions. Similarly, there is currently no requirement for veterinary prescriptions for Controlled Drugs or copies of such prescriptions to be submitted to the relevant NHS agency.

A written prescription for a Schedule 1-4 CD is valid for 28 days. A repeat of a Schedule 2 or 3 CD is not acceptable.

1.8.2 Prescribing cascade

The Veterinary Medicines Regulations 2009 make it an offence to place on the market (which includes sale or supply by wholesale or retail) or to administer (or cause or permit to be administered) any medicinal product for use in an animal unless it is an authorised veterinary medicinal product.

Where no authorised veterinary medicinal product exists in the UK for a condition, the veterinary surgeon responsible for the animal may treat the animal concerned by invoking the "cascade", and prescribing as follows:

(a) A veterinary medicinal product authorised in the UK for use in another animal species or for another condition in the same species (off-label use);
(b) If no product as described in (a) exists, either;
(i) a human medicinal product authorised in the UK, or
(ii) a veterinary medicinal product not authorised in the UK but authorised in another member State for use with any animal species (in the case of a food-producing animal, it must be a food-producing species); or
(c) If no product as described in (b) is suitable, a veterinary medicinal product prepared extemporaneously (i.e. made up at the time of need by a registered pharmacist, a veterinary surgeon or the holder of an appropriate manufacturer's licence in accordance with a veterinary prescription.
(NB: Pharmacists who are asked to provide medicines, eg, against a prescription, for animal treatment under the circumstances used in (a), (b) or (c) above should ensure that the veterinary surgeon has prescribed that product specifying that it is to be used under the "cascade".)

The supply and administration of medicines under the "cascade" is permitted only if it is in accordance with a prescription issued by a veterinary surgeon under whose care the animal has been placed.

Requests to purchase human licensed medicinal products over the counter for use in animals

Under the Regulations, it is an offence to supply an authorised human medicinal product (human licensed General Sale List [GSL] or Pharmacy [P] medicine for administration to an animal, except in accordance with a prescription under the cascade from a veterinary surgeon.

Pharmacists must not supply human GSL or P medicines over the counter if they are intended for animal administration, even where oral authorisation from a veterinary surgeon has been given.

Human licensed products (Prescription Only Medicine [POM], P or GSL) may only be supplied for use in an animal

against a prescription under the cascade as described above. The prescription must specifically state words to the effect that the medicinal product is for use and administration under the cascade, either by that veterinary surgeon or under his direction and responsibility.

1.8.3 Records

Pharmacists must keep records of the receipt and supply of POM-V and POM-VPS products. They must keep all documents relating to the transaction. All documents and records must be retained for at least five years. The information retained must include:

(a) the date;
(b) the name of the VMP;
(c) the batch number (NB: in the case of a VMP for a non-food-producing animal, the batch number need only be recorded either on the date that batch is received or on the date that the VMP from that batch is first supplied);
(d) the quantity received or supplied;
(e) the name and address of the supplier or recipient; and
(f) if there is a written prescription, the name and address of the person who wrote the prescription and a copy of the prescription.

If the document relating to the transaction (for example, the prescription) does not include all of this information, the pharmacist must make a record of the missing information as soon as is reasonably practicable following the transaction.

Audit

It is a legal requirement for a detailed audit to be carried out at least once a year by every person who is entitled to supply a VMP on prescription. All incoming and outgoing VMPs must be reconciled with products currently held in stock, with any discrepancies being recorded.

The Veterinary Medicines Directorate (VMD) has stated that the legal requirement to audit VMPs applies to products licensed as POM-V and POM-VPS. It would be good practice to audit stocks of NFA-VPS, however this is not mandatory. There is no requirement to audit stocks of AVM-GSL.

Proof of purchase

The keeper of a food-producing animal must keep proof of purchase of all veterinary medicinal products acquired for the animal (or, if they were not bought, documentary evidence of how they were acquired). An itemised EPOS till receipt or handwritten receipt would constitute proof of purchase.

1.8.4 Labelling

The label of a veterinary medicine supplied against a prescription for administration under the cascade should contain the following information:

(i) the name and address of the pharmacy, veterinary surgery or approved premises supplying the VMP;
(ii) the name of the veterinary surgeon who prescribed it;
(iii) the name and address of the animal owner;

(iv) the identification (including the species) of the animal or group of animals;

(v) the date of supply;

(vi) the expiry date of the product, if applicable;

(vii) the name or description of the product which should at least include the name and quantity of active ingredients;

(viii) dosage and administration instructions;

(ix) any special storage precautions;

(x) any necessary warnings for the user, target species, administration or disposal of the product;

(xi) the withdrawal period, if relevant; and

(xii) the words "Keep out of the reach of children" and "For animal treatment only".

Manufacturers' labelling

The following are labelling and leaflet requirements for manufacturers.

All labels and package leaflets of authorised veterinary medicinal products must be in English and may contain in legible characters "UK authorised veterinary medicinal product" or other wording as specified in the marketing authorisation to indicate that the product is authorised in the UK. The labels and package leaflets may contain other languages provided that all the information is identical in all the languages.

Where it is reasonably practicable, the following information must be present on the immediate packaging, in legible characters:

(1)

(a) the name, strength and pharmaceutical form of the veterinary medicinal product;

(b) the name and strength of each active substance, and of any excipient if this is required under the summary of product characteristics;

(c) the route of administration (if not immediately apparent);

(d) the batch number;

(e) the expiry date;

(f) the words "For Animal Treatment Only" and if appropriate "To be supplied only on veterinary prescription";

(g) the contents by weight, volume or number of dose units;

(h) the marketing authorisation number;

(i) the name and address of the marketing authorisation holder or, if there is a distributor authorised in the marketing authorisation, that distributor;

(j) a suitably labelled space to record discard date (if relevant);

(k) the target species;

(l) the distribution category;

(m) the words "Keep out of reach of children";

(n) storage instructions;

(o) the in-use shelf-life (if appropriate);

(p) for food-producing species, the withdrawal period for each species or animal product concerned;

(q) any warning specified in the marketing authorisation;

(r) disposal advice;

(s) full indications;

(t) dosage instructions;

(u) contraindications;

(v) further information required in the marketing authorisation;

(w) if the product is one that requires a dose to be specified for the animal being treated, a space for this.

Where all of this information is present on the immediate packaging there is no need for a package leaflet or any outer packaging. Where it is not reasonably practicable to have all of the above information on the immediate packaging, then the immediate packaging must at least have the following:

(2)

(a) the name of the veterinary medicinal product, including its strength and pharmaceutical form;

(b) the name and proportion of each active substance, and of any excipient if knowledge of this excipient is needed for safety reasons;

(c) the route of administration (if not immediately apparent);

(d) the batch number;

(e) the expiry date;

(f) the words "For Animal Treatment Only" and if appropriate "To be supplied only on veterinary prescription";

(g) the words "Keep the container in the outer carton".

The outer package must also contain as much of the information as possible set out above in list (2), but where this is not reasonably practicable, a package leaflet must be supplied with the product.

The package leaflet must relate solely to the VMP with which it is included, and be approved in the marketing authorisation for that product.

The package leaflet must be written in plain English.

The leaflet must contain the information set out above in list (1), except for the batch number and the expiry date, and include the name of both the marketing authorisation holder and, if different, the name of the distributor named in the marketing authorisation.

If there is a package leaflet, the immediate packaging and the outer packaging must both refer the user to it.

1.8.5 Wholesale dealing

There are specific restrictions on wholesale dealing. However, there is provision for a person lawfully conducting a retail pharmacy business to wholesale to another retailer (eg, a veterinary practitioner) provided that in any one year the amount supplied does not exceed five per cent in terms of value of turnover of the retail pharmacy business. Human licensed medicines may be wholesaled to a veterinary practitioner for their use in their practice (*see* Section 1.2.4 for requirements that must be followed when a retail pharmacy business wholesales medicines).

The holder of a wholesale dealer's authorisation must record, as soon as is reasonably practicable after each incoming or outgoing transaction (including disposal), the following:

(a) the date and nature of the transaction;

(b) the name of the VMP;

(c) the manufacturer's batch number;

(d) the expiry date;

(e) the quantity; and

(f) the name and address of the supplier or recipient.

The records retained in respect of wholesale dealing must be kept for at least three years.

1.8.6 Sheep dips

The supply must be to a person (or a person acting on that person's behalf) who is qualified to use it, i.e. a person who holds either:

(a) a Certificate of Competence in the Safe Use of Sheep Dips showing that Parts 1 and 2 or units 1 and 2 of the assessment referred to in the Certificate have been satisfactorily completed; or

(b) a National Proficiency Tests Council (NPTC) level 2 Award in the Safe Use of Sheep Dip (QCF).

The certificate must be issued:

(a) in England, Wales, and Northern Ireland by:
  (i) the National Proficiency Tests Council;
  (ii) NPTC Part of the City & Guilds Group; or
  (iii) City and Guilds NPTC;

(b) in Scotland, by one of those organisations or the Scottish Skills Testing Service.

The supplier must make a record of that person's certificate or award number as soon as is reasonably practicable and keep it for three years.

If the active ingredient of the VMP is an organophosphorus compound, the supplier must give the buyer:

(a) a double sided laminate notice. (NB: This is not necessary where the notice has been provided to the buyer within the previous twelve months and the supplier knows or has reasonable cause to believe that the buyer still has it available for use.)

The notice must meet the following specifications.

The notice must be at least A4 size with a laminated cover and must tell the user of the sheep dip:
  (i) to read and act in accordance with the label, including instructions on measuring and diluting concentrate;
  (ii) that sheep dip is absorbed through the skin;
  (iii) always to wear the recommended protective clothing, including gloves, and have spare protective clothing available;
  (iv) always to wash protective clothing before taking it off; and
  (v) to direct any questions to the supplier or manufacturer.

The notice must contain a diagram showing recommended protective clothing.

(b) two pairs of gloves as specified in the above notice or providing demonstrably superior protection to the user against exposure to the sheep dip.

1.8.7 Medicated feedingstuffs prescriptions (MFS)

The supply of a feedingstuff containing a VMP can only be supplied in accordance with a written prescription. The prescription must include:

(a) the name and address of the person prescribing the product;

(b) the qualifications enabling the person to prescribe the product;

(c) the name and address of the keeper of the animal(s) to be treated;

(d) the species of animal, identification and number of animals;

(e) the premises at which the animals are kept if different from the address of the keeper;

(f) the date of the prescription;

(g) the signature or other authentication of the person prescribing the product (NB: "other authentication" is not acceptable for a CD);

(h) the name and amount of the product prescribed;

(i) the dosage and administration instructions (NB: the VMD have advised that a dosage of "as directed" is not acceptable):

(j) any necessary warnings;

(k) the withdrawal period;

(l) the manufacturer or distributor of the feedingstuffs (who must be approved for the purpose);

(m)if the validity exceeds one month, a statement that not more than 31 days supply may be provided at any time;

(n) the name, type and quantity of feedingstuffs to be used;

(o) the inclusion rate of the veterinary medicinal product and the resulting inclusion rate of the active substance;

(p) any special instructions;

(q) the percentage of the prescribed feedingstuffs to be added to the daily ration; and

(r) if it is prescribed under the cascade, a statement to that effect.

A prescription for a feedingstuff is valid for three months or shorter if specified on the prescription, and should be sufficient for only one course of treatment. Where a prescription is for longer than one month, the supplier cannot provide more than one month's supply at a time.

The person supplying the feedingstuff must keep the prescription for five years.

1.8.8 Medicated animal feedingstuffs

Pharmacists who wish to supply VMPs or specified feed additives for incorporation into feedingstuffs or premixtures/feedingstuffs containing such products should consult the Animal Medicines Inspectorate (AMI) of the VMD for advice (see contact details below).

For further information regarding medicated/specified feed additives or products, contact the AMI:

Animal Medicines Inspectorate
Veterinary Medicines Directorate
Avenue A
Stoneleigh Park
Warwickshire CV8 2LG
Tel: 024 7684 9260
Fax: 024 7684 9261
e-mail: *amienquiries@vmd.defra.gsi.gov.uk*

1.8.9 Advertising

A VMP may be advertised provided that the advertisement is not misleading, and does not make a medicinal claim that is not in the SPC. There are additional requirements for advertisements for VMPs which are only available on prescription, POM-V and POM-VPS.

A POM-V cannot be advertised except as a price list, or where the advertisement is aimed at veterinary surgeons, pharmacists, veterinary nurses, or professional keepers of animals.

A POM-VPS cannot be advertised except as a price list, or where the advertisement is aimed at veterinary surgeons, pharmacists, professional keepers of animals, owners or keepers of horses, other veterinary healthcare professionals (includes veterinary nurses) and suitably qualified persons.

It is an offence to advertise a VMP that contains psychotropic drugs or narcotics, except where this is aimed at a veterinary surgeon or a pharmacist. It is also an offence to advertise an authorised human medicinal product for administration to animals. This includes sending a price list of or including authorised human medicinal products to a veterinary surgeon or veterinary practice, except in certain circumstances.

1.8.10 Small Animal Exemption Scheme (SAES)

There is an exemption in the Regulations in relation to VMPs intended solely for the following animals: aquarium fish; cage birds; ferrets; homing pigeons; rabbits; small rodents; and terrarium animals, where the animal is kept exclusively as a pet. This exemption allows those VMPs, intended solely for these animals and which comply with the requirements of Schedule 6 of the Regulations to be placed on the market, imported or administered without a marketing authorisation. For further information on the SAES contact the VMD.

1.8.11 Suspected adverse reactions

The Suspected Adverse Reaction Surveillance Scheme (SARSS) is a national surveillance scheme run by the Veterinary Medicines Directorate (VMD). The scheme aims to record and monitor reports of suspected adverse reactions to veterinary medicines and human medicines in both animals (any species) and humans. A human SAR may occur in a person administering a veterinary medicinal product, or a person exposed to a recently treated animal. The scheme also records lack of efficacy, adverse environmental effects, and suspected residues in milk and meat.

Suspected adverse reactions in animals or humans should be reported on Form MLA 252A to:
The Suspected Adverse Reactions Surveillance Scheme,
FREEPOST KT 4503,
Veterinary Medicines Directorate,
Woodham Lane,
Addlestone,
Surrey KT15 3BR

Forms are available on request from the VMD (tel 01932 338427; fax 01932 336618) and from the VMD website *www.vmd.gov.uk*. Tear-out copies are included in the *The Veterinary Formulary* and *NOAH Compendium of Data Sheets for Animal Medicines*.

1.8.12 Contacts

For further information on the Veterinary Medicines Regulations 2009 please contact the Veterinary Medicines Directorate, (tel 01932 336911; *www.vmd.gov.uk*; e-mail enquiries: postmaster@vmd.defra.gsi.gov.uk). In addition, the VMD's website contains Veterinary Medicines Guidance Notes (VMGN) on various aspects of the Regulations: *www.vmd.gov.uk/General/VMR/vmgn.htm*, which may be of assistance.

1.9: Alphabetical list of medicines for veterinary use

This list of medicines for veterinary use brings together specified feed additives (SFA) and veterinary medicines. Where INNs differ from BANs, these are indicated in square brackets. For current lists of prescription only medicines-veterinarian (POM-V), prescription only medicines-veterinarian, pharmacist, suitably qualified person (POM-VPS), non-food animal medicine-veterinarian, pharmacist, suitably qualified person (NFA-VPS), authorised veterinary medicine-general sale list (AVM-GSL), small animal exemption scheme (SAES), see the Veterinary Medicines Directorate (VMD) website, *www.vmd.gov.uk*. The Royal Pharmaceutical Society welcomes, in writing, details of any errors or omissions.

A

Acetarsol: for Poisons Act 1972 restrictions see poisons section
Aconite tablets 2c-MM AVM-GSL
ACP preparations POM-V
Acticam preparations POM-V
Action Actodine New Formulation AVM-GSL
Action Actodip Supreme RTU teat dip and teat spray AVM-GSL
Action Super teat dip 1:3 AVM-GSL
Actodip Supreme Concentrate for teat dip and teat spray AVM-GSL
Adequan preparations POM-V
Adocam oral suspension POM-V
Adrenocaine injection POM-VPS
Advantage preparations POM-V
Advantix preparations POM-V
Advocate preparations POM-V
Advocin preparations POM-V
Aftopur preparations POM-V
Aivlosin preparations POM-V
Alamycin preparations POM-V
Albacert oral suspension POM-VPS
Albenil preparations POM-VPS
Albensure preparations POM-VPS
Albex preparations POM-VPS
Alcide Uddergold PM Concentrate for teat dip AVM-GSL
Alfamed spray POM-V
Alfaxan injection POM-V
Alizin injection POM-V
Allverm oral suspension POM-VPS
Alphaject 2-2 vaccine POM-V
Alstomec pour on POM-VPS
Altresyn oral solution POM-V

Alvegesic Vet injection POM-V
Aludex solution POM-V
Amfipen LA injection POM-V
Amoxicure POM-V
Amoxinsol preparations POM-V
Amoxival tablets POM-V
Amoxycare preparations POM-V
Amoxycillin [Amoxicillin] tablets POM-V
Amoxygen preparations POM-V
Amoxypen preparations POM-V
Amoxyvet capsules POM-V
Ampibrittin injection POM-V
Ampicaps capsules POM-V
Ampicare capsules POM-V
Ampicillin vet capsules POM-V
AMX concentrate for solution for Fish Treatment POM-V
Anarthron injection POM-V
Animalintex Hoof Treatment poultice AVM-GSL
Animalintex poultice AVM-GSL
Animec preparations POM-VPS
Animedazon spray POM-V
Animeloxan oral suspension POM-V
Anivit B12 injection POM-VPS
Anivit 4BC injection POM-VPS
Anti-Crustacean for aquariums SAES
Anti-Fungus & Bacteria for ponds SAES
Anti-Fungus & Finrot for aquariums SAES
Anti-Internal Bacteria for aquariums SAES
Anti-Parasite for ponds SAES
Antirobe capsules POM-V
Antisedan injection POM-V
Anti-Slime & Velvet for aquariums SAES

Anti-Ulcer for ponds SAES
Anti-Whitespot for aquariums SAES
Anti-Whitespot for ponds SAES
Anxt-F oral solution AVM-GSL
Apiguard gel AVM-GSL
Apistan AVM-GSL
Appertex tablets AVM-GSL
Apralan preparations POM-V
Aquarium Bactocide SAES
Aquarium Diseasolve SAES
Aquarium Ichcide SAES
Aquatet premix POM-V
AquaVac ERM vaccines POM-VPS
AquaVac FNM Plus vaccine POM-V
AquaVac Furovac 5 vaccine POM-V
AquaVac RELERA vaccines POM-V
AquaVac Vibrio vaccines POM-V
Aqupharm preparations POM-V
Armitage Pet Care Felt Flea collar AVM-GSL
Armitage Pet Care Flea and Tick spot on AVM-GSL
Armitage Pet Care Flea shampoo for Dogs AVM-GSL
Armitage Pet Care Flea spray for Cats/Dogs AVM-GSL
Armitage Pet Care Insecticidal Flea shampoo + conditioner AVM-GSL
Armitage Pet Care Protect Flea collar for Cats AVM-GSL
Armitage Pet Care Protect Flea and Tick collar for Dogs AVM-GSL
Arnica Montana tablets 2c-MM AVM-GSL
Arsanilic acid: for Poisons Act 1972 restrictions see poisons section
Arsenicum Album tablets 4c-MM AVM-GSL

Artervac vaccine POM-V
Atipam injection POM-V
Atopica capsules POM-V
Atrocare injection POM-V
Aureomycin preparations POM-V
Auriplak ear tag POM-VPS
Aurizon ear drops POM-V
Aurofac preparations POM-V
Aurogran premix POM-V
Auroto ear drops POM-V
Autoworm preparations POM-VPS
Avatec 15% CC premix SFA
Avatec 150G CC (Game Birds) premix POM-V
Avian Tuberculin PPD POM-V
Aviax 15% SFA
Avicas tablets AVM-GSL
Avinew vaccine POM-V
AviPro vaccines POM-V

B

Badger BCG POM-V
Banacep vet tablets POM-V
Barricade 5% concentrate for spray POM-VPS
Battle's Ketosis drench AVM-GSL
Baycox preparations POM-V
Baymec pour on POM-VPS
Baytril preparations POM-V
Bayvarol strips AVM-GSL
BBraun Vet Care Hypertonic NaCl solution POM-V
BCK granules AVM-GSL
Beaphar Cat Flea powder/ spray AVM-GSL

KEY TO ANNOTATIONS

CD Lic: A substance controlled by the Misuse of Drugs Act 1971 to which the restrictions of the Regulations apply and, in addition, the production, possession and supply of which is limited in the public interest to purposes of research or other special purposes. A Home Office licence is required for such purposes

CD: A substance controlled by the Misuse of Drugs Act 1971 to which the principal restrictions of the Misuse of Drugs Regulations 2001 apply

CD No Register: A substance controlled by the Misuse of Drugs Act 1971 to which the restrictions of the Regulations apply except that no entry in the Controlled Drugs Register is required and invoices must be retained for two years

CD Benz : A substance controlled by the Misuse of Drugs Act 1971 to which the restrictions of the Regulations apply but with the following relaxation: no restriction on import and export and labelling requirements (except those under the Veterinary Medicines Regulations 2009), prescription requirements, except for the validity of a prescription being limited to 28 days, do not apply, except those falling under the controls of the Veterinary Medicines Regulations 2009, records need not be kept by retailers, destruction requirements apply only to importers, exporters and manufacturers, there are no safe custody requirements

CD Anab: A substance controlled by the Misuse of Drugs Act 1971 to which the restrictions of the Regulations apply but with the following relaxation: no restriction on possession and labelling requirements (except those under the Veterinary Medicines Regulations 2009), prescription requirements, except for the validity of a prescription being limited to 28 days, do not apply, except

those falling under the controls of the Veterinary Medicines Regulations 2009, records need not be kept by retailers, destruction requirements apply only to importers/exporters and manufacturers, there are no safe custody requirements

CD Inv: A substance controlled by the Misuse of Drugs Act 1971 but which is exempt from all restrictions under the Regulations except that the invoice or a copy of it must be kept for two years

POM-V: A substance that may be sold or supplied to the public by a veterinary surgeon or pharmacist but only in accordance with a veterinary surgeon's prescription as described in the Veterinary Medicines Regulations 2009

POM-VPS: A substance that may be prescribed and supplied by a veterinary surgeon, pharmacist or suitably qualified person as described in the Veterinary Medicines Regulations 2009

NFA-VPS: A substance for a non-food producing animal that may supplied by a veterinary surgeon, pharmacist or suitably qualified person as described in the Veterinary Medicines Regulations 2009

AVM-GSL: A substance to which there are no restrictions on the retail supply

SAES: A substance for use in certain animals kept exclusively as pets under the Small Animal Exemption Scheme as described in the Veterinary Medicines Regulations 2009

SFA: A specified feed additive incorporated in feed as authorised by an individual Commission Regulation in accordance with Regulation 1831/2003/EC

Beaphar Dog Flea and Tick drops AVM-GSL

Beaphar Dog Flea powder/ shampoo/ spray AVM-GSL

Beaphar Ear drops AVM-GSLBeaphar Flea and Tick collar for Dogs AVM-GSL

Beaphar Flea collar for Cats AVM-GSL

Beaphar Flea spray AVM-GSL

Beaphar Soft Cat Flea collar Twin Pack AVM-GSL

Beaphar Worming Cream AVM-GSL

Beaphar Worming granules AVM-GSL

Belladonna tablets 2c-MM AVM-GSL

Benazecare tablets POM-V

Benazepril Hydrochloride Novartis tablets POM-V

Betamox preparations POM-V

Bexepril tablets POM-V

Big Cat Wormer tablets NFA-VPS

Bilosin injection POM-V

Bimamix oral suspension POM-V

Bimectin preparations POM-VPS

Bimotrim Co injection POM-V

Bimoxyl preparations POM-V

Binixin injection POM-V

BioTech's Anti-Flea and Anti-Tick drops for Dogs AVM-GSL

BioTech's Flea and Tick drops for Dogs AVM-GSL

BioTech's Flea shampoo for Dogs AVM-GSL

Biozine AVM-GSL

Birnagen Forte AS vaccine POM-V

Birp AVM-GSL

Bisolvon preparations POM-V

Blackleg vaccine POM-VPS

Bloat Guard drench POM-VPS

Bloat Guard premix POM-V

Blockade teat dip AVM-GSL

Blu-Gard teat dip AVM-GSL

Blu-Gard teat spray AVM-GSL

Bob Martin 2 in 1 Dewormer tablets for Cats AVM-GSL

Bob Martin All-In-One Dewormer tablets for Dogs AVM-GSL

Bob Martin Dog spot on AVM-GSL

Bob Martin Double Action spot on for Cats/Dogs AVM-GSL

Bob Martin Easy to Use Dewormer granules for Cats/Dogs AVM-GSL

Bob Martin Flea and Tick collar for Cats/Dogs AVM-GSL

Bob Martin Flea and Tick spot on AVM-GSL

Bob Martin Flea Killing Mousse Plus for Cats AVM-GSL

Bob Martin Flea powder for Cats and Dogs AVM-GSL

Bob Martin Flea shampoo for Dogs AVM-GSL

Bob Martin Flea spray for Dogs AVM-GSL

Bob Martin Flea tablets AVM-GSL

Bob Martin Permethrin Dog spot on AVM-GSL

Bob Martin Permethrin Reflective Flea collar AVM-GSL

Bob Martin Silent Flea spray for Cats AVM-GSL

Bob Martin Spot on Dewormer AVM-GSL

Bob Martin Velvet Flea collar Twin Pack AVM-GSL

Bob Martin Vetcare spot-on for Cats/Dogs AVM-GSL

Bolfo Flea spray AVM-GSL

Bonocarp tablets POM-V

Bovaclox preparations POM-V

Bovex preparations POM-VPS

Bovidec vaccine POM-V

Bovidip preparations AVM-GSL

Bovilis vaccines POM-V

Bovine Tuberculin PPD POM-V

Bovivac S vaccine POM-V

Bravoxin vaccine POM-VPS

Bronchi-Shield vaccine POM-V

BTVPUR Alsap 8 POM-V

Buprecare injection CD No Register POM-V

Bupregesic injection POM-V

Buprenodale injection POM-V

Buscopan preparations POM-V

Busol injection POM-V

Butox Swish pour on POM-VPS

C

C Dip teat dip and teat spray AVM-GSL

Calciject preparations POM-VPS

Calcium borogluconate 40% POM-VPS

Calcium borogluconate 40% CM POM-VPS

Calicide premix POM-V

Canac Dog Flea and Tick collar AVM-GSL

Canac One Dose Worming tablets for Dogs AVM-GSL

Canac Soft Flea collar for Cats AVM-GSL

Canaural ear drops POM-V

Canidryl tablets POM-V

Canigen vaccines POM-V

Caninsulin injection POM-V

Canovel Insecticidal Conditioning collar for Dogs AVM-GSL

Canovel Insecticidal Flea and Tick shampoo and conditioner AVM-GSL

Canovel Long Acting Flea and Tick spray AVM-GSL

Capstar tablets AVM-GSL

Carprieve preparations POM-V

Carprodyl tablets POM-V

Carprogesic preparations POM-V

Cartrophen Vet injection POM-V

Casofend oral suspension POM-VPS

Catovel Insecticidal Conditioning collar for Cats AVM-GSL

Cazitel Plus tablets NFA-VPS

Cefadale tablets POM-V

Cefalexin tablets POM-V

Cefaseptin tablets POM-V

Cefenil injection POM-V

Ceftiomax injection POM-V

Cephacare tablets POM-V

Cephaguard intramammary preparations POM-V

Cephorum tablets POM-V

Ceporex preparations POM-V

Cepravin intramammary preparations POM-V

Cerenia preparations POM-V

Cestem tablets NFA-VPS

Cevac vaccines POM-V

Cevaxel injection POM-V

Chanaverm oral solution POM-VPS

Chanazine preparations POM-V

Chloromed preparations POM-V

Chlorsol 50 oral solution POM-V

Chorulon CD Anab POM-V

Chronogest vaginal sponge POM-V

CIDR vaginal delivery system for Cattle POM-V

Circovac vaccine POM-V

Clamoxyl preparations POM-V

Clavaseptin tablets POM-V

Clavucill tablets POM-V

Clavudale tablets POM-V

Clik pour on POM-VPS

Clinacin tablets POM-V

Clinacox premix SFA

Clinagel Vet POM-V

Clindacyl tablets POM-V

Clinidip L Concentrate AVM-GSL

Clinidip Superconcentrate AVM-GSL

Clomicalm tablets POM-V

Closamectin preparations POM-VPS

Closiver injection POM-VPS

Cobactan preparations POM-V

Coliscour oral solution POM-V

Colombo Morenicol Alparex SAES

Colombo Morenicol FMC-50 SAES

Colombovac vaccines POM-VPS

Colvasone injection POM-V

Combiclav preparations POM-V

Combimox preparations POM-V

Combinex preparations POM-VPS

Combisyn preparations POM-V

Combivit injection POM-VPS

Comforion Vet injection POM-V

Compagel POM-V

Companazone 25 tablets POM-V

1:3 Concentrate teat dip/teat spray and udderwash (03940/4074) AVM-GSL

Convenia injection POM-V

Coopers Ectoforce sheep dip POM-VPS

Coopers Fly Repellent Plus for horses AVM-GSL

Coopers Head to Tail Veterinary Flea powder AVM-GSL

Coopers Head to Tail Veterinary Flea shampoo AVM-GSL

Coopers Spot On Insecticide POM-VPS

Copasure 24G capsules AVM-GSL

Copinox preparations AVM-GSL

Copper sulphate MA 02987/4005 POM-V

Copprite preparations POM-VPS

Cortavance spray POM-V

Corvental-D capsules POM-V

Cosecure bolus POM-VPS

Co-Trimazine tablets POM-V

Cotrimoxgen tablets POM-V

Countdown 1:4 Concentrate for teat dip and spray AVM-GSL

Countdown Extra RTU teat dip and spray AVM-GSL

Countdown He RTU teat dip AVM-GSL

Countrywide Farmers Concentrate Iodine teat dip and teat spray AVM-GSL

Countrywide Farmers RTU teat dip and teat spray AVM-GSL

Covexin 8 vaccine POM-VPS

Covexin 10 vaccine POM-VPS

Coxi Plus oral powder POM-V

Coxidin premix SFA

CPF Dairyclene Iodine RTU teat dip and spray AVM-GSL

Cronyxin injection POM-V

Crovect pour on POM-VPS

Cryomarex Rispens vaccine POM-VPS

Crystapen 5 Mega for injection POM-V

CTC Blue spray POM-V

Cyclio spot on preparations AVM-GSL

Cyclix preparations POM-V

Cyclo spray POM-V

Cycloprost POM-V

Cyclosol LA injection POM-V

Cycostat 66G premix SFA

Cydectin preparations POM-VPS

Cygro 1% premix SFA

Cylap vaccine POM-V

CynoVAX vaccines POM-V

CZV Avian Tuberculin PPD POM-V

D

Dairyclene Chlorhexidine RTU teat dip and spray AVM-GSL

Dairyclene Iodine Concentrate for teat dip and spray AVM-GSL

Dalmazin POM-V

Dalocain injection POM-VPS

Dalophylline gel POM-VPS

Danilon Equidos oral granules POM-V

Deccox preparations POM-V

Dectomax preparations POM-VPS

Defencare shampoo AVM-GSL

Defendog AVM-GSL

Delvosteron injection POM-V

Denagard preparations POM-V

Deosan Iodip Concentrate AVM-GSL

Deosan Summer Teatcare Plus AVM-GSL

Deosan Super Excel teat dip and spray AVM-GSL

Deosan Super Iodip Concentrate teat dip and spray AVM-GSL

Deosan Teatcare Plus teat dip and spray AVM-GSL

Deosan Thixodip teat dip AVM-GSL

Deosect spray POM-VPS

Depidex preparations POM-VPS

Depocillin injection POM-V

Depo-Medrone V injection POM-V

Deposel injection POM-V

Dermisol preparations POM-VPS

Dermobion Clear POM-V

Dermobion Green POM-V

Dermoline preparations AVM-GSL

Detogesic injection POM-V

Devomycin preparations POM-V

Dexadreson injection POM-V

Dexafort injection POM-V

Dexdomitor injection POM-V

Diaproof K AVM-GSL

Dichlorophen tablets BP AVM-GSL

Dicural preparations POM-V

Dilumarex POM-V

Diluvac Forte POM-V

Dimazon injection POM-V

Dinalgen preparations POM-V

Dipal Concentrate teat dip and spray AVM-GSL

Dog Wormer tablets NFA-VPS

Dolagis tablets POM-V

Dolethal injection CD No Register POM-V

Dolorex injection POM-V

Dolpac tablets NFA-VPS

Domidine injection POM-V

Domitor injection POM-V

Domosedan injection POM-V

Dopram-V drops POM-VPS

Dopram-V injection POM-V

Dorbene Vet injection POM-V

Dormilan injection POM-V

Downland Calcium Borogluconate 20% PMD POM-VPS

Downland Calcium Borogluconate 40% CM POM-VPS

Downland Fluke and Worm drench POM-VPS

Downland Levamisole injection POM-VPS

Downland Low Volume Calcium POM-VPS

Doxyseptin tablets POM-V

Draxxin injection POM-V

Droncit injection POM-V

Droncit spot on AVM-GSL

Droncit tablets AVM-GSL

Drontal preparations NFA-VPS

Dual Action Worming tablets for Cats/Dogs AVM-GSL

Dunlop's 20 PMD POM-VPS

Dunlop's 40 CB POM-VPS

Dunlop's 40 CM POM-VPS

Dunlop's 4BC Vitamin injection POM-VPS

Dunlop's Water for injection POM-V

Duofast intramammary preparation POM-V

Duowin spray POM-V

Duphacillin injection POM-V

Duphacort Q injection POM-V

Duphacycline preparations POM-V

Duphafral Extravite injection POM-VPS

Duphafral Multivitamin 9 injection POM-VPS

Duphalyte solution POM-V

Duphamox preparations POM-V

Duphapen preparations POM-V

Duphapen + Strep injection POM-V

Duphatrim preparations POM-V

Duramune vaccines POM-V

Durateston injection CD Anab POM-V

Duvaxyn vaccines POM-V

Dynaclav injection POM-V

Dysect preparations POM-VPS

E

Easotic ear drops POM-V

Eazi-Breed CIDR vaginal delivery system POM-V

Ecomectin preparations POM-VPS

Econor preparations POM-V

Effipro spot on NFA-VPS

Effipro spray POM-V
Effydral solution AVM-GSL
Eficur injection POM-V
Elancoban G100/G200 SFA
Embotape oral paste POM-VPS
Emprasan Extracare RTU teat dip and spray AVM-GSL
Emprasan Lanolin teat dip concentrate AVM-GSL
Emprasan Sovereign teat dip AVM-GSL
Emprasan Summer Guard teat dip and teat spray AVM-GSL
Enacard tablets POM-V
Endofluke 10 oral suspension POM-VPS
Endospec preparations POM-VPS
Endoworm oral suspension POM-VPS
Energaid AVM-GSL
Engemycin preparations POM-V
Enovex preparations POM-VPS
Enrocare preparations POM-V
Enrox preparations POM-V
Enroxil preparations POM-V
Enterisol Ileitis vaccine POM-V
Enurace tablets POM-V
Enzaprost injection POM-V
Enzovax vaccine POM-V
Epiphen preparations CD No Register POM-V
Eprinex pour on POM-VPS
Equest preparations POM-VPS
EquibactinVet oral paste POM-V
Equifulvin granules POM-V
Equilis vaccines POM-V
Equimax preparations POM-VPS
Equimidine injection POM-V
Equinixin granules POM-V
Equioxx POM-V
Equip vaccines POM-V
Equipalazone preparations POM-V
Equiparin preparations POM-V
Equipaste POM-VPS
Equitape paste POM-VPS
Equitrim preparations POM-V
Eqvalan preparations POM-VPS
Eraquell oral paste POM-VPS
Ermogen vaccine POM-V
Erythrocin preparations POM-V
EstroPlan injection POM-V
Estrumate injection POM-V
Eurican vaccines POM-V
Euthatal solution CD No Register POM-V
Excenel preparations POM-V
Excis solution POM-V
Exelpet Wormer for Cats/Dogs AVM-GSL
Exitel Plus tablets NFA-VPS
Exodus oral paste POM-VPS
Exspot Insecticide for Dogs AVM-GSL

F

Farmcare Concentrated teat dip AVM-GSL
Farmcare RTU teat dip AVM-GSL
Fasimec Duo oral suspension POM-VPS
Fasinex preparations POM-VPS
Feligen RCP vaccine POM-V
Felimazole tablets POM-V
Feline 3 vaccine POM-V
Felocell CVR vaccine POM-V
Fenflor preparations POM-V
Fenoflex preparations POM-V
Fenzol 5% solution POM-VPS
Fertagyl injection POM-V
Fertipig HCG injection POM-V
Fevaxyn vaccines POM-V
Finadyne preparations POM-V
Fiproline spot on NFA-VPS
Fiproline spray POM-V
Flea spot on preparations POM-V
4Fleas Fipronil spot on preparations NFA-VPS
Flectron Fly tags POM-VPS
Fleegard preparations POM-V
Flexicam oral suspension POM-V
Florkem injection POM-V
Florocol premix POM-V

Florvetol injection POM-V
Flubenol preparations POM-VPS
Flubenvet premix POM-VPS
Flukiver suspension POM-VPS
Flunixin injection POM-V
Flypor solution POM-VPS
Folliplan oral solution POM-V
Folltropin POM-V
Footrot aerosol AVM-GSL
Footvax vaccine POM-VPS
Forgastrin AVM-GSL
Forketos AVM-GSL
Formi LHS SFA
Fortekor tablets POM-V
Forthyron tablets POM-V
Foston injection POM-V
Framomycin injection POM-V
Frontline Combo spot on preparations POM-V
Frontline spot on NFA-VPS
Frontline spray POM-V
Frusecare tablets POM-V
Frusedale 40 tablets POM-V
Frusemide [Furosemide] tablets POM-V
Fuciderm gel POM-V
Fucithalmic Vet POM-V
Furnidil B AVM-GSL
Furexel Combi oral paste POM-VPS
Furogen 2 vaccine POM-V
Furosemide tablets BP POM-V

G

Galastop oral solution POM-V
Galaxy vaccines POM-V
Gallimune vaccines POM-V
Gallivac vaccines POM-V
Garlic and Fenugreek tablets AVM-GSL
Garlic tablets AVM-GSL
Gastrogard oral paste POM-V
Gelofusine Veterinary POM-V
General Tonic for Aquariums SAES
General Tonic for Ponds SAES
Genestran injection POM-V
Genta Equine injection POM-V
Genus teat dip and spray concentrate AVM-GSL
Genus teat dip and spray solution RTU AVM-GSL
Gestavet preparations CD Anab POM-V
Gleptosil injection POM-VPS
Gletvax 6 vaccine POM-VPS
Glucose 40% w/v injection POM-VPS
Gold Glycodip teat dip and teat spray AVM-GSL
Golden-Hoof AVM-GSL
Golden-Hoof Plus AVM-GSL
Golden RTU teat dip and teat spray AVM-GSL
Golden-Udder gel AVM-GSL
Goldfish Disease Safe for Aquariums SAES
Goldfish Start Up Pack SAES
Goldfish Treatment for Ponds SAES
Gonazon preparations POM-V
Granofen Wormer for Cats and Dogs NFA-VPS
Greenleaf tablets AVM-GSL
Gripovac vaccine POM-V
Grisol-V preparations POM-V

H

Haemaccel infusion solution (Veterinary) POM-V
Halocur solution POM-V
Halothane-Vet POM-V
Hamra Blue teat dip and teat spray AVM-GSL
Harkers Pigeon Coccidiosis Treatment AVM-GSL
Hartz Control Pet Care System One Spot Flea and Tick Remedy AVM-GSL
HatchPak Avinew vaccine POM-V
HatchPak Avinew IB120 vaccine POM-V
HatchPak IB120 vaccine POM-V
Hemovet dressings AVM-GSL
Hemove swabs AVM-GSL

Heptavac vaccines POM-VPS
Hexamine and sodium acid phosphate tablets POM-V
Hexasol LA injection POM-V
Hexodip Extra RTU teat dip and teat spray AVM-GSL
Hi-Craft Flea & Tick collar for Dogs AVM-GSL
Hi-Craft Flea collar for Cats AVM-GSL
High Emollient RTU teat dip and teat spray AVM-GSL
Hiprabovis Pneumos vaccine POM-V
Hipracox Broilers vaccine POM-V
Hipragumboro GM97 vaccine POM-V
Hornex Calf Dehorning paste POM-VPS
Hy-50 Vet injection POM-V
Hyalovet 20 injection POM-V
HydroDoxx POM-V
Hydrogen cyanide: for Poisons Act 1972 restrictions see poisons section
Hylartil Vet injection POM-V
Hyonate injection POM-V
Hyoresp vaccine POM-V
Hypercard 10 tablets POM-V
Hyperdrug Veterinary Flea and Tick drops AVM-GSL
Hypermune preparations POM-V
Hypnorm CD POM-V

I

Ibaflin preparations POM-V
Ibraxion vaccine POM-V
Imaverol POM-VPS
Imizol injection POM-V
Imposil injection POM-VPS
Improvac vaccine POM-V
Imuresp RP vaccine POM-V
Incurin tablets POM-V
Ingelvac vaccines POM-V
Insuvet preparations POM-V
Intradine injection POM-V
Intra-Epicaine injection POM-V
Intravit 12 injection POM-VPS
Intubeaze spray POM-V
Iodactiv teat dip AVM-GSL
Iodine Concentrate for teat dip and teat spray AVM-GSL
Iodine Glycerine RTU teat dip and teat spray AVM-GSL
Iodypro AVM-GSL
Iosan preparations AVM-GSL
Isoba POM-V
Isocare POM-V
Isofane POM-V
IsoFlo POM-V
IsoFlo Vet POM-V
Isoflurane Vet POM-V
Isolec POM-V
Isovet POM-V
Isoxetol POM-V
Itrafungol oral solution POM-V
Ivermectin Virbac 18.7 mg/g oral paste POM-VPS
Ivertin Cattle POM-VPS
Ivomec preparations POM-VPS

J

Johnson's 4fleas powder for Cats and Dogs AVM-GSL
Johnson's 4fleas Protector spot-on for Cats/Dogs AVM-GSL
Johnson's 4fleas shampoo for Dogs AVM-GSL
Johnson's 4fleas 11 4 mg, 57 mg tablets for Cats and Dogs AVM-GSL
Johnson's Anti-Mite & Insect spray AVM-GSL
Johnson's Anti-Pest Insect spray AVM-GSL
Johnson's Anti-Scratch powder AVM-GSL
Johnson's Antiseptic Wound powder AVM-GSL
Johnson's Cat Easy Worm syrup AVM-GSL
Johnson's Cat Flea powder AVM-GSL

Johnson's Cat Flea pump spray AVM-GSL
Johnson's Cat Flea spray AVM-GSL
Johnson's Diarrhoea tablets AVM-GSL
Johnson's Dog Flea powder AVM-GSL
Johnson's Dog Flea pump spray AVM-GSL
Johnson's Dog Flea shampoo AVM-GSL
Johnson's Dog Flea spray AVM-GSL
Johnson's ear drops AVM-GSL
Johnson's Easy Roundwormer AVM-GSL
Johnson's Easy Tapewormer for Cats/Dogs AVM-GSL
Johnson's Easy Wormer granules for Cats/Dogs AVM-GSL
Johnson's Felt Cat Flea collar AVM-GSL
Johnson's Flea & Tick spot on AVM-GSL
Johnson's Flea Guard collar for Cats AVM-GSL
Johnson's Flea Guard Waterproof Flea and Tick collar for Dogs AVM-GSL
Johnson's Insecticidal Flea and Tick drops AVM-GSL
Johnson's Kil-Pest Insect powder AVM-GSL
Johnson's One Dose Easy Wormer for Dogs AVM-GSL
Johnson's Pigeon Insect powder AVM-GSL
Johnson's Pigeon Insect spray AVM-GSL
Johnson's Puppy Easy Worm syrup AVM-GSL
Johnson's Puppy Flea powder AVM-GSL
Johnson's Rid-Mite Insect powder AVM-GSL
Johnson's Scaly lotion AVM-GSL
Johnson's Twin-Wormer for Cats/Dogs AVM-GSL
Juramate injection POM-V

K

K dip teat dip and teat spray AVM-GSL
Kaogel VP oral suspension AVM-GSL
Karidox oral solution POM-V
Katavac vaccines POM-V
Kenocidin preparations AVM-GSL
Kenostart teat dip and teat spray AVM-GSL
Ketaset injection CD Benz POM-V
Ketodale injection POM-V
Ketofen preparations POM-V
Ketol oral solution AVM-GSL
KetoProPig POM-V
Ketosaid oral solution AVM-GSL
Kidney tablets AVM-GSL
Killitch AVM-GSL
King British Bacteria Control SAES
King British Disease Clear SAES
King British Fin Rot & Fungus Control SAES
King British Methylene Blue SAES
King British Original Formula WS3 White Spot Terminator SAES
King British Pond Fish Treatment SAES
King British Professional Fin Rot & Fungus Control SAES
King British Professional Original Formula WS3 White Spot Terminator SAES
King British Professional Pond Fish Treatment SAES
King British Professional Ulcer & Open Wound Treatment SAES
King British Professional White Spot Control SAES
King British Revitaliser Tonic SAES
King British Ulcer & Open Wound Treatment SAES
King British Velvet Control SAES
King British White Spot Control SAES
Kitzyme Flearid Insecticidal spray AVM-GSL
KL One Minute poultice AVM-GSL

Kloxerate preparations POM-V
Koi Anti-fungus and Bacteria for Ponds SAES
Koi Anti-Parasite for Ponds SAES
KoiCare Acriflavin SAES
KoiCare B-D-S Fluke Treatment SAES
KoiCare Ex-5 SAES
KoiCare F-M-G SAES
KoiCare Formaldehyde SAES
KoiCare Koi Calm SAES
KoiCare Malachite SAES
KoiCare Permanganate dip SAES
Kokcisan 120G SFA

L

Lactaclox intramammary preparation POM-V
Lactatrim MC intramammary preparation POM-V
Lactovac vaccine POM-V
Lambivac vaccine POM-VPS
Lanodip preparations AVM-GSL
Lapinject VHD vaccine POM-V
Large Animal Diprevon injection POM-V
Large Animal Etorphilon injection CD POM-V
Large Animal Immobilon CD POM-V
Large Animal Revivon POM-V
Laurabolin preparations CD Anab POM-V
Lectade preparations AVM-GSL
Leptavoid-H vaccine POM-V
Lethobarb CD No Register POM-V
Leucogen vaccine POM-V
Leucofeligen vaccine POM-V
Leukocell 2 vaccine POM-V
Levacide preparations POM-VPS
Levacur oral solution POM-VPS
Levadren oral solution POM-VPS
Levafas oral suspension POM-VPS
Levasure oral solution POM-VPS
Leventa oral solution POM-V
Levitape oral suspension POM-VPS
Leyodip Concentrate teat dip and teat spray AVM-GSL
Libromide tablets POM-V
Lice Killing shampoo AVM-GSL
Life-Aid preparations AVM-GSL
Lignocaine and adrenaline injection POM-VPS
Lignol injection POM-VPS
Lincocin preparations POM-V
Lincoject injection POM-V
Linco-Spectin preparations POM-V
Liquid Fungus Care SAES
Liquid Life-Aid AVM-GSL
Liquidox oral solution POM-V
Locaine injection POM-VPS
Locatim oral solution POM-V
Locovetic injection POM-V
Louping lll vaccine POM-VPS
Loxicam oral suspension POM-V
Lutalyse injection POM-V
Luteosyl injection POM-V
Luxspray 50V RTU teat dip and teat spray AVM-GSL

M

Magnidown POM-VPS
Magniject injection POM-VPS
Malaseb shampoo POM-V
Mamyzin injection POM-V
Maprelin injection POM-V
Marbocyl preparations POM-V
Marbokem injection POM-V
Masivet tablets POM-V
Masocare preparations AVM-GSL
Masodine preparations AVM-GSL
Masodip preparations AVM-GSL
Mastex AVM-GSL
Mastiplan LC intramammary preparation POM-V
Maxiban G160 SFA
Maximec Horse oral paste POM-VPS
Maxxene spot on NFA-VPS

Mebadown Super oral suspension POM-VPS
Medesedan injection POM-V
Medetor injection POM-V
Medicinal Oxygen POM-V
Medrone V tablets POM-V
Meflosyl injection POM-V
Megacal-M injection POM-VPS
Megodine preparations AVM-GSL
Megorex RTU teat dip and teat spray AVM-GSL
Melafix SAES
Melafix Cichlid SAES
Melafix Marine SAES
Melovem injection POM-V
Meloxidyl preparations POM-V
Meloxivet preparations POM-V
Mesalin injection POM-V
Metacam preparations POM-V
Methylene Blue for Aquariums SAES
Metricure intrauterine preparation POM-V
Micotil injection POM-V
Milbemax tablets POM-V
Milbotyl injection POM-V
Milk-Line Teat Plus teat dip and spray AVM-GSL
Millophyline-V preparations POM-V
Mixed Vegetable tablets AVM-GSL
Monteban G100 SFA
Monzaldon injection POM-V
M+PAC vaccine POM-V
MS222 POM-VPS
Multiject IMM intramammary preparation POM-V
Multivitamin injection (MA 02000/4131) POM-VPS
Multiworm tablets for Cats NFA-VPS
MV Chlorhexidine RTU teat dip and spray AVM-GSL
MV Iodine RTU teat dip and spray AVM-GSL
Mycen injection POM-V
Mydiavac vaccine POM-V
Myolaxin POM-V
Mypravac suis vaccine POM-V

N

Nafpenzal intramammary preparation POM-V
Nandoral tablets CD Anab POM-V
Nandrolin preparations CD Anab POM-V
Nargesic injection POM-V
Narketan 10 injection CD Benz POM-V
Natura Insecticidal collars AVM-GSL
Natural Herb tablets AVM-GSL
Navilox preparations POM-V
Naxcel injection POM-V
Nelio tablets POM-V
Nemovac vaccine POM-V
Neocolipor vaccine POM-V
Neopen injection POM-V
Netvax vaccine POM-V
Nisamox preparations POM-V
Nobilis AE 1143 vaccine POM-VPS
Nobilis CAV-P4 vaccine POM-V
Nobilis diluent CA POM-VPS
Nobilis diluent Oculonasal POM-V
Nobilis E coli inac vaccine POM-V
Nobilis Erysipelas vaccine POM-VPS
Nobilis Gumboro 228E vaccine POM-V
Nobilis Gumboro D78 vaccine POM-V
Nobilis IB 4-91 vaccine POM-V
Nobilis IB H-120 vaccine POM-VPS
Nobilis IB-Ma5 vaccine POM-VPS
Nobilis IB Multi+ND+EDS vaccine POM-V
Nobilis IB+ND+EDS vaccine POM-VPS
Nobilis Influenza vaccine POM-V
Nobilis Influenza H5N2 vaccine POM-V
Nobilis Ma5 + Clone 30 vaccine POM-VPS
Nobilis Marexine CA126 vaccine POM-VPS
Nobilis MG 6/85 vaccine POM-V

Nobilis ND C2 vaccine POM-V
Nobilis ND Clone 30 Live vaccine POM-VPS
Nobilis ORT inac vaccine POM-V
Nobilis Paramyxo P201 vaccine POM-VPS
Nobilis Reo ERS inac POM-V
Nobilis Reo inac vaccine POM-V
Nobilis Reo+IB+G+ND vaccine POM-V
Nobilis Rhino CV vaccine POM-V
Nobilis Rismavac vaccine POM-VPS
Nobilis Rismavac + CA126 vaccine POM-VPS
Nobilis RT+IB Multi+G+ND vaccine POM-V
Nobilis RT+IB Multi+ND+EDS vaccine POM-V
Nobilis Salenvac vaccine POM-V
Nobilis Salenvac T vaccine POM-V
Nobilis TRT inac vaccine POM-V
Nobilis TRT live vaccine POM-V
Nobilis TRT+ND vaccine POM-V
Nobivac Bb for Cats vaccine POM-V
Nobivac DHP vaccine POM-V
Nobivac DHPPi vaccine POM-V
Nobivac Ducat vaccine POM-V
Nobivac Ducat-Chlam vaccine POM-V
Nobivac FeLV vaccine POM-V
Nobivac KC vaccine POM-V
Nobivac Lepto 2 vaccine POM-V
Nobivac Myxo vaccine POM-V
Nobivac Parvo-C vaccine POM-V
Nobivac Pi vaccine POM-V
Nobivac Piro vaccine POM-V
Nobivac Rabies vaccine POM-V
Nobivac solvent for vaccines POM-V
Nobivac Tricat Trio vaccine POM-V
Noramp injection POM-V
Norbet tablets POM-V
Norcal preparations POM-VPS
Norixin injection POM-V
Norobrittin injection POM-V
Norocarp preparations POM-V
Norocillin preparations POM-V
Noroclav preparations POM-V
Noroclox preparations POM-V
Norodine preparations POM-V
Norodyl preparations POM-V
Norofas injection POM-VPS
Norofol injection POM-V
Norofulvin preparations POM-V
Noromectin preparations POM-VPS
Noroprost injection POM-V
Norotyl LA injection POM-V
Norvax Compact PD vaccine POM-V
Norworm preparations AVM-GSL
Novem preparations POM-V
Nuflor preparations POM-V
Nux Vomica tablets 2c-MM AVM-GSL

O

Occrycetin preparations POM-V
Octacillin WSP POM-V
Onsior preparations POM-V
Opticlox eye ointment POM-V
Optimmune eye ointment POM-V
Oralject preparations POM-V
Oramec oral solution POM-VPS
Orbax preparations POM-V
Orbenin preparations POM-V
Orbeseal intramammary preparation POM-V
Ornicure powder POM-V
Orojet Lamb oral solution POM-V
Osmonds Gold Fleece sheep dip POM-VPS
Otodex Skin cream AVM-GSL
Otodex Veterinary ear drops AVM-GSL
Otomax ear drops POM-V
Ovagen POM-V
Ovarelin injection POM-V
Ovarid tablets POM-V
Ovidown oral suspension POM-VPS
Ovipast Plus vaccine POM-VPS
Ovispec S&C preparations POM-VPS
Ovivac P Plus vaccine POM-VPS

Ovuplant implant POM-V
Oxycare preparations POM-V
Oxycomplex NS injection POM-V
Oxytetrin preparations POM-V
Oxytocin-S injection POM-V

P

Pabac vaccine POM-VPS
Palladia tablets POM-V
Panacur preparations POM-VPS; but if Panacur 2.5%, 10% Small Animal oral suspension, Panacur granules, Panacur 18.75% oral paste NFA-VPS
Pangram 5% injection POM-V
Panomec injection POM-VPS
Paracide dip POM-VPS
Paracox vaccines POM-V
Parafend preparations POM-VPS
Paramectin preparations POM-VPS
Parasitex Insecticidal collar AVM-GSL
Pardale-V tablets NFA-VPS
Parvovax vaccine POM-V
Pastobov vaccine POM-V
Pathocef intramammary preparation POM-V
Paxcutol shampoo POM-V
Pedigree Care Flea and Tick collar AVM-GSL
Pen & Strep injection POM-V
Penacare injection POM-V
Penbenocillin injection POM-V
Pentobarbital Solution 20% for Euthanasia CD No Register POM-V
Pentoject injection CD No Register POM-V
Peridale preparations AVM-GSL
Pet Star Cat Flea collar AVM-GSL
Pet Star Dog Flea and Tick collar AVM-GSL
Pethidine injection CD POM-V
Pfizer Scour Formula AVM-GSL
PG 600 injection CD Anab POM-V
Pharmasin oral solution POM-V
Phenoxypen POM-V
Phenylbutazone tablets POM-V
Phenoleptil tablets CD No Register POM-V
Phosphorus Supplement injection POM-V
Pigzin premix POM-V
Pimafix SAES
Piperazine Citrate tablets BP 500 mg AVM-GSL
Piperazine Citrate Worm tablets AVM-GSL
Pirsue intramammary preparation POM-V
Planate injection POM-V
Planipart injection CD Anab POM-V
Plerion tablets NFA-VPS
PLT tablets POM-V
Pluset injection POM-V
PMSG-Intervet POM-V
Pond Aid All You Need Health SAES
Pond Aid Bacterad SAES
Pond Aid Eradick SAES
Pond Care Melafix SAES
Pond Care Pimafix SAES
Pond Care Stress Coat SAES
Porcilis AR-T vaccine POM-VPS
Porcilis AR-T DF vaccine POM-V
Porcilis Begonia DF vaccine POM-V
Porcilis Begonia IDAL vaccine POM-V
Porcilis Coli 6C POM-VPS
Porcilis Ery vaccine POM-VPS
Porcilis Ery + Parvo vaccine POM-V
Porcilis Glässer vaccine POM-V
Porcilis M Hyo vaccine POM-V
Porcilis PCV vaccine POM-V
Porcilis Porcoli vaccines POM-V
Porcilis Porcoli Diluvac Forte POM-VPS
Porcilis PRRS vaccine POM-V
Posatex ear drops POM-V
Potencil POM-V
Poulvac AE vaccine POM-VPS
Poulvac Bursa Plus vaccine POM-V
Poulvac Bursine 2 vaccine POM-V

Poulvac Flufend H5N3RG vaccine POM-V

Poulvac Hitchner B1 vaccine POM-VPS

Poulvac IB H120 vaccine POM-VPS

Poulvac IB Primer vaccine POM-V

Poulvac IBMM vaccine POM-VPS

Poulvac IBMM + ARK vaccine POM-V

Poulvac i-IB,ND,EDS,IBD,SHS vaccine POM-V

Poulvac ILT vaccine POM-VPS

Poulvac iSE vaccine POM-V

Poulvac Marek CVI vaccine POM-VPS

Poulvac Marek CVI + HVT vaccine POM-VPS

Poulvac MD-Vac lyophilised vaccine POM-VPS

Poulvac NDW vaccine POM-VPS

Poulvac Pabac vaccine POM-V

Poulvac SHS vaccine POM-V

Poulvac TRT vaccine POM-V

Powerflox injection POM-V

Pracetam preparations POM-V

Prac-Tic spot on POM-V

Prascend tablets POM-V

Prazitel Plus tablets NFA-VPS

Prednicare tablets POM-V

Prednidale tablets POM-V

Prednisolone tablets BP (Vet) POM-V

Pregsure BVD vaccine POM-V

Premadex preparations POM-VPS

Preventef Insecticidal collar for Dogs AVM-GSL

Previcox preparations POM-V

Prid intrauterine device POM-V

Prilactone tablets POM-V

Prilben Vet tablets POM-V

Prilenal tablets POM-V

Prilium preparations POM-V

Proactive teat dip and spray AVM-GSL

Procare injection POM-V

Procyon vaccines POM-V

Pro-dynam oral powder POM-V

Profender preparations POM-V

Program injection POM-V

Program Plus tablets POM-V

Program oral suspension for Cats AVM-GSL

Program tablets for Dogs AVM-GSL

Progressis vaccine POM-V

Promeris spot on POM-V

Promone-E injection POM-V

Propalin syrup POM-V

Propisderm teat dip AVM-GSL

PropoClear injection POM-V

PropoFlo injection POM-V

PropoFlo Vet injection POM-V

Prosolvin injection POM-V

Prostavet injection POM-V

Protect spot Flea and Tick drops for Dogs AVM-GSL

ProteqFlu vaccines POM-V

Protocon Gold gel AVM-GSL

Provita Protect for Newborn Calves POM-VPS

Pulmodox preparations POM-V

Pulmotil preparations POM-V

Purevax vaccines POM-V

Pyceze POM-V

Pyratape P Horse Wormer POM-VPS

Pyriproxyfen premix POM-V

Pyroflam injection POM-V

Q

Quadrisol oral gel POM-V

Qualimec preparations POM-VPS

Qualmintic injection POM-VPS

Quantum vaccines POM-V

QuarterMate teat dip and teat spray AVM-GSL

R

Rabigen SAG2 vaccine POM-V

Rabisin vaccine POM-V

Radiol Insecticidal Soapless shampoo with Conditioner AVM-GSL

Rapidexon injection POM-V

Rapinovet injection POM-V

Raspberry Leaf tablets AVM-GSL

Readymix Gold teat dip and spray AVM-GSL

Rearguard solution POM-V

Receptal injection POM-V

Reconcile tablets POM-V

Regulin implant POM-VPS

Regumate preparations POM-V

Release injection CD No Register POM-V

Renegade pour on POM-VPS

Reprocine injection POM-V

Reproval injection POM-V

Resflor injection POM-V

Respiporc Flu3 vaccine POM-V

Retarbolin CD Anab POM-V

Revertor injection POM-V

Revivon (Large Animal) POM-V

Rexxan spot on NFA-VPS

Rheumocam tablets POM-V

RhusTox tablets 2c-MM AVM-GSL

Rilexine tablets POM-V

Rimadyl preparations POM-V

Rimifin tablets POM-V

Ripercol oral solution POM-VPS

Rispoval vaccines POM-V

Romidys injection POM-V

Rompun preparations POM-V

Ronaxan tablets POM-V

Rotavec Corona vaccine POM-V

RTU teat dip and spray (MA 21357/4012) AVM-GSL

Ruby Teatguard AVM-GSL

Rumbul Rumen Bullet Cattle POM-VPS

Rumbul Rumen Bullet Sheep POM-VPS

Rycoben oral suspension POM-VPS

S

Sacox 120 SFA

Salinomax 120G premix SFA

Salmosan POM-V

Saniphor spray AVM-GSL

Sapphire RTU teat dip and teat spray AVM-GSL

Savlon Veterinary Antiseptic Concentrate AVM-GSL

Scabivax vaccine POM-V

Scalibor collar NFA-VPS

Scullcap and Valerian tablets AVM-GSL

Sebolyse shampoo POM-V

Sedalin gel POM-V

Sedator injection POM-V

Sedaxylan injection POM-V

Sededorm injection POM-V

Sedivet injection POM-V

Selectan injection POM-V

Seleen shampoo AVM-GSL

Selgian tablets POM-V

Sensospray RTU teat dip and teat spray AVM-GSL

Sergeants Pet Patrol AVM-GSL

Seven Seas Kitzyme Flea Rid Reflective Flea collar AVM-GSL

Seven Seas Vetzyme Flea Rid Reflective Flea collar AVM-GSL

Sevoflo POM-V

Sheptaclox DC intramammary preparation POM-V

Sherley's Easy Treat Wormer tablets AVM-GSL

Sherley's Easy Treat Worming cream AVM-GSL

Sherley's Felt Flea collar AVM-GSL

Sherley's Flea and Tick collar for Dogs AVM-GSL

Sherley's Flea collar for Cats AVM-GSL

Sherley's Flea spray AVM-GSL

Sherley's Insecticidal Dog shampoo AVM-GSL

Sherley's Multiwormer for Cats/Dogs AVM-GSL

Sherley's One Dose Wormer for Dogs AVM-GSL

Sherley's Rheumatine Tablets for Adult Dogs AVM-GSL

Sherley's Worming granules for Cats/Dogs AVM-GSL

Sherley's Worming syrup AVM-GSL

Shotaflor injection POM-V

Silkidip teat dip and teat spray AVM-GSL

Slentrol oral solution POM-V

Slice premix POM-V

Sodium calciumedetate injection POM-V

Sodium salicylate POM-V

Solacyl POM-V

Soloxine tablets POM-V

Solubenol POM-VPS

Soludox POM-V

Solu-Medrone V injection POM-V

Solupraz SAES

Somulose injection CD POM-V

Spartrix tablets AVM-GSL

Spectam preparations POM-V

Spirovac vaccine POM-V

Spunhill Gold AVM-GSL

Sputolosin powder POM-V

Stabox preparations POM-V

Star Iodocare Concentrate for teat dip and teat spray AVM-GSL

Star Ready-Dip teat dip and teat spray AVM-GSL

Star Teat-ex AVM-GSL

Startvac injection POM-V

Stellamune vaccines POM-V

Stenoral premix SFA

Sterile water for injections BP POM-V

SteroVet POM-V

Stomorgyl tablets POM-V

Streptacare injection POM-V

Stresnil injection POM-V

Stress Coat SAES

Stress Coat Marine SAES

Strinacin II tablets POM-V

Stronghold preparations POM-V

Strongid Caramel POM-VPS

Strongid P preparations POM-VPS

Suiseng vaccine POM-V

Sulphur Colecton preparations AVM-GSL

Sumex pour on POM-VPS

Summer C dip AVM-GSL

Supaverm oral suspension POM-VPS

Super Concentrate teat dip and teat spray AVM-GSL

Supercare Summer Tg AVM-GSL

Superteat teat dip and teat spray AVM-GSL

Suprelorin implant POM-V

Supremadex injection POM-VPS

Suredip teat dip and teat spray AVM-GSL

Surolan ear drops POM-V

Suvaxyn Aujeszky 783+O/W vaccine POM-V

Suvaxyn Ery vaccine POM-V

Suvaxyn M. hyo vaccine POM-V

Suvaxyn M. hyo-Parasuis vaccine POM-V

Suvaxyn MH One POM-V

Suvaxyn Parvo/E vaccine POM-V

Suvaxyn Parvo ST POM-V

Suvaxyn PCV vaccine POM-V

Swaycop injection POM-VPS

Swimbladder Treatment for Aquariums SAES

Switch pour on AVM-GSL

Synulox preparations POM-V

Synutrim preparations POM-V

Syvazul 1 POM-V

T

Tapewormer tablets for Cats/Dogs AVM-GSL

Tardak injection POM-V

Telmin preparations POM-VPS

Tensolvet gel POM-VPS

Terramycin preparations POM-V

Terrexine intramammary preparation POM-V

Tetanus Antitoxin Behring POM-V

Tetanus Toxoid Concentrated POM-V

Tetcin spray POM-V

Tetra Delta intramammary preparation POM-V

TetraMedica ContraSpot SAES

TetraMedica FungiStop SAES

TetraMedica General Tonic SAES

TetraMedica Gold Med SAES

TetraMedica Lifeguard SAES

TetraMedica Marine Oopharm SAES

Tetramin premix POM-V

TetraPond MediFin SAES

Tetroxy LA injection POM-V

Tetsol 800 POM-V

Therios tablets POM-V

Thyroxyl tablets POM-V

Tiacil Ophthalmic solution POM-V

Tiamvet POM-V

Tildren POM-V

Tilmovet preparations POM-V

Tivafol injection POM-V

Tolfedine preparations POM-V

Tolfine injection POM-V

Top Drop preparations POM-V

Torbugesic injection POM-V

Torbutrol tablets POM-V

Torphasol injection POM-V

Tracherine vaccine POM-V

Tramazole oral suspension POM-VPS

Tri Lyte Plus AVM-GSL

Tribex preparations POM-VPS

Tribovax-T vaccine POM-VPS

Tribrissen preparations POM-V

Triclacert preparations POM-VPS

Triclafas oral suspension POM-VPS

Trimacare preparations POM-V

Trimediazine preparations POM-V

Trimedoxine preparations POM-V

Trinacol injection POM-V

Trivacton 6 vaccine POM-VPS

Trocoxil tablets POM-V

Trodax injection POM-VPS

Tropical Fish Start Up Pack SAES

Troscan tablets AVM-GSL

Tryplase capsules AVM-GSL

TUR 3 vaccine POM-V

Twin Pack Two Collars Bob Martin Flea and Tick for Dogs AVM-GSL

Twinox tablets POM-V

3TX 1:3 Concentrate for teat dip and spray AVM-GSL

Tylan preparations POM-V

Tyluvet-20 injection POM-V

U

Ubro Red Dry Cow POM-V

Ubro Yellow Milking Cow POM-V

Ubrolexin POM-V

Udder Guard AVM-GSL

Ultrapen LA injection POM-V

Uniferon injection POM-VPS

Uniprim preparations POM-V

Unisolve POM-VPS

Urilin syrup POM-V

V

Valbazen oral suspension POM-VPS

Vanguard vaccines POM-V

Vasotop tablets POM-V

Vaxxitek HVT + IBD vaccine POM-V

Vecoxan suspension POM-VPS

Vectin preparations POM-VPS

Ventipulmin preparations CD Anab POM-V

Venture 321 teat dip and teat spray AVM-GSL

Venture Io-care RTU teat dip and teat spray AVM-GSL

Venture Satinex teat dip and teat spray AVM-GSL

Veramix Sheep Sponge and cream POM-V
VersifelCVR vaccine POM-V
Vetalar V injection CD Benz POM-V
Vetergesic injection CD No Register POM-V
Veterinary Wound powder AVM-GSL
Vetflurane POM-V
Vetical 40+M injection POM-VPS
Veticop injection POM-VPS
Vetivex preparations POM-V
Vetmedin preparations POM-V
Vetmulin preparations POM-V
Vetofol injection POM-V
Vetoryl preparations POM-V
Vetrazin pour on POM-VPS
Vetremox preparations POM-V
Vetzyme Antiseptic cutaneous powder AVM-GSL
Vetzyme Antiseptic ointment AVM-GSL
Vetzyme Flearid Insecticidal spray AVM-GSL
Vetzyme Flearid shampoo for Dogs AVM-GSL
Vetzyme JDS Insecticidal shampoo AVM-GSL

Vetzyme Kitzyme Ear drops AVM-GSL
Vetzyme One Dose Wormer for Dogs AVM-GSL
VevoVitall SFA
Vexitor spot on for Cats NFA-VPS
Vidalta tablets POM-V
Virbac Ivermectin & Praziquantel oral gel for Horses POM-VPS
Virbacef injection POM-V
Virbagen preparations POM-V
Virbagest oral solution POM-V
Virbamec preparations POM-VPS
Virbaxyl preparations POM-V
Vitamin B1 injection POM-V
Vitamin K1 injection POM-V
Vitbee preparations POM-VPS
Vitenium injection POM-V
Vitesel injection POM-V
Vivitonin preparations POM-V
Voren preparations POM-V

W

Walpole's Buffer solution POM-V
Water for injection POM-V
Whiskas Care Flea collar AVM-GSL
Whiskas Wormer for Cats AVM-GSL

White Spot Cure SAES
Wilko Cat Felt Flea collar AVM-GSL
Wilko Cat Flea powder AVM-GSL
Wilko Cat Flea spray AVM-GSL
Wilko Dog Flea drops AVM-GSL
Wilko Dog Flea powder AVM-GSL
Wilko Dog Flea spray AVM-GSL
Wilko Dual Action Worming tablets for Cats AVM-GSL
Wilko Insecticidal Dog shampoo AVM-GSL
Wilko Long Lasting Flea and Tick collar for Dogs AVM-GSL
Wilko Long Lasting Flea collar for Cats AVM-GSL
Wilko Silent Action Dog Flea spray AVM-GSL
Wilko Single Dose Wormer for Dogs AVM-GSL
Wilko Vinyl Cat Flea collar AVM-GSL
Wilko Vinyl Dog Flea and Tick collar AVM-GSL
Wilko White Spot Control SAES
Willcain injection POM-VPS
Wormer tablets for Cats/Dogs NFA-VPS
Wormazole preparations NFA-VPS

X

Xeden tablets POM-V
Xylacare injection POM-V
Xylapan injection POM-V

Y

Yarvitan oral solution POM-V
Ypozane tablets POM-V

Z

Zactran injection POM-V
Zanil Fluke drench POM-VPS
Zermasect preparations POM-VPS
Zermex preparations POM-VPS
Zerofen preparations POM-VPS; but if Zerofen 22% granules (small animals) AVM-GSL
Zincoped solution AVM-GSL
Zincotec Zinc Oxide premix POM-V
Zitac Vet tablets POM-V
Zolan tablets POM-V
Zolvix oral solution POM-V
Zubrin preparations POM-V
Zulvac 8 vaccines POM-V

2: Code of Ethics and Professional Standards and Guidance

Introduction

In 2010 The Royal Pharmaceutical Society of Great Britain (RPSGB) will transfer its regulatory function to The General Pharmaceutical Council (GPhC) – a new, independent pharmacy regulator. While the exact date for the transfer is still subject to parliamentary process, it is important to note that, following transfer of the Society's regulatory activities, two new organisations will exist, each with a specific remit:

- *The General Pharmaceutical Council* will regulate pharmacists, pharmacy technicians and pharmacy premises.
- *The Royal Pharmaceutical Society* will assume the role of the professional leadership body for the profession

To avoid confusion, and in acknowledgement of the forthcoming changes, the RPSGB is not publishing any regulatory standards in this edition of *Medicines, Ethics and Practice*.

Pre-transfer of regulatory activities

Until the two new organisations come into existence, both the RPSGB's existing Code of Ethics and its professional standards and guidance documents will continue to be the standards with which pharmacists and pharmacy technicians must comply.

These documents can be found in *MEP* number 33, published in July 2009, and also on the web at *www.rpsgb.org/ protectingthepublic/ethics/*

Post-transfer of regulatory activities

When the General Pharmaceutical Council becomes the regulator it will set its own standards for pharmacists, pharmacy technicians and premises. At that time the GPhC standards will replace the Society's current Code of Ethics and professional standards and guidance documents.

The GPhC has already consulted on and will publicise its regulatory standards in advance of the formal transfer date. Its standards will only come into effect once the transfer of regulatory activities has taken place. In the meantime you should continue to adhere to the RPSGB Code of Ethics and the professional standards and guidance documents as already described.

For further information please visit *www.rpsgb.org* or *www.pharmacyregulation.org*

3: Professional Development and Training

3.1 Continuing professional development

The Society has two clear functions within continuing professional development (CPD); as the pharmacy regulator it sets standards for CPD and has been calling in your CPD records for review. In its role as the professional leadership body, the Society provides advice and support for practice development, offers CPD materials, events and access to specialist groups and networks in facilitating CPD.

All pharmacists and pharmacy technicians are currently expected to make a declaration that they are either practising or non-practising when they renew their membership of the Society. (N.B While this applies to the current registration status, there will be no provision under the General Pharmaceutical Council to join the non-practising or the overseas register). You are practising as a pharmacist or a pharmacy technician if, whilst acting in the capacity of or holding yourself out as a pharmacist or a pharmacy technician, you undertake any work or give any advice in relation to the dispensing or use of medicines, the science of medicines, the practice of pharmacy or the provision of health care. Guidance on making the practising/non-practising declaration is available on the Society's website at *www.rpsgb.org/registrationandsupport/registration*. The main points covered in the guidance are shown in the panel.

As a practising pharmacist or pharmacy technician you have a mandatory obligation to maintain a record of your CPD. In March 2009 the Society issued professional standards and guidance for CPD under the Code of Ethics. The Society also provides CPD support materials and facilities for recording CPD online, on paper or on a freestanding personal computer.

If you are currently on the non-practising register or if you are a pharmacist registered as an overseas member of the Society, you are not required to maintain a CPD record. However, if you wish to do so, you can keep a record of your CPD on the Society's online CPD recording facility by logging into *www.uptodate.org.uk* and registering as a user.

You may also find it useful to access the CPD Plan and Record, the guidance document that is available to all practising pharmacists and pharmacy technicians on the CPD website at *http://www.uptodate.org.uk/home/PlanRecord.shtml*

Main points

A person practises as a pharmacist or pharmacy technician if, while acting in the capacity of or holding himself out as a pharmacist or pharmacy technician, he undertakes any work, or gives any advice, in or in relation to the dispensing or use of medicines, the science of medicines or the practice of pharmacy or the provision of healthcare. Key points to note are:

- When you consider your practising status, it may be helpful to ask yourself whether you or others feel that the work you undertake or advice you give has added value or credibility because you are a pharmacist. If so, you are practising.
- It is possible still to be practising if you are retired or not working if, for example, you continue to provide advice on pharmacy matters.
- It is a misconception that a pharmacist who is not dispensing can place themselves in the non-practising category. Even if you do not dispense, you are not automatically non-practising.
- Most working pharmacists are practising, not only those who dispense, or work or provide advice in a clinical context. It includes, for example, those working in industry, academia and administration.
- Just because you undertake work or give advice that could be provided by someone who is not a pharmacist, does not mean that you are non-practising. The facts that those you work with or advise know you are a pharmacist adds professional credibility to your work and advice.
- If you are in doubt, the fact that something has made you question whether you are a practising pharmacist probably means that you are.
- To assume that you are practising is a good place to start. Only those pharmacists who have truly retired from work, or those who have moved on to other non-related careers, have the non-practising route open to them.

The same guidance applies to registered pharmacy technicians.

Following demerger of the Society's regulatory functions there will be no provision under the General Pharmaceutical Council to join the non-practising or overseas registers.

What is CPD?

Continuing professional development (CPD) is a framework you can use to maintain your competence as a professional. The Society's framework applies equally to pharmacists and pharmacy technicians. CPD is a cyclical process of reflection, planning, action and evaluation. It includes everything that you as a pharmacist or a pharmacy technician learn, which makes you better equipped to carry out your role within the pharmacy profession. The RPSGB provides support and access to materials for development as part of our professional development portfolio.

CPD Standards

The CPD Standards state that as a practising pharmacist or pharmacy technician you must keep a CPD record that complies with the good practice criteria for CPD recording, either electronically by logging into the Society's CPD website *www.uptodate.org.uk*, on a PC with the desktop program, or on paper using the Society's Plan & Record system. They also state that as a practising pharmacist or pharmacy technician you must make a minimum of nine entries in each twelve month period which reflect the context and scope of your practice and submit these to the Regulator when requested.

The CPD cycle enables you to update, maintain and develop your capabilities by:

- Helping you identify your individual learning needs
- Recognising the contribution of workplace learning
- Acknowledging that we learn in a variety of ways, so there may be a variety of preferred choices
- Linking your learning to your own practice and development
- Avoiding the need to complete a fixed number of hours of continuing education with the emphasis of your CPD being on quality, rather than quantity.

It is important to distinguish CPD from the more familiar term continuing education (CE). CE refers to traditional methods of learning such as attending workshops, following diploma or distance learning courses, or structured reading. These activities can be very useful and will inevitably feature as part of most pharmacists and pharmacy technicians' CPD, but professional development also occurs through activities such as:

- Learning by doing
- Dealing with problems/situations in the workplace or elsewhere (including incidents outside your professional responsibilities from which you learn something that is applicable to them)
- Participating in group activities, e.g. specialist groups, virtual networks, stakeholder/professional body activities, internal staff meetings and staff training events, involvement in projects and professional audits
- Preparation for lecturing, doing presentations or training others
- Work shadowing
- Secondment to another department.

This list is not exhaustive and could include any other activities that develop your professional capabilities.

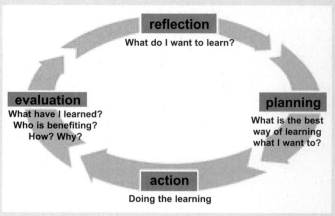

The CPD cycle

Advice on making a CPD entry

The CPD Standards state that you must make a minimum of nine CPD entries per year.

You are likely to find your own pattern of recording CPD, perhaps two entries every other month, for example. Evidence from the Society's pilots indicates that pharmacists and pharmacy technicians are learning all the time, and need to be selective about what they choose to enter in their CPD record. We advise you to keep a portfolio of all your learning activities and work towards choosing a balanced CPD record that complies with the Society's Professional Standards and Guidance for CPD and that you keep this record up to date. The guidance suggests a range of learning activities that could be included in your CPD record. While you can start a CPD entry at any of the four phases of the CPD cycle, you should make some CPD entries that start at reflection. You may also want to record a combination of CPD entries that demonstrate the importance of your learning to different parties (yourself, colleagues, your organisation and, particularly, on users of your products and/or services). Likewise, you may choose to illustrate the range of activities you participate in as part of your CPD (such as reading, workshops and discussion with peers).

The Society, as the Regulator, has been calling in CPD records for review since July 2009 and the process of calling in and reviewing CPD records will transfer to the General Pharmaceutical Council when appropriate. If your CPD record is called for review, you may select for review completed CPD entries that you have found to be most meaningful in the work you undertake as a pharmacist or pharmacy technician. You must ensure that you include a minimum of nine entries in each twelve month period from March 2009 when the CPD Standards were implemented. You will be required to submit a proportion of the required nine entries for the current year, depending on when your record is called for review. If you have registered as a pharmacist or pharmacy technician since March 2009 the same will apply to the submission of entries covering the year in which you joined the register.

Assistance and support

CPD assistance and support is available from the professional support team at the new Professional Leadership Body. If you wish to discuss how you can develop your practice and record your CPD, please email support@rpsgb.org, call 020 7572 2302 or contact the team using the online enquiry form available on *www.rpharms.com*

3.2 Pharmacy support staff

The Society has a range of policies covering minimum training and competence requirements for pharmacy support staff. For pharmacy technicians a regulatory framework is now in place and this became statutory on 1 July 2009.

Further information on policies for medicines counters assistants and dispensing/pharmacy assistants can be found in the pharmacy support staff section of the Society's website *www.rpsgb.org*.

Further information on pharmacy technician registration can be found on the pharmacy technician page of the Society's website *www.rpsgb.org*.

Medicines counter assistants

Since 1996 it has been a professional requirement that any assistant who is given delegated authority to sell medicines under a protocol should have undertaken, or be undertaking, an accredited course relevant to their duties.

The Society's requirement is that courses should cover the knowledge and understanding associated with units 2.04 and 2.05 of the Pharmacy Services S/NVQ level 2, entitled

- *Assist in the Sale of OTC medicines and provide information to customers on symptoms and products* and
- *Assist in the supply of prescribed items (taking in a prescription and issuing prescribed items).*

Medicines counter assistants should be enrolled on a training programme within three months of commencing their role (or as soon as practical within local training arrangements) and the programme should be completed within a three-year time period.

A list of accredited medicines counter assistant courses is available on the support staff training programmes page of the Society's website *www.rpsgb.org*.

Dispensing/pharmacy assistants

Since January 1 2005 pharmacists have had a professional obligation to ensure that dispensing/pharmacy assistants are competent in the areas in which they are working to a minimum standard equivalent to the Pharmacy Services / S/NVQ level 2 qualification or undertaking training towards this. This policy applies to staff working in the following areas:

- Sale of over the counter medicines and the provision of information to customers on symptoms and products *
- Prescription receipt and collection *
- The assembly of prescribed items (including the generation of labels)
- Ordering, receiving and storing pharmaceutical stock
- The supply of pharmaceutical stock
- Preparation for the manufacture of pharmaceutical products (including aseptic products)
- Manufacture and assembly of medicinal products (including aseptic products)

---

* Medicines counter assistants are exempt from further training in these units provided they have successfully completed an accredited MCA course or have previously been considered to have met the Society's requirements for MCAs.

The requirement can be met by completing a training programme relevant to the job role and there are four acceptable ways of doing this:

- Successful achievement of Pharmacy Services S/NVQ level 2
- Successful achievement of relevant units of the Pharmacy Services S/NVQ level 2
- Successful achievement of a training programme accredited to be of an equivalent level to S/NVQ level 2
- Successful achievement of relevant units of an accredited training programme of an equivalent level to Pharmacy Services S/NVQ level 2.

Dispensing/pharmacy assistants should be enrolled on a training programme within three months of commencing their role (or as soon as practical within local training arrangements) and the programme should be completed within a three-year time period.

A list of accredited training programmes for dispensing and pharmacy assistants is available on the support staff training programmes page of the Society's website *www.rpsgb.org*.

Pharmacy technician registration

The Society opened a voluntary register of pharmacy technicians in January 2005. The voluntary register became a statutory register across Great Britain on 1 July 2009. Registration will continue to be voluntary for two years after this date. On 1 July 2011 registration will become mandatory (compulsory) and the title "pharmacy technician" will become protected in law. All those currently practising as pharmacy technicians will need to apply to register by midnight on 30 June 2011 to continue working as pharmacy technicians.

Until this date transitional arrangements for entry onto the register will apply (this is sometimes referred to as grandparenting) and a range of pharmacy technician qualifications will be accepted. These arrangements enable those with the responsibilities, experience and training background of pharmacy technicians (though this may have predated S/NVQs and/or been delivered through a company scheme) to apply for registration. Evidence of recent work experience under the supervision, direction or guidance of a pharmacist as a pharmacy technician or trainee pharmacy technician is also required.

From 1 July 2011 those wanting to register as pharmacy technicians must have:

- A UK qualification (or qualifications) meeting the long term registration requirements. The current requirement is S/NVQ level 3 in Pharmacy Services plus an accredited underpinning knowledge programme,
- Work experience as a pharmacy technician, or student technician, carried out under the supervision, direction or guidance of a pharmacist of an accountable pharmacist for at least 14 hours per week for at least two years.

Contact:
Pharmacy technicians
  Tel: 020 7572 2610
  e-mail: pharmacytechnician@rpsgb.org
Medicines Counter Assistants or dispensing/pharmacy assistants
  Tel: 0207 572 2604
  e-mail: supportstaff@rpsgb.org

4: References

4.1 Council Members and National Pharmacy Boards Members 2010-2011

Council (see panel below)

President
Mr Steve Churton

Vice-President
Professor Nicholas Barber

Treasurer
Mr John Gentle

Mr Steve Acres
Ms Seema Agha
Mr Gerald Alexander
Mrs Margaret Allan
Mr Martin Astbury
Mrs Kay Blair
Mr David Carter
Mrs Dorothy Drury
Dr Phillida Entwistle
Mr Graeme Hall
Mrs Sylvia Hikins
Mrs Lorna Jacobs
Mr John Jolley
Mr Alan Kershaw
Mrs Sue Kilby
Dr Tristan Learoyd
Miss Yvonne Liddell
Professor Alistair Michell
Mrs Alison Moore
Ms Marcia Saunders
Mr David Thomson
Mrs Valerie Turner

English Pharmacy Board

Chairman
Mrs Lindsey Gilpin

Vice-Chairman
Mr Sultan "Sid" Dajani

Ms Seema Agha
Mrs Catherine Armstrong
Mr Martin Astbury
Dr David Branford
Mr David Carter
Mr John Gentle
Miss Shilpa Gohil
Mrs Sue Kirby
Dr Tristan Learoyd
Mr Graham Phillips
Mr Graeme Stafford
Miss Rachael Lemon

Scottish Pharmacy Board

Chairman
Mrs Sandra Melville

Vice-Chairman
Mr Alistair Jack

Mr Ewan Black
Dr Anne Boyter
Professor John Cromarty
Ms Evelyn Mackenzie
Mrs Fiona MacLean
Mrs Alpana Mair
Mrs Janine Milne
Dr Derek Stewart
Mr Charles Tait
Mr William Templeton
Mr David Thomson

Welsh Pharmacy Board

Chairman
Miss Nuala Brennan

Vice-Chairman
Mrs Mair Davies

Mr Keith Davies
Mrs Wendy Davies
Mr Marc Donovan
Mr Richard Evans
Mr Robert Gartside
Mr Brian Hawkins
Ms Diane Heath
Mr Don Hughes
Mr Phillip Parry
Mrs Fiona Price

The Council

In late 2010 it is expected that the Society's regulatory function will trasfer to the General Pharmaceutical Council and its professional leadership functions will be governed by a new Royal Charter. The General Pharmaceutical Council has its own separate Council and the Society will be governed by a new Assembly and the three existing National Board. These governance structures will supersede the Society's Council as listed on this page.

4.2 Support for pharmacists

Pharmacist Support is an independent welfare charity working for pharmacists and their families, preregistration trainees and pharmacy students in times of need.

Our support services include a variety of programmes developed in consultation with pharmacists to offer a helping hand to colleagues who find themselves confronted by difficult circumstances for whatever reason. Our services include:

- Listening Friends
- Specialist advice services
- Health Support Programme
- Financial assistance
- Information and Signposting

Many of the services are delivered directly by volunteer pharmacists. Because there is a shared professional background, our volunteers are uniquely able to understand the specific pressures affecting pharmacists and their families.

If you are currently affected by any issues, please do not hesitate to contact us by ringing our freephone number on 0808 168 2233. Your enquiry will be dealt with promptly and in complete confidence

More information about our range of services

Listening Friends offers free listening services to pharmacists suffering from stress. The service is confidential and anonymous, and provides the opportunity to talk to a pharmacist trained to offer support regarding the particular pressures that apply to the pharmacy profession. The service is not restricted to work related problems, but offers support for all causes of stress such as ill health, family issues, and bereavement.

To access the Listening Friends service call 0808 168 5133

Specialist advice services in the areas of benefits, debt and employment law are provided completely free of charge and are confidential. Specially trained advisers will help you by offering a range of advice in response to your particular problem. Examples of this support include 'benefit checks' to ensure you are receiving the correct amount of benefits and tax credits, preparation of financial statements, rescheduling of payments to creditors if you have multiple debts, and advice in connection with your employment.

To access the specialist advice services call 0808 168 2233

The Health Support Programme exists to help pharmacists who experience problems with alcohol, drug, or other types of dependency. The programme is delivered by Action on Addiction - one of the country's top addiction support providers. Fully qualified addiction specialists staff the helpline 24/7, and all calls to this service are entirely confidential.

To access the Health Support Programme call 0808 168 5132

Financial assistance is provided to cover a range of circumstances:

- to support mental or physical quality of life, for example, respite care for a family member, counselling and therapies, convalescence after an illness or accident, purchasing a particular disability aid or care home fees

- to meet a specific cost, for example, to purchase a washing machine, to carry out essential car or household repairs, or to pay winter fuel bills. Often these applicants have been affected by an unforeseen loss of work due to redundancy or ill health, or are living on a very low income and can't afford to pay an unexpected bill

- to provide a regular 'top-up' for people who have a very low income and are finding it difficult to make ends meet without getting into debt. Applicants are often widows/widowers or retired pharmacists, and this regular assistance can help them to maintain a quality of life which they would otherwise lose

- to support students facing particular hardship due to unforeseen circumstances such as family issues, ill health or bereavement. We realise that most students leave university with significant debt, however a one-off payment can be made available to students who are bearing particular hardship.

To find out more about the financial assistance provided call our freephone number on 0808 168 2233

Information and Signposting - Our information and signposting service has been developed in response to enquiries. There is a growing collection of information on our website including fact sheets and a directory of useful organisations. We also provide a telephone and email enquiry service and have access to a range of information resources. If we are unable to deal with your query ourselves, we will signpost you on to an appropriate source.

To access our Information and Signposting service call 0808 168 2233 or check out our online Directory at www.pharmacistsupport.org

Who is eligible?

If you are a pharmacist, a widow or widower of a pharmacist, a retired pharmacist, a pharmacy student, or a preregistration trainee you are eligible to apply for support; as long as you or your partner have been on the register at some point. If you have a friend who is a pharmacist, or a colleague who needs support, please contact us, and you can be sure of complete confidentiality in making your enquiry.

Grants and financial assistance applications are granted on a case-by-case basis, and eligibility is assessed based on the level of income against the level of outgoings; therefore, your income need not be exceptionally low to apply, and you may still be eligible if you have savings. As a rule, most people who receive means tested benefits, including pension credit, are automatically eligible for consideration.

Contact us

For more information on Pharmacist Support and our services, contact a member of the support team on 0808 168 2233. Alternatively, visit our website *www.pharmacistsupport.org*, where you will find a number of useful factsheets and a directory listing the details of a wide range of organisations who can give help, advice and support in a number of different subject areas.

Pharmacist Support is a registered charity, Number 221438, and is funded by donations from pharmacists.

4.3 Headquarters enquiries guide

The Royal Pharmaceutical Society of Great Britain is currently the professional body for pharmacists and the regulatory body for pharmacists and pharmacy technicians in England, Scotland and Wales.

Later this year a dedicated professional body for pharmacy will be created when the Society's regulatory functions transfer to the General Pharmaceutical Council. The expected date of transfer is 27 September 2010, Parliamentary processes permitting.

The contact details below are for the three main functions of the current Royal Pharmaceutical Society:

- Professional body functions
- Publishing
- Regulatory functions

Professional body functions

New website

The professional body functions now have a new website, **www.rpharms.com**, which, following demerger, will become the website for the Royal Pharmaceutical Society. All of the services of the new Society are available through this user-friendly website.

Members will have exclusive access to content such as our support service, information on continuing professional development, networking opportunities through our online groups and local practice forums and the latest practice guidance.

For enquiries before 27 September 2010

RPS Support

Information, advice and support for members with pharmacy practice, CPD, professional, legal and ethical enquiries.

Tel 020 7572 2302
Email support@rpsgb.org
Online enquiry form *www.rpharms.com/support*

For library resource enquiries and literature searches

Tel 020 7572 2300
Email library@rpsgb.org

For museum and historical services
Tel 020 7572 2210
Email museum@rpsgb.org

Scottish office

Headquarters of the Society in Scotland

Tel 0131 556 4386
Fax 0131 558 8850
Email scotinfo@rpsgb.org

Welsh office

Headquarters of the Society in Wales

Tel 029 2073 0310
Fax 029 2073 0311
Email wales@rpsgb.org

For enquiries after 27 September 2010:

The main contact number for all enquiries for the new professional body will be **0845 257 2570**

For RPS Support

Information, advice and support for members with pharmacy practice, CPD, professional, legal and ethical enquiries
Tel 0845 257 2570
Email support@rpharms.com

For membership enquiries

Tel 0845 257 2570
Email membership@rpharms.com

Pharmaceutical Press
The publishing division of the Royal Pharmaceutical Society

The Pharmaceutical Journal

Editor and Editing Director	020 7572 2414
Editorial content	020 7572 2414
Distribution	
pharmacists and technicians	020 7572 2266
other	0203 318 3141

Pharmaceutical Press

Customer Services	01256 302692
Editorial	020 7572 2207
Sales and marketing	020 7572 2663

Regulatory functions
The regulatory functions of the Royal Pharmaceutical Society of Great Britain (regulation of pharmacists, pharmacy technicians and pharmacy premises) will transfer to the General Pharmaceutical Council in September 2010, Parliamentary processes permitting. For further information please visit **www.pharmacyregulation.org** or contact the GPhC at info@pharmacyregulation.org or on 020 3365 3400.

Registration

Registration	020 7572 2322
Overseas Registration	020 7572 2317
Pharmacy Technician Registration	020 7572 2610

Accreditation:	020 7572 2685
Pre-registration	020 7572 2370
Continuing Professional Development	020 7572 2540
Legal and Ethical Advisory Service	020 7572 2308
Complaints about Pharmacies/Pharmacists	020 7572 2308

Inspectors

Chief Inspector (Vacant)	020 7572 2311/2312

Northern Region

Lynsey Cleland (Regional Lead Inspector)	020 7572 2661
Stan Brandwood	020 7572 2550
Paula Gardner	020 7572 2577
Alison Hopkins	020 7572 2557
John Russ Liddell	020 7572 2561
Helen Jackson	020 7572 2558
Rachel O'Callaghan	020 7572 2573
Stewart Waugh	020 7572 2570
Deborah Zuckert	020 7572 2555

Central Region

Jill Williams (Regional Lead Inspector)	020 7572 2572
Helen Boniface	020 7572 2635
Nicola Carlisle	020 7572 2553
Richard Chapman	020 7572 2522
Barry Cohen	020 7572 2551
Annie Garton	020 7572 2541
Steven Gascoigne	020 7572 2554
Deborah Hylands	020 7572 2567
Akhtar Malik	020 7572 2574
Noor Mohamed	020 7572 2533

Southern Region

Tim Snewin [Regional Lead Inspector]	020 7572 2568
Simon Denton	020 7572 2565
Peter Gibbs	020 7572 2559
Susan Melvin	020 7572 2562
Sharon Monks	020 7572 2515
Carole Muir	020 7572 2516
Martin Packham	020 7572 2569
Jacqueline Riley	020 7572 2566
Eilean Robson	020 7572 2552
Andrew Smith	020 7572 2408

Emergency connection to ex-directory telephone numbers

Community pharmacists can be connected to ex-directory, no-connection telephone numbers if they need to contact patients in a real emergency.

This privilege, which is also available to doctors, hospitals and emergency authorities, was granted to pharmacists by British Telecom in February 1998 as a result of representation to BT by the then National Pharmaceutical Association.

It is important that pharmacists use the privilege appropriately and only exercise their right of access when stricly necessary. The following guidelines must be adhered to:

- Pharmacists should only consider asking for connection to an ex-directory, no-connection number in a "life and death" situation. This can be interpreted as an emergency which is likely to pose a very serious threat to the health of the patient if information cannot be passed on immediately and when the patient's telephone number cannot be found from another source (eg, the GP's surgery).
- A pharmacist needing to contact an ex-directory, no-connection number should dial 100, explain the situation and request connection to the ex-directory number.
- The pharmacist will only be connected when the following criteria are met:
  - the pharmacist must be calling from community pharmacy premises
  - the pharmacist must explain the reason for the emergency connection request and advise the operator that it is a life and death situation (the operator will not judge the nature of the emergency but will accept the word of the pharmacist)
  - the pharmacist must give his or her name and the name of the pharmacy premises from which he or she is calling.

BT will monitor all requests for emergency connection. If the privilege is abused it is likely that this important facility for community pharmacists will be withdrawn.

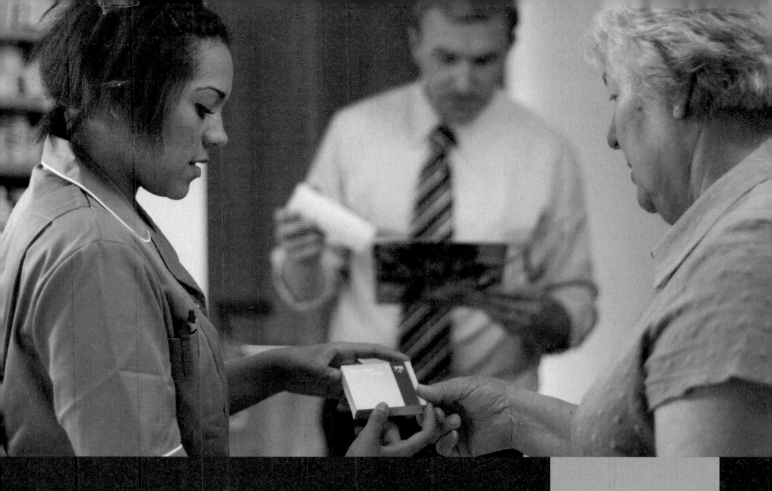
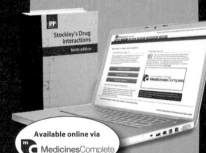
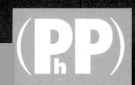

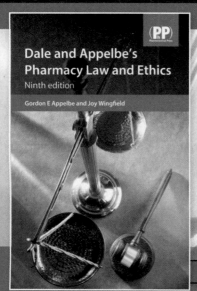

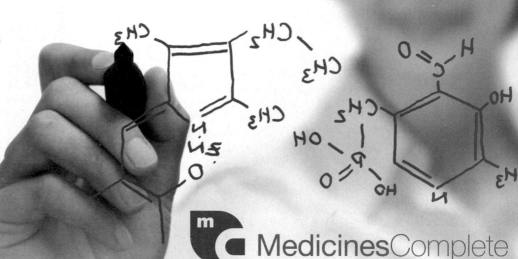